1992
YEAR BOOK OF
ONCOLOGY®

The 1992 Year Book® Series

Year Book of Anesthesia and Pain Management: Drs. Miller, Abram, Kirby, Ostheimer, Roizen, and Stoelting

Year Book of Cardiology®: Drs. Schlant, Collins, Engle, Frye, Kaplan, and O'Rourke

Year Book of Critical Care Medicine®: Drs. Rogers and Parrillo

Year Book of Dentistry®: Drs. Meskin, Currier, Kennedy, Leinfelder, Matukas, and Rovin

Year Book of Dermatologic Surgery: Drs. Swanson, Salasche, and Glogau

Year Book of Dermatology®: Drs. Sober and Fitzpatrick

Year Book of Diagnostic Radiology®: Drs. Federle, Clark, Gross, Madewell, Maynard, Sackett, and Young

Year Book of Digestive Diseases®: Drs. Greenberger and Moody

Year Book of Drug Therapy®: Drs. Lasagna and Weintraub

Year Book of Emergency Medicine®: Drs. Wagner, Burdick, Davidson, Roberts, and Spivey

Year Book of Endocrinology®: Drs. Bagdade, Braverman, Horton, Kannan, Landsberg, Molitch, Morley, Odell, Rogol, Ryan, and Sherwin

Year Book of Family Practice®: Drs. Berg, Bowman, Davidson, Dietrich, and Scherger

Year Book of Geriatrics and Gerontology®: Drs. Beck, Abrass, Burton, Cummings, Makinodan, and Small

Year Book of Hand Surgery®: Drs. Amadio and Hentz

Year Book of Health Care Management: Drs. Heyssel, Brock, King, and Steinberg, Ms. Avakian, and Messrs. Berman, Kues, and Rosenberg

Year Book of Hematology®: Drs. Spivak, Bell, Ness, Quesenberry, and Wiernik

Year Book of Infectious Diseases®: Drs. Wolff, Barza, Keusch, Klempner, and Snydman

Year Book of Infertility: Drs. Mishell, Paulsen, and Lobo

Year Book of Medicine®: Drs. Rogers, Bone, Cline, Braunwald, Greenberger, Utiger, Epstein, and Malawista

Year Book of Neonatal and Perinatal Medicine®: Drs. Klaus and Fanaroff

Year Book of Nephrology: Drs. Coe, Favus, Henderson, Kashgarian, Luke, Myers, and Strom

Year Book of Neurology and Neurosurgery®: Drs. Currier and Crowell

Year Book of Neuroradiology: Drs. Osborn, Harnsberger, Halbach, and Grossman

Year Book of Nuclear Medicine®: Drs. Hoffer, Gore, Gottschalk, Sostman, Zaret, and Zubal

Year Book of Obstetrics and Gynecology®: Drs. Mishell, Kirschbaum, and Morrow

Year Book of Occupational and Environmental Medicine: Drs. Emmett, Brooks, Harris, and Schenker

Year Book of Oncology®: Drs. Young, Longo, Ozols, Simone, Steele, and Weichselbaum

Year Book of Ophthalmology®: Drs. Laibson, Adams, Augsburger, Benson, Cohen, Eagle, Flanagan, Nelson, Reinecke, Sergott, and Wilson

Year Book of Orthopedics®: Drs. Sledge, Poss, Cofield, Frymoyer, Griffin, Hansen, Johnson, Simmons, and Springfield

Year Book of Otolaryngology–Head and Neck Surgery®: Drs. Bailey and Paparella

Year Book of Pathology and Clinical Pathology®: Drs. Gardner, Bennett, Cousar, Garvin, and Worsham

Year Book of Pediatrics®: Dr. Stockman

Year Book of Plastic, Reconstructive, and Aesthetic Surgery: Drs. Miller, Cohen, McKinney, Robson, Ruberg, and Whitaker

Year Book of Podiatric Medicine and Surgery®: Dr. Kominsky

Year Book of Psychiatry and Applied Mental Health®: Drs. Talbott, Frances, Freedman, Meltzer, Perry, Schowalter, and Yudofsky

Year Book of Pulmonary Disease®: Drs. Bone and Petty

Year Book of Sports Medicine®: Drs. Shephard, Eichner, Sutton, and Torg, Col. Anderson, and Mr. George

Year Book of Surgery®: Drs. Schwartz, Jonasson, Robson, Shires, Spencer, and Thompson

Year Book of Transplantation: Drs. Ascher, Hansen, and Strom

Year Book of Ultrasound: Drs. Merritt, Mittelstaedt, Carroll, and Nyberg

Year Book of Urology®: Drs. Gillenwater and Howards

Year Book of Vascular Surgery®: Dr. Bergan

Roundsmanship®: '92–'93: A Student's Survival Guide to Clinical Medicine Using Current Literature: Drs. Dan, Feigin, Quilligan, Schrock, Stein, and Talbott

Editor

Robert C. Young, M.D., F.A.C.P.

President, Fox Chase Cancer Center, Philadelphia

Associate Editors

Eli Glatstein, M.D.

Professor and Chair, Department of Radiation Oncology, University of Texas Southwestern Medical Center, Dallas

Dan L. Longo, M.D., F.A.C.P.

Director, Biological Response Modifiers Program, National Cancer Institute, Frederick Cancer Research and Development Center

Robert F. Ozols, M.D., Ph.D.

Chairman, Medical Oncology, Fox Chase Cancer Center, Philadelphia

Joseph V. Simone, M.D.

Physician-in-Chief, Memorial Sloan-Kettering Cancer Center, New York

Glenn D. Steele, Jr., M.D.

The William V. McDermott Professor of Surgery, Harvard Medical School; Chairman, Department of Surgery, New England Deaconess Hospital, Boston

1992
The Year Book of ONCOLOGY®

Editor
Robert C. Young, M.D., F.A.C.P.

Associate Editors
Eli Glatstein, M.D.
Dan L. Longo, M.D., F.A.C.P.
Robert F. Ozols, M.D., Ph.D.
Joseph V. Simone, M.D.
Glenn D. Steele, Jr., M.D.

Mosby Year Book

St. Louis Baltimore Boston Chicago London Philadelphia Sydney Toronto

Editor-in-Chief, Year Book Publishing: Kenneth H. Killion
Sponsoring Editor: Kelly Blossfeld
Manager, Literature Services: Edith M. Podrazik
Senior Information Specialist: Terri Santo
Senior Medical Writer: David A. Cramer, M.D.
Assistant Director, Manuscript Services: Frances M. Perveiler
Assistant Managing Editor, Year Book Editing Services: Tamara L. Smith
Senior Production/Desktop Publishing Manager: Max F. Perez
Proofroom Manager: Barbara M. Kelly

A Year Book Medical Publishers imprint of Mosby–Year Book, Inc.

Mosby–Year Book, Inc.
11830 Westline Industrial Drive
St. Louis, MO 63146

Printed in the United States of America.

Editorial Office:
Mosby–Year Book, Inc.
200 North LaSalle St.
Chicago, IL 60601

International Standard Serial Number: 1040-1741
International Standard Book Number: 0-8151-9754-3

Contributing Editors

Jeffrey S. Dover, M.D.
Chief, Dermatology Section, New England Deaconess Hospital, Boston; Assistant Professor of Dermatology, Harvard Medical School, Boston

Thomas C. Hamilton, Ph.D.
Associate Member, Fox Chase Cancer Center, Philadelphia

J. Milburn Jessup, M.D.
Staff Surgeon, New England Deaconess Hospital, Boston; Associate Professor of Surgery, Harvard Medical School, Boston

Gary Kruh, M.D., Ph.D.
Associate Member, Fox Chase Cancer Center, Philadelphia

Paul J. Martin, M.D.
Member, Fred Hutchinson Cancer Research Center; Professor, University of Washington, Seattle

James L. Sherley, M.D., Ph.D.
Associate Member, Fox Chase Cancer Center, Philadelphia

Joseph R. Testa, Ph.D.
Member, Director of Molecular Cytogenetics, Fox Chase Cancer Center, Philadelphia; Adjunct Professor, Fels Institute for Cancer Research and Molecular Biology, Temple University School of Medicine, Philadelphia

Table of Contents

Journals Represented

Mosby–Year Book subscribes to and surveys nearly 900 U.S. and foreign medical and allied health journals. From these journals, the Editors select the articles to be abstracted. Journals represented in this YEAR BOOK are listed below.

American Journal of Clinical Pathology
American Journal of Clinical Oncology
American Journal of Epidemiology
American Journal of Medicine
American Journal of Neuroradiology
American Journal of Pediatric Hematology/Oncology
American Journal of Preventive Medicine
American Journal of Public Health
American Journal of Roentgenology
American Journal of Surgery
American Surgeon
Annals of Internal Medicine
Annals of Surgery
Annals of Thoracic Surgery
Archives of Dermatology
Archives of Disease in Childhood
Archives of Internal Medicine
Archives of Otolaryngology—Head and Neck Surgery
Archives of Pathology and Laboratory Medicine
Archives of Surgery
Blood
British Journal of Cancer
British Journal of Haematology
British Journal of Obstetrics and Gynaecology
British Journal of Radiology
British Medical Journal
Cancer
Cancer Research
Chest
Clinical Orthopaedics and Related Research
Clinical Otolaryngology
Digestive Diseases and Sciences
European Heart Journal
European Journal of Cancer
Gastroenterology
Gynecologic Oncology
Head and Neck
Hepatology
International Journal of Cancer
International Journal of Radiation, Oncology, Biology, and Physics
Journal of Advanced Nursing
Journal of Bone and Joint Surgery (American Volume)
Journal of Clinical Investigation
Journal of Clinical Oncology
Journal of Family Practice
Journal of Infectious Diseases
Journal of Investigative Dermatology
Journal of Neurology

Journal of Neurosurgery
Journal of Nuclear Medicine
Journal of Pathology
Journal of Pediatric Surgery
Journal of Pediatrics
Journal of Thoracic and Cardiovascular Surgery
Journal of Urology
Journal of the American Medical Association
Journal of the National Cancer Institute
Lancet
Medical Journal of Australia
Modern Pathology
Nature
New England Journal of Medicine
Obstetrics and Gynecology
Pediatric Dermatology
Pediatric Infectious Disease Journal
Pediatric Nursing
Pediatrics
Plastic and Reconstructive Surgery
Postgraduate Medical Journal
Proceedings of the National Academy of Sciences
Psychological Medicine
Radiology
Radiotherapy and Oncology
Science
Surgery
Urology

Standard Abbreviations

The following terms are abbreviated in this edition: acquired immunodeficiency syndrome (AIDS), the central nervous system (CNS), cerebrospinal fluid (CSF), computed tomography (CT), electrocardiography (ECG), human immunodeficiency virus (HIV), and magnetic resonance (MR) imaging (MRI).

Publisher's Preface

As a publishers, we feel challenged to seek ways of presenting complex information in a clear and readable manner. To this end, the 1992 YEAR BOOK OF ONCOLOGY now provides structured abstracts in which the various components of a study can easily be identified through headings. These headings are not the same in all abstracts, but rather are those which most accurately designate the content of each particular journal article. We are confident that our readers will find the information contained in our abstracts to be more accessible than ever before. We welcome your comments.

1 Cancer Etiology

Introduction

The causes of cancer range from the purely genetic (e.g., congenital retinoblastoma, Li-Fraumeni syndrome) to the purely environmental (e.g., choriocarcinoma), but most cancers involve the action of both genetic and environmental mechanisms working in concert. Carcinogenesis generally requires both the induction of a genetic change and a stimulus to divide. Efforts to identify carcinogenic substances generally rely very heavily on the induction of mutation to indict a particular agent. However, the evidence is quite persuasive that mutations alone are generally not sufficient to lead to cancer. Indeed, it appears that most cell types must accumulate a variety of genetic defects before autonomous growth results.

Although carcinogenesis testing of chemicals tends to produce false positives (the identification of substances that do not actually cause cancer in humans), 1 important factor contributing to cancer incidence and mortality that goes relatively free of investigation is poverty. What is carcinogenic about poverty?

Dan L. Longo, M.D., F.A.C.P.

Molecular Biology of Cancer

Relationship Between K-*ras* Oncogene Activation and Smoking in Adenocarcinoma of the Human Lung

Slebos RJC, Hruban RH, Dalesio O, Mooi WJ, Offerhaus GJA, Rodenhuis S (Netherlands Cancer Inst, Amsterdam; Johns Hopkins Univ Hosp, Baltimore, Md)

J Natl Cancer Inst 83:1024–1027, 1991 1–1

Background.—Mutational activation of K-*ras* is frequent in cancers of the pancreas, colon, and lung. Point mutations in K-*ras* codon 12, which are found in approximately one third of pulmonary adenocarcinomas, might result from direct mutation by carcinogenic components of tobacco smoke.

Study Design.—Smoking was related to *ras* mutations in a series of 54 patients with adenocarcinoma of the lung, 27 of whom were smokers. The activating point mutations in K-*ras* and N-*ras* were determined by the polymerase chain reaction, using oligonucleotide hybridization to detect mutated sequences.

Findings.—Eight cancers from smokers and 2 from nonsmokers harbored a point mutation in codon 12 of K-*ras*. The respective frequencies were 30% and 7%, a significant difference. There was a trend toward more frequent *ras* activation with the intensity of smoking (table).

Distribution of Point Mutations in Codon 12 of K-*ras* Among Nonsmokers, Smokers Who Had Smoked For as Many as 50 Pack-Years, and Smokers Who Had Smoked More Than 50 Pack-Years

	K-ras negative	K-ras positive	Total
Nonsmokers	25	2	27
Smokers			
15-50 pack-years	11	4	15
51-120 pack-years	8	4	12
Total	44	10	54

Note: Chi-square test for trend: $P = .037$.
(Courtesy of Slebos RJC, Hruban RH, Dalesio O, et al: *J Natl Cancer Inst* 83:1024–1027, 1991.)

Conclusion.—Exposure to tobacco smoke may be an important factor inducing point mutations in K-*ras* in human lung adenocarcinomas. Similar mutations may also occur infrequently in the tumors of nonsmokers.

▶ Activation of *ras* oncogenes has been demonstrated in animal tumors induced by chemical carcinogens. The *ras* oncogenes code for 21-kd proteins *(p21-ras)* that have a role in signal transduction by virtue of their binding to GTD, guanosine diphosphate, and guanosine triphosphate activity. The point mutations in the *ras* genes that result in amino acid substitutions in *p21-ras* lead to uncontrolled cell proliferation and oncogenesis. The results of this study help close the loop from strong epidemiologic associations of cigarette smoking and lung cancer to the actual molecular carcinogenesis of cigarette smoke. Carcinogenesis in cigarette smoke can lead to point mutations in the *ras* genes of 30% of the adenocarcinomas in smokers.

There are other mutations, presumably induced by carcinogenesis in cigarette smoke, that are also likely to have an etiologic role in lung cancer. For example, single point mutation can lead to abnormal function of the suppressor *p53* gene, a gene that frequently is altered in lung cancer (and in many other tumors as well).— R.F. Ozols, M.D., Ph.D.

Transduction and Expression of the Human Carcinoembryonic Antigen Gene in a Murine Colon Carcinoma Cell Line

Robbins PF, Kantor JA, Salgaller M, Hand PH, Fernsten PD, Schlom J (Natl Cancer Inst, Bethesda, Md)

Cancer Res 51:3657–3662, 1991 1–2

Background.—Tumor-associated antigens may be important targets for active immunotherapy. One of these antigens is carcinoembryonic antigen (CEA), which is present on the surface of nearly all gastrointestinal tumors; however, CEA is not expressed in rodent tumors. Two clones of mouse colon adenocarcinoma cells that express high levels of human CEA were developed and analyzed.

Methods.—The cell line studied, MC-38, was transduced with a retroviral construct that contained complementary DNA encoding human CEA. This cell line, which causes tumors in syngeneic C57BL/6 mice, has been the target of many studies of active immunotherapy. Individual transduced clones expressing high levels of cell surface CEA were isolated, and 2 clones—MC-38-cea1 and MC-38-cea2—were extensively characterized.

Results.—Both MC-38-cea1 and MC-38-cea2 expressed CEA levels that were considerably higher than those of the moderately differentiated WiDr human colon carcinoma cell line and similar to those expressed by the GEO and CBS lines, which express some of the highest reported levels of CEA. The CEA expressed by MC-38-cea1 had a molecular weight similar to that of native CEA (M_r 180,000), whereas MC-38-cea2 expressed a relative molecular mass 70,000 glycosylated immunoreactive product. Sequencing of this clone revealed a deletion of 2 of the 3 repeated domains seen in CEA. Both clones showed a reaction with 7 anti-CEA monoclonal antibodies.

Discussion.—The development of a mouse tumor cell line that expresses human CEA provides a basis for both the mapping of the immunodominant epitopes of CEA and the development of a syngeneic model to study immunotherapy directed against this antigen. In addition, a matched control tumor that does not express CEA will also be available.

▶ Thus far, the usefulness of nonspecific, partially specific, or specific immunotherapy in the treatment of bowel cancers has, if anything, been disproven. The major problems with human studies include the fact that specific active immunotherapy protocols have not been directed at specific epitopes; have not been monitorable by precise definitions of the patient's immune status before, during, and after therapy; and have most often been performed using vaccines that are composed of impossible-to-identify immunogen gemisches. Not surprisingly, with such a lack of available specific resources and/or the ability to analyze specific effect, the experimental results have been and will undoubtedly continue to be negative. However, the presence of CEA among all transformed gastrointestinal phenotypes and its increased expression (when compared with CEA family members present in normal crypt cells) have long offered the opportunity of a more precise target for the immunotherapy of colon and rectum cancers.

A number of problems must be surmounted. First of all, with the exception of the results of some very early studies in the CEA literature (which were not subsequently confirmed), CEA does not appear to be immunogenic in the autologous host. Second, no animal models of CEA producing gastrointestinal tumors have been demonstrated (again, with the exception of 1 investigator's work on rodent CEA, which has not been reproducible). In this study, Robbins (in Schlom's laboratory) has begun the task of defining precisely (using a transfected human CEA gene) a potentially applicable rodent gastrointestinal cancer model with a precise CEA epitope that could be used as a target for interesting immunotherapy syngeneic constructs. This may be the first in a series of analyzable models that could allow for a rational approach to using human immunotherapy in gastrointestinal cancers.—G.D. Steele, Jr., M.D.

Promoter Deletion and Loss of Retinoblastoma Gene Expression in Human Prostate Carcinoma

Bookstein R, Rio P, Madreperla SA, Hong F, Allred C, Grizzle WE, Lee W-H (Univ of California at San Diego, La Jolla, Calif; Univ of Texas Health Sciences Ctr at San Antonio, San Antonio; Univ of Alabama at Birmingham, Birmingham)

Proc Natl Acad Sci U S A 87:7762–7766, 1990 1–3

Introduction.—All retinoblastomas and some other neoplasms, such as bone or soft-tissue sarcomas and lung or breast carcinomas, show mutational inactivation of the retinoblastoma gene (RB). In several types of tumor cells with these mutations, including a prostatic carcinoma line, tumorigenicity is suppressed by exogenous copies of wild-type RB. Prostatic carcinoma specimens were investigated for RB mutation to provide further evidence of RB inactivation in the genesis of prostate cancer.

Methods.—Primary or metastatic prostate carcinoma specimens that were obtained at operation or autopsy were studied. The RB protein expression was studied by use of immunoblot analysis and immunostaining of histologic sections.

Results.—There were definite signs of RB-encoded protein in the tumor cells of 5 specimens; 1 had equivocal signs and 1 had no signs. In the latter specimen, the RB mutations were characterized both by deletion of 103 nucleotides containing transcriptional start sites and by the loss of the second RB allele. The promoter activity of upstream DNA sequences in a heterologous expression system was effectively abolished by the 103–base-pair deletion.

Conclusion.—Mutation of the RB promoter appears to inactivate the gene in vivo. In humans, some prostate carcinomas may have RB mutations; screening for these mutations can be done using immunohistochemical methods. Based on preliminary observations, the RB mutations may be present in 10% to 30% of prostate cancers.

▶ Prostate cancer has been added to the evergrowing list of human tumors in which inactivation of the suppressor genes appears to play a significant role in tumor formation in a subset of patients. As in other tumors in which mutational inactivation of the RB (or other suppressor gene) has been demonstrated, there is little information regarding any impact on biological behavior or prognosis in tumors with such a genetic abnormality. Tumor formation is likely the result of the interaction between tumor-promoting genes (oncogenes) and tumor suppressor genes. The development of more sensitive assays to determine the status of both suppressor and promoter genes in clinical specimens will permit the evaluation of their clinical usefulness in comparison with other prognostic factors, including stage, tumor volume, tumor markers, and DNA content.—R.F. Ozols, M.D., Ph.D.

Suppression of Tumorigenicity in Wilms Tumor by the p15.5-p14 Region of Chromosome 11

Dowdy SF, Fasching CL, Araujo D, Lai K-M, Livanos E, Weissman BE, Stanbridge EJ (Univ of California, Irvine; Univ of North Carolina Chapel Hill)

Science 254:293–295, 1991 1–4

Background.—Wilms' tumor, a nephroblastoma found in children, originates from embryonal renal stem cells and has been associated with genomic changes at both the 11p13 and 11p15 regions. Some studies have ruled out involvement of both these regions in some familial Wilms' tumors, implying a role for a third genetic locus.

Objective.—To distinguish between involvement at 11p13 and 11p15, a chromosome 11 was constructed that had 1 or the other region deleted. This chromosome was introduced into the tumorigenic Wilms' tumor-cell line G401. Tumor-forming activity was assayed in nude mice.

Findings.—The 11p13-deleted chromosome retained the ability to inhibit tumor formation in nude mice, but an 11p15.5-p14.1–deleted chromosome did not. A second genetic locus, residing in the p15.5-p14.1 region of chromosome 11, suppresses the tumorigenic phenotype of the G401 Wilms' tumor-cell line.

Interpretation.—There may be at least 2 genetic subtypes of Wilms' tumor, 1 involving inactivation of a key element of a negative growth-regulating pathway at 11p13 (WT1), and the other involving inactivation of a separate negative growth regulator at 11p15.5-p14.1 (WT2). The WT2 gene may be an important growth regulator in other malignancies (e.g., adrenocortical carcinoma, bladder carcinoma, breast cancer, testicular cancer, and pulmonary cancers).

▶ One of the more exciting observations relative to the etiology of cancer has been the discovery of tumor suppressor genes. Their existence had been suspected for some time, but it is only in recent years that they have been identified and their functions explored. The importance of the discovery of suppressor genes and the precise identification of the function of each of them simply doubles the potential for genetic intervention in the control of cancer. Indeed, if one cannot remove a cancer-causing gene, one might be able to enhance the effect of a tumor suppressor gene.—J.V. Simone, M.D.

Overexpression and Mutation of *p53* in Epithelial Ovarian Cancer

Marks JR, Davidoff AM, Kerns BJ, Humphrey PA, Pence JC, Dodge RK, Clarke-Pearson DL, Iglehart JD, Bast RC Jr, Berchuck A (Duke Univ)

Cancer Res 51:2979–2984, 1991 1–5

Background.—The gene *p53* has been implicated as a proto-oncogene producing a nuclear phosphoprotein. It frequently acquires mutations during the development of human malignancies, including colon, breast, and lung cancers. The loss of wild-type *p53* function may have a role in malignant transformation.

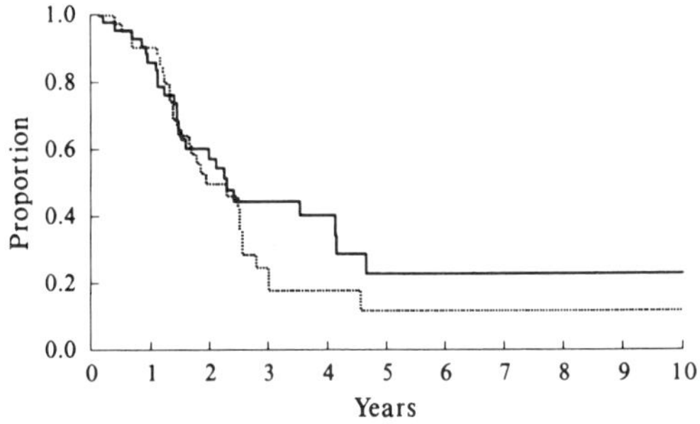

Fig. 1–1.—Relationship between *p53* overexpression and survival in ovarian cancer. Survival in 92 patients with advanced-stage disease with *p53* overexpression is indicated by the *dotted line*, and that of patients with normal *p53* expression is indicated by the *solid line*. $P > .2$. (Courtesy of Marks JR, Davidoff AM, Kerns BJ, et al: *Cancer Res* 51:2979–2984, 1991.)

Study Design.—The expression of p53 was examined in 107 epithelial ovarian cancers, using immunohistochemical methods with monoclonal antibody PAb1801. Sixty-nine tumor samples were obtained at initial surgery, and 38 were obtained at second-look or subsequent laparotomy. Thirteen samples of nonmalignant gynecologic tissue also were examined.

Findings.—None of the benign tissues stained positively, but half the cancers exhibited strong nuclear immunoreactivity in a majority of the malignant epithelial cells. Similar proportions of early-stage and advanced-stage cancers stained for *p53*. The median survival did not differ significantly in patients with and without p53 overexpression (Fig 1–1). Mutation of *p53* alone probably is not sufficient to induce epithelial ovarian malignancy, but *p53* may contribute to the development of these cancers.

▶ The *p53* anti-oncogene is the most commonly altered genetic locus in human cancers. Because of this unique status, many laboratories are actively exploring the usefulness of *p53* as a diagnostic and/or prognostic cancer marker. The study reported in this research article is an important contribution to this effort. The authors examined a series of 107 epithelial ovarian carcinomas with respect to their *p53* expression status and correlated clinical features. They established that *p53* overexpression is a specific characteristic of malignant gynecologic tissues, occurring in 50% of the examined ovarian cancers. Additionally, they demonstrated that immunohistochemical detection of *p53* overexpression is a sensitive test for the presence of *p53* mutations. The most important aspect of the paper is that, in general, *p53* mutations (as detected by protein overexpression) showed no significant correlation with any important clinical feature. The authors suggest that their results may indicate that *p53* mutations alone are insufficient to induce epithelial ovarian malignancies. More to the point, the data indicate that, at least for this particular disease, *p53* expression status is not likely to be a useful predictor of disease status or treatment outcome.—J.L. Sherley, M.D., Ph.D.

Follow-up Study of Twenty-Four Families With Li-Fraumeni Syndrome
Garber JE, Goldstein AM, Kantor AF, Dreyfus MG, Fraumeni JF Jr, Li FP (Natl Cancer Inst, Bethesda, Md; Dana Farber Cancer Inst, Boston)
Cancer Res 51:6094–6097, 1991 1–6

Background.—The previously described Li-Fraumeni cancer family syndrome comprises susceptibility to breast cancer, sarcomas, and other neoplasms in children and young adults. Follow-up was made of 24 families (blood relatives) previously identified as having the Li-Fraumeni syndrome, in the expectation that findings would allow calculation of cancer frequencies and the possibility of identifying a gene carrier state.

Methods.—Individuals in 24 kindreds that demonstrated the characteristics of the Li-Fraumeni syndrome participated in the study. Pedigrees were constructed for each family, with 864 blood relatives identified. An autosomal-dominant inherited susceptibility was hypothesized for particular cancers in the syndrome, and it was tested in 545 previously unaffected relatives. A second hypothesis, that tumors would occur excessively in those family members at higher risk for carrying a gene for the syndrome, also was tested.

Results.—The 545 family members who were free of cancer were followed for 2–20 years. Any excess malignancies during this period occurred among the younger members of the population, with the relative risk of cancer decreasing with age (table). The test for trend in relative risk was significant. Individual neoplasm excess for breast cancer, adrenocortical carcinomas, brain tumors, and leukemia before age 45, and for osteosarcomas and soft tissue sarcomas at any age also was significant for the study population. For those younger than 45 years, using the restrictive model analysis, 87% of the neoplasms occurred in individuals who had a greater probability of carrying the gene for the syndrome.

Implications.—These results indicate that the characteristics of the Li-Fraumeni syndrome continue to appear in specific families. Once the de-

Observed and Expected Numbers of Cancers During Follow-up, by Age at Diagnosis

Age (yr)	Persons at risk*	No. of cancers: Observed	No. of cancers: Expected	RR (95% CI)
0–19	249	6	0.3	21.1 (7.7–46.0)
20–44	375	17	2.8	6.2 (3.6–9.9)
45–59	154	14	5.8	2.4 (1.3–4.1)
60+	101	15	15.7	1.0 (0.5–1.6)
All ages	545	52	24.5	2.1 (1.6–2.8)

*Number of individuals contributing person-years of observation within the age catagory. During the follow-up period, some individuals contributed to more than 1 age category; therefore, the sum of the numbers is not 545. (Courtesy of Garber JE, Goldstein AM, Kantor AF, et al: *Cancer Res* 51:6094–6097, 1991.)

fective gene becomes known, a clearer understanding of the syndrome will occur. Germ-line mutations of the tumor suppressor gene *p53* were noted in several of the families who had this syndrome.

▶ The Li-Fraumeni syndrome is 1 of the most important discoveries in cancer epidemiology, because of the susceptibility to so many types of cancer. Once again, the importance of this information is that it sets the stage for the increasingly powerful molecular biology tools that are being developed for the precise identification of those individuals who are at risk. As physicians, of course, we hope this will translate into an opportunity for intervention—at the least, early stage therapy and, at best, prevention of the last step in the carcinogenesis cascade.—J.V. Simone, M.D.

Germ-Line Transmission of a Mutated *p53* Gene in a Cancer-Prone Family With Li-Fraumeni Syndrome

Srivastava S, Zou Z, Pirollo K, Blattner W, Chang EH (Uniformed Services Univ of the Health Sciences, Bethesda Natl Cancer Inst, Bethesda, Md)

Nature 348:747–749, 1990 1–7

Background.—Tumor suppressor genes are implicated in many inherited and sporadic forms of neoplasia. There is considerable evidence that tumors form through loss-of-function mutations in suppressor genes, as predicted by the 2-hit model. Mutations in the suppressor gene *p53* are found in various human tumors. They usually represent the loss of 1 allele and the substitution of a single base in the other.

Objective.—The *p53* gene was analyzed in a family with Li-Fraumeni syndrome, a rare autosomal dominant disorder characterized by diverse epithelial and mesenchymal neoplasms at multiple sites. Some of the tumors appeared to be related to exposure to carcinogens, including ionizing radiation.

Findings.—The family studied had noncancerous skin fibroblasts exhibiting a radiation-resistant phenotype. The DNA from the skin fibroblasts of 4 family members (of 2 generations) had the same point mutation in codon 245 (GGC --> GAC) of the *p53* gene. Aspartic acid is substituted for glycine in a region known to be a frequent target of point mutations in *p53*. The affected fibroblast cell lines retained the normal *p53* allele. All 4 affected individuals had cancer. The mutation was absent from fibroblast DNA from 2 individuals who married into the cancer-prone lineage.

Discussion.—The *p53* mutation found in noncancerous cells may predispose to carcinogenesis in this family.

▶ Based on the work of numerous laboratories, it is now clear that somatic mutations in the *p53* anti-oncogene are important in the development of many diverse human tumors. Given the designation of *p53* as a tumor suppressor gene, whether germline mutations in the gene predispose to cancer is an important question. This issue is addressed by the authors, who used molecular genetic techniques to study the genotype of *p53* in a family of patients with features of the familial cancer syndrome described by Li and Fraumeni in 1969 (1). A primary feature of this syndrome suggests the involvement of *p53* mutations, namely the occurrence of cancers of diverse tissues.

The authors examined the *p53* genotype of 10 members from 3 generations of 1 family with Li-Fraumeni. A single mutated *p53* allele that showed almost perfect transmission with the phenotype of cancer was detected. There was only 1 case in which an examined family member with primary Li-Fraumeni features did not carry the *p53* mutation. This exception may be an indication that there are other, yet undefined, factors that are also critical elements in the Li-Fraumeni syndrome. The data presented are consistent with the hypothesis that the detected *p53* mutation is an important genetic factor in the development of cancer in the members of this family, thereby suggesting that germline *p53* mutations can predispose individuals to cancer.—J.L. Sherley, M.D., Ph.D.

Reference

1. Li FP, Fraumeni JF Jr: *Ann Intern Med* 71:747, 1969.

Prognostic Significance of Proliferation Associated Nucleolar Antigen P120 in Human Breast Carcinoma

Freeman JW, McGrath P, Bondada V, Selliah N, Ownby H, Maloney T, Busch RK, Busch H (Univ of Kentucky Med Ctr, Lexington; American Red Cross, Detroit; Michigan Cancer Found, Detroit; Baylor College of Medicine, Houston, Tex)

Cancer Res 51:1973–1978, 1991 1–8

Background.—Nucleolar antigen P120 is found in rapidly proliferating cells but not in normal resting cells. It is also absent from many benign and slowly growing malignant tumors. Preliminary immunocytochemical studies suggest that many, but not all, breast tumors express the P120 antigen.

Objective.—An attempt was made, by analyzing 120 primary breast tumors, to determine whether expression of P120 correlates with prognostic features of the tumor. Most of the tumors were also stained for *erb*B-2 protein. The P120 protein was detected by indirect immunofluorescence.

Findings.—Whereas P120 was identified in 69% of breast cancers, 25% stained positively for *erb*B-2. Twenty-six of the latter 28 tumors were also positive for P120 protein. Fifty-five patients eventually died of recurrent breast cancer; P120 was identified in 89% of their tumors. More than 80% of the patients with P120-negative tumors lived longer than 7 years without recurrent disease (Fig 1–2). Those patients whose tumors expressed P120 and involved the lymph nodes had the worst outlook, but those with P120-negative tumors did well regardless of node status.

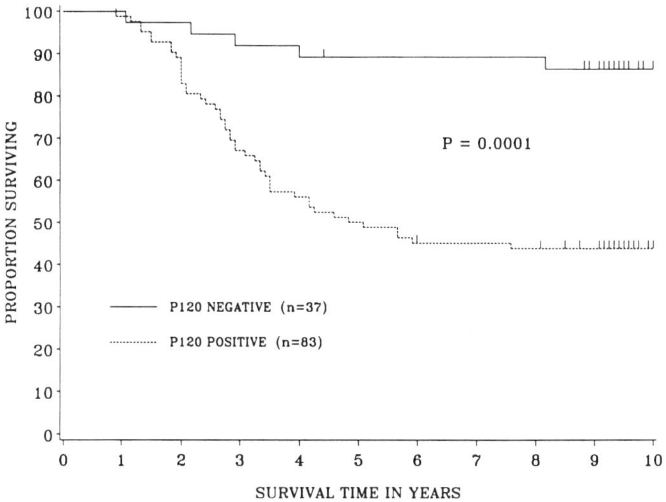

Fig 1–2.—Kaplan-Meier plot of survival from breast cancer in patients with P120-negative tumors *(solid line)* or with P120-positive tumors *(dashed line)*. The *P* value represents the significance for survival for patients with P120-negative tumors. (Courtesy of Freeman JW, McGrath P, Bondada V, et al: *Cancer Res* 51:1973–1978, 1991.)

Conclusion.—The level of expression of P120 by breast cancers has prognostic significance. Further studies will show whether P120 expression correlates with other proliferative parameters such as the S-phase cell percentage.

▶ The P120 antigen is found neither in normal resting tissues nor in benign tumors, but it has been detected in most tumors. The level of P120 antigen is associated with the proliferative state of the cell resulting from an as yet undefined role in producing a hyperactive nucleolus. This study suggests that increased P120 antigen levels are associated with a worse prognosis in breast cancer. This antigen can be added to the growing list of putative prognostic factors (c-*erb*-2, cathespin, *nm*23, *p53,* etc) recently identified in breast cancer biopsy specimens. The clinical usefulness of these newer molecular prognostic factors compared with the more traditional clinical measurements (tumor size, grade, receptor status, ploidy, and nodal status) remains to be determined.—R.F. Ozols, M.D., Ph.D.

Hydroxyurea Accelerates Loss of Extrachromosomally Amplified Genes From Tumor Cells

Von Hoff DD, Waddelow T, Forseth B, Davidson K, Scott J, Wahl G (Univ of Texas, San Antonio; Salk Inst for Biological Studies, La Jolla, Calif)
Cancer Res 51:6273–6279, 1991 1–9

Objective.—Gene amplification is 1 mechanism by which tumor cell resistance to antineoplastic drugs and overexpression of several oncogenes in diverse tumors are mediated. It seems likely that acentric extrachromosomal elements, such as double minute chromosomes, play an intermediary role in the amplification process. These elements, which partition unequally at mitosis, can be lost if selection is not present. Drug-resistant genes were studied to determine whether cells could be made more sensitive to drug treatment by enhancing the loss rate of extrachromosomally amplified genes.

Methods.—The cell lines investigated were vinblastine-resistant human squamous tumor cells; carbamylphosphate synthetase, aspartate transcarbamylase, dihydroorotase genes from *N*-(phosphonacetyl)-L-aspartic acid-resistant Chinese hamster ovary cells, and dihydrofolate reductase genes from methotrexate-resistant human squamous tumor cells. All contained extrachromosomally amplified drug resistance genes. The elimination of multidrug resistance gene 1 from each of these cell lines was measured.

Findings.—Hydroxyurea treatment hastened the loss of extrachromosomally amplified drug resistance genes in each cell line. There was a corresponding increase in drug sensitivity with the loss of these genes. No differential effect on the replication of extrachromosomal DNA sequences appeared to be involved in the mechanism of accelerated loss.

Conclusions.—Hydroxyurea may be helpful in accelerating the elimination of extrachromosomally amplified genes. Although the mechanism is unclear, it does not involve inhibition of DNA synthesis. The results of this study are qualitatively similar to those of previous studies, thus documenting the reproducibility of the protocol.

▶ The process of somatic genetic evolution in tumors is of great significance in the development of the fully malignant phenotype as well as drug resistance. This process can result in double minute chromosomes carrying genes of importance to tumor growth and drug resistance. The amplification and rearrangement of the epidermal growth factor receptor in glioblastomas is an example of the former, whereas the amplification of dihydrofolate reductase in methotrexate-resistant cells, carbamylphosphate synthetase in *N*-(phosphonacetyl)-L-aspartic acid cells, and multidrug resistance gene 1 in vinblastine resistant cells are examples of the latter.

This report confirms a phenomenon first reported in 1983 (1)—that hydroxyurea treatment accelerates the loss of extrachromosomally amplified drug-resistant genes. With the current emphasis on the development of drug strategies aimed at circumventing resistance mechanisms, the possibility of using hydroxyurea or other agents to decrease genetic elements carrying resistance genes is a consideration. Most importantly, this work illustrates the complex interplay between drug therapy and genetic instability in cancer.—G. Kruh, M.D., Ph.D.

Reference

1. Snapka RM, Varshavsky A: *Proc Natl Acad Sci U S A* 80:7533, 1983.

Human Immunodeficiency Virus Induction of Malignant Transformation in Human B Lymphocytes

Laurence J, Astrin SM (Cornell Univ, New York; Fox Chase Cancer Ctr, Philadelphia)

Proc Natl Acad Sci U S A 88:7635–7639, 1991 1–10

Background.—Patients with HIV infection have an increased risk of aggressive B-cell lymphomas developing. Many of these tumors are related to Epstein-Barr virus (EBV) and c-*myc* activation. The interactions among EBV, c-*myc*, and HIV were studied in primary B cells.

Methods.—Peripheral mononuclear cells were isolated from heparinized venous blood, and these cells were exposed to EBV or HIV. Membrane immunofluorescence assays; in situ hybridization for EBV, HIV, and c-*myc;* and transformation assays both in vitro and in vivo were then performed.

Results.—Human immunodeficiency virus was capable of infecting the nonimmortalized peripheral B lymphocytes from EBV-seropositive, HIV-seronegative donors. A subset of the lymphocytes then became transformed according to several criteria. The cells propagated in 1% serum and cloned in soft agar, displaying their altered growth properties. After subcutaneous injection into mice with severe combined immunodeficiency, they formed invasive tumors of the Burkitt's lymphoma phenotype. Epstein-Barr virus DNA and RNA were markedly enhanced in these cells, as were endogenous c-*myc* transcripts and protein. A similar upregulation of EBV and c-*myc* transcripts occurred when previously immortalized B-cell lines were infected with HIV-1.

Conclusions.—Human immunodeficiency virus mediates deregulation of c-*myc* and activation of EBV, 2 events that are linked to B-cell neoplasia. It therefore has properties of a transforming retrovirus. Human immunodeficiency virus may play a part in the pathogenesis of B-cell lymphoma in patients with AIDS, beyond inducing immune suppression.

▶ Although this paper demonstrates that HIV apparently can infect and induce genetic changes in B cells that are latently infected with EBV, there are several puzzling aspects about it. It is not clear how HIV enters B cells and whether the virus requires CD4 expression to bind to the cells. It might be possible that only those B cells expressing surface immunoglobulin with specificity for HIV-envelope protein would be able to bind and internalize the virus. Unfortunately, this prediction was not evaluated in this study. Because many or most of the lymphomas that occur in patients with AIDS show no evidence of involvement by EBV, and because these in vitro effects of HIV were dependent on the presence of the EBV genome in the B cells, it is not clear whether these experiments accurately reflect the in vivo genesis of lymphoma in patients with AIDS. Another potential stumbling block is that HIV sequences have not been detected in B-cell lymphomas from patients with AIDS, but they would be expected if this mechanism occurred in vivo. Finally, the B cells that were transformed in vitro by HIV were not analyzed for the presence of the t(8;14) that is found regularly in patients with AIDS-related lymphoma. Nevertheless, this interesting work may suggest that HIV or fragments of its genome may lead to the activation of certain genes in B cells, which could lead to the development of lymphoma. Whether this occurs in patients with AIDS will require elucidation by further study.

Another lymphoid malignancy that occurs with higher-than-expected frequency in patients with AIDS is Hodgkin's disease. Since we first reported this complication in 1984 (1), a number of reports of patients with AIDS and Hodgkin's disease have appeared. These patients usually have mixed cellularity histology and stage IV disease, and they respond poorly to the usually effective combination chemotherapy programs. Either the disease is refractory or the treatment increases the risk of opportunistic infections, or both. One of the largest experiences with Hodgkin's disease in patients with AIDS was recently published by Zalusky and colleagues (2); they were so pleased with their work that they published it twice (3). It is of interest that Hodgkin's disease in this setting does not obey the rules of contiguous nodal-based spread seen in Hodgkin's disease in patients without AIDS. The involvement of HIV in the transformation of Reed-Sternberg cells or the activation of latent EBV has not yet been carefully examined in patients with AIDS who have Hodgkin's disease.—D.L. Longo, M.D., F.A.C.P.

References

1. Longo DL: *Ann Intern Med* 100:96–98, 1984.
2. Ree HJ, et al: *Cancer* 67:1614, 1991.
3. Gold JE, et al: *Am J Hematol* 36:93, 1991.

Expression of Cathepsin L in Human Tumors

Chauhan SS, Goldstein LJ, Gottesman MM (Natl Cancer Inst, Bethesda, Md)
Cancer Res 51:1478–1481, 1991 1–11

Background.—Cathepsin L is a lysosomal acid cysteine protease found in all types of cells. It acts in the degradation and turnover of intracellular proteins. Malignantly transformed mouse fibroblasts produce large amounts of cathepsin L, but little is known about expression of the protease in human cancer. Proteases secreted by cancer cells could facilitate tumor invasion and metastasis by degrading the components of extracellular membranes.

Objective.—The expression of cathepsin L was examined by quantitative RNA slot-blot analysis in approximately 100 human tumor samples. The assay uses a specific human cathepsin L complementary DNA probe.

Findings.—In general, the cancers expressed higher levels of cathepsin L than did the normal tissues. Renal and testicular tumors expressed the highest levels, followed by nonsmall cell cancers of the lung. Most of the breast, ovarian, colon, bladder, prostatic, and thyroid neoplasms that were examined also expressed increased levels of cathepsin L. Very little messenger RNA for cathepsin L was present in Wilms' tumor, fibrosarcoma, leukemia, or lymphoma.

Conclusions.—The expression of cathepsin L may prove to be a helpful diagnostic or prognostic marker for human neoplasms. These findings complement reports that cathepsin D may serve as a prognostic marker for breast cancer.

▶ Cathepsin is a potent protease that can degrade the basement membrane and thereby facilitate the metastatic process. Previous reports have suggested that increased levels of cathepsin expression may be associated with a poorer prognosis in breast cancer. This study demonstrated that most common solid tumors had increased levels of cathepsin, suggesting that measurements of cathepsin levels may aid in the diagnosis of certain cancers, in addition to having prognostic significance.—R.F. Ozols, M.D., Ph.D.

Cancer Causation

Epipodophyllotoxin-Related Leukemia: Identification of a New Subset of Secondary Leukemia

Whitlock JA, Greer JP, Lukens JN (Vanderbilt Univ, Nashville, Tenn)

Cancer 68:600–604, 1991 1–12

Background.—Chemotherapeutic regimens involving alkylating agents can be complicated by acute nonlymphocytic leukemia (ANLL). In a patient who was successfully treated for a sacrococcygeal germ-cell tumor with a regimen that included etoposide and cisplatin, acute monocytic leukemia developed subsequently.

Case Report.—Girl, 22 months, was seen with a rapidly increasing sacral mass. A biopsy specimen showed a yolk sac tumor, and staging assessment showed lung metastases. Treatment consisted of 8 15-day cycles of vinblastine, bleomycin, cisplatin, and etoposide. The total cumulative etoposide dose was 3,000 mg/m^2. There was no evidence of disease 5 months later. One year later, however, the patient was found to have lymphadenopathy and splenomegaly. The diagnosis of acute monoblastic leukemia was confirmed by bone marrow examination. Cytosine arabinoside and daunomycin produced a remission. High-dose cytosine arabinoside and daunomycin comprised the consolidation therapy. Fifteen months later, the patient remained in remission.

Literature Review.—Identification was made of 36 additional cases of secondary ANLL occurring after etoposide-containing chemotherapeutic regimens were used for a variety of neoplasms. The secondary leukemia occurring in these patients could be distinguished from the secondary leukemia occurring after treatment with alkylating agents by a shorter latency period, a predominance of monocytic or myelomonocytic features, and frequent cytogenetic abnormalities involving 11q23.

Conclusion.—Those patients who are given an epipodophyllotoxin are at risk for a secondary leukemia developing that is distinct from the syndrome of secondary leukemia associated with alkylating agents. In the former, ANLL typically has monocytic features and is frequently associated with 11q23 abnormalities.

▶ Etoposide and teniposide are topo-isomerase II inhibitors that are active in a wide range of tumor types, including lymphoma, Hodgkin's disease, leukemia, testicular cancer, and small cell lung cancer. Pui and colleagues (1) from St. Jude Children's Research Hospital also found an increased incidence of secondary acute myelogenous leukemia (12% at 6 years) occurring in their patients who received teniposide with or without etoposide on a weekly or twice-weekly chronic administration schedule. The schedule was critical, because the incidence was zero in patients who had more than 2 weeks between doses of the epipodophyllotoxin. The leukemia associated with administration of teniposide or etoposide has a characteristic cytogenetic defect involving chromosome 11 at the locus (11q23) of a putative oncogene called acute lymphocytic leukemia-1 (ALL-1), and it occurs with a shorter latency than does secondary leukemia occurring after administration of chronic alkylating agents or combined modality therapy.

Etoposide is too valuable a drug to abandon, especially because more recent data suggest that the activity may be greater if the drug is administered daily by the oral route or by continuous intravenous infusion. Will these schedules be leukemogenic? Is the leukemia related to achieving a high peak-serum dose with a bolus injection and then not allowing time between injections to repair the damage to the stem cell induced by the first dose? Is area under the curve a critical variable? We do not yet have satisfactory answers to these questions.

A recent study by Malkin and colleagues (2) suggests that, in some young patients treated for 1 cancer in whom a second cancer subsequently develops, underlying familial defects in the *p53* gene may be present, creating a susceptibility to subsequent cancers. Such changes were found in only a small fraction of such patients. Numerically, in children, the greatest risk of developing a second cancer is related to having undergone radiation therapy in the course of treatment of the first cancer.—D.L. Longo, M.D., F.A.C.P.

References

1. Pui C-H, et al: *N Engl J Med* 325:1682, 1991.
2. Malkin D, et al: *N Engl J Med* 326:1309, 1992.

Helicobacter Pylori **Infection and the Risk of Gastric Carcinoma**

Parsonnet J, Friedman GD, Vandersteen DP, Chang Y, Vogelman JH, Orentreich N, Sibley RK (Stanford Univ, Stanford, Calif; Kaiser Permanente Med Care Program, Oakland, Calif; Orentreich Found for the Advancement of Science, New York)
N Engl J Med 325:1127–1131, 1991 1–13

Background.—The incidence of gastric carcinoma has decreased in the United States and western Europe in the past 50 years, but it is still estimated to be the world's second most common cancer. Its incidence is hypothesized to be determined by environmental rather than genetic factors. Recently, *Helicobacter pylori* has been linked to chronic atrophic gastritis, an established precursor of the intestinal type of gastric carcinoma. *Helicobacter pylori* infection was investigated as a risk factor for gastric carcinoma in a nested case-control study.

Methods.—From a cohort of 128,992 individuals followed at a health maintenance organization since the mid-1960s, 186 individuals with gastric carcinoma were selected and matched with 186 controls according to age, sex, and race. Frozen serum samples were tested by enzyme-linked immunosorbent assay for *H. pylori* IgG antibodies. Biopsy reports and tissue specimens were reviewed to confirm the histologic reports. Data on cigarette use, blood group, ulcer disease, and gastric surgery were obtained from questionnaires administered at enrollment.

Findings.—Of 109 patients with confirmed gastric adenocarcinoma, 84% had previously been infected with *H. pylori,* compared with 61% of the controls. In women and blacks, *H. pylori* was a particularly strong risk factor for stomach cancer. *Helicobacter pylori* infection and gastric surgery were independent risk factors for cancer, but peptic ulcer disease was negatively associated with the subsequent development of cancer.

Conclusion.—Infection with *H. pylori,* especially beginning in childhood, is associated with an increased risk of gastric adenocarcinoma. Individuals who were seropositive for *H. pylori* were approximately 3 times more likely than matched controls to have gastric adenocarcinoma during follow-up lasting as long as 24 years.

▶ Bacterial carcinogenesis? The data are amazingly convincing that peptic ulcer disease is substantially less likely to recur if patients infected with *H. pylori* are treated for that infection with bismuth subcitrate for 4 weeks, amoxicillin for 4 weeks, and metronidazole for 2 weeks (1). Indeed, therapy for peptic ulcer disease is not complete without a vigorous attempt to eradicate *H. pylori.* The evidence is mounting that chronic gastritis with this bacterium is a premalignant lesion. In addition to this report, 3 others published this year reach the same conclusion (2–4). The problem is that the infection is highly prevalent. At the same time and for unexplained reasons, the incidence of gastric cancer in the United States is declining without a clear similar trend in *H. pylori* prevalence. Huge numbers of people (possibly 180 million) have the infection, yet few go on to have gastric cancer develop.

The epidemiologic findings present us with a quandary. Therapy for the infection is pretty effective and not terribly expensive, but it is impractical to try to eradicate the infection entirely in every citizen. However, the eradication of the infection in individuals who are at high risk might prevent cancer in a simple and relatively cheap manner. How do we determine who is at high risk and who should receive therapy? A simple blood test to detect antibodies to the organism can reliably detect infected individuals; however, other features that can identify individuals who are at risk are not yet clear.—D.L. Longo, M.D., F.A.C.P.

References

1. Rauws EAJ, Tytgat GNJ: *Lancet* 335:1233, 1990.
2. Nomura A, et al: *N Engl J Med* 325:1132, 1991.
3. Forman D, et al: *Br Med J* 302:1302, 1991.
4. Talley NJ, et al: *J Natl Cancer Inst* 83:1734, 1991.

Risk Factors

Smoking-Attributable Cancer Mortality in 1991: Is Lung Cancer Now the Leading Cause of Death Among Smokers in the United States?

Shopland DR, Eyre HJ, Pechacek TF (Natl Cancer Inst, Bethesda, Md; American Cancer Society, Atlanta)

J Natl Cancer Inst 83:1142–1148, 1991 1–14

Objective.—This report summarizes the findings from 2 new reports (in 1989 and 1990) on the health consequences of smoking as reported by the Surgeon General. Emphasis was placed on the new relative risk estimates for the major smoking-related cancer sites, the estimate of total 1991 cancer mortality burden attributed to smoking, and the implication of these findings in relation to other serious diseases to which smoking contributes (e.g., coronary heart disease).

Data Analysis.—The prospective study by the American Cancer Society involved 1.2 million men and women in the United States. For most of the 8 major cancer sites causally associated with cigarette smoking, the mortality risks among smokers increased substantially compared with nonsmokers. The lung cancer risk doubled among male smokers and increased more than fourfold in female smokers, whereas the lung cancer risk for those who never smoked remained virtually unchanged. On the basis of these new relative risks, it was projected that smoking alone would contribute to 157,226 of the 514,000 total cancer deaths expected to occur in 1991. Of these, 123,111 excess cancer deaths resulted from lung cancer. Cigarette smoking accounted for 86.1% of the 1991 projected lung cancer deaths and 30.6% of the total cancer deaths. Smoking directly contributed to 21.5% of all cancer deaths in women and 45% of all cancer deaths in men. Given the declining pattern of deaths resulting from coronary heart disease and overall death rates, lung cancer has now displaced coronary heart disease as the single leading cause of excess mortality among smokers in the United States.

Discussion.—Lung cancer is now the leading cause of death among smokers in the United States. These findings provide new impetus to efforts to reduce smoking prevalence.

▶ This provocative paper suggests that lung cancer is now the leading cause of death among smokers in the United States. The tragedy of lung cancer is that it is so disgustingly preventable, and we must work harder at educating our patients about the hazards of smoking and the benefits of cessation. The time to stop smoking is as soon as possible, not after the diagnosis of cancer has been made.—E. Glatstein, M.D.

Prenatal Exposure to Parents' Smoking and Childhood Cancer

John EM, Savitz DA, Sandler DP (Univ of North Carolina, Chapel Hill; Stanford Univ, Stanford, Calif; Natl Inst of Environmental Health Sciences, Research Triangle Park, NC)

Am J Epidemiol 133:123–132, 1991 1–15

Introduction.—Many studies have reported increased risks of adverse pregnancy outcome as an effect of maternal smoking, and such exposure may also increase the child's risk of cancer. There have been no studies of the risk of childhood cancer associated with paternal smoking. Data from a childhood cancer study of data on both parents' tobacco smoking during the prenatal period were reviewed.

Methods.—The data were drawn from a case-control study of childhood cancer and exposure to electromagnetic fields. All children 14 years of age and younger in whom cancer was diagnosed in Denver between 1976 and 1983 served as incident cases. The controls, who were matched for age, sex, and geographic area, were selected by random-digit dialing. Data on smoking by the parents and other members of the household were obtained by personal interviews. A total of 223 cases and 196 controls was analyzed.

Results.—Maternal smoking during the first trimester of pregnancy was associated with an increased risk for all cancers combined (odds ratio [OR], 1.3) after adjustment for the father's level of education. The risks of acute lymphocytic leukemia (OR, 1.9) and lymphoma (OR, 2.3) were also increased. Again after adjustment for the father's education, associations with the father's smoking (in the absence of maternal smoking) were found for all cancers combined (OR, 1.2), acute lymphocytic leukemia (OR, 1.4), lymphomas (OR, 1.6), and brain cancer (OR, 1.6). Associations with maternal smoking alone tended to be stronger than those with paternal smoking alone.

Conclusion.—Prenatal exposure to parents' smoking may have an effect on childhood cancer. The risk estimates are limited by the small number of cases. Prenatal exposure may have different effects on male and female fetuses.

▶ If we needed any further evidence that smoking is bad, here it is. Not only is smoking bad for the smoker and for those who inhale ambient smoke, but there is now evidence that maternal or paternal smoking increases an infant's risk of having cancer later in life. Maternal smoking during the first trimester of pregnancy substantially increased the risk of acute lymphocytic leukemia and lymphoma. The same is true of paternal smoking during the first trimester of an offspring's gestation. Although the data are only suggestive, the increased risk is great enough to give any parent pause about taking the chance of increasing the risk of cancer in the child. Physicians should counsel parents-to-be about these data.—J.V. Simone, M.D.

A Meta-Analysis of the Effect of Estrogen Replacement Therapy on the Risk of Breast Cancer

Steinberg KK, Thacker SB, Smith SJ, Stroup DF, Zack MM, Flanders WD, Berkelman RL (Ctrs for Disease Control, Atlanta; Emory Univ)
JAMA 265:1985–1990, 1991 1–16

Effect of Estrogen Replacement Therapy on the Relative Risk of Breast Cancer in Women, Stratified by Risk Factors

Type or Stratification	Strata	Number of Values*	Mean Relative Risk (95% confidence interval)	P Value for Equality of	References
Family History of Breast	Yes	7	3.4 (2.0 - 6.0)	0.003	23, 32, 33, 38, 42, 62
	No	7	1.5 (1.2 - 1.7)		23, 32, 33, 38, 42, 62
Parity	Nulliparous	7	1.5 (1.1 - 2.1)	0.40	23, 32, 33, 38, 42, 62
	Parous	10	1.3 (1.0 - 1.7)		23, 33, 42, 62
Benign Breast Disease	Yes	9	1.7 (1.2 - 2.3)	0.50	23, 32, 33, 37, 38, 42, 62
	No	8	1.4 (1.2 - 1.7)		23, 32, 33, 37, 38, 42, 62
Age at First Full Term Pregnancy (years)	< 20	3	1.1 (0.6 - 2.0)	0.38	23, 33, 38
	20 - 30	5	1.1 (0.9 - 1.5)		23, 33, 38, 42
	> 30	3	1.7 (1.0 - 3.0)		23, 38, 42

*Some studies used 2 durations of estrogen use, which were assumed to include different women.
(Courtesy of Steinberg KK, Thacker SB, Smith SJ, et al: *JAMA* 265:1985–1990, 1991.)

Objective.—Although understanding of the risks and benefits of estrogen replacement therapy has improved, its effect on the risk of breast cancer is still uncertain. A meta-analysis was done to ascertain the impact of the duration of estrogen replacement therapy on the risk of breast cancer.

Methods.—The dose-response slopes of the relative risk of breast cancer against the duration of estrogen use obtained from 16 studies were combined. This summary dose-response slope was then used to calculate the proportional increase in breast cancer risk for each year of estrogen use.

Findings.—The risk of cancer apparently did not increase until after at least 5 years of use among women with any type of menopause. There was a 30% increase in risk after 15 years of estrogen therapy, for a relative risk of 1.3. The increased risk was primarily attributable to the results of studies that included premenopausal women or women receiving estradiol. In these studies, the relative risk was 2.2 after 15 years. Those women with a family history of breast cancer had a significantly higher risk if they had ever used estrogen replacement compared with those who had not (table).

Discussion.—This analysis shows that, in women experiencing any type of menopause, the breast cancer risk increases after at least 5 years of estrogen use. The risk increases to 1.3 after 15 years of use.

▶ There has been enormous concern about the potential effect of estrogen replacement on the risk of breast cancer. Most of the earlier studies suggested either no risk or a minimal increase in breast cancer risk. This large meta-analysis of 16 studies suggests that breast cancer risk does increase after at least 5 years of estrogen exposure. After 15 years of exposure, the relative risk is 1.3, suggesting a 30% increase in breast cancer risk. This appears to be particularly true in women with a family history of breast cancer; in these women, the relative risk was increased threefold. The table documents the relative risks of estrogen in particular groups of women with known risk factors. The study is confounded by the inability to distinguish between the effects of premenopausal and postmenopausal estrogens, different estrogen preparations, and estrogen-progesterone combinations. Nevertheless, the analysis suggests that prolonged estrogen exposure does increase breast cancer risk, particularly in women with a family history of breast cancer.—R.C. Young, M.D., F.A.C.P.

Service in Vietnam and Risk of Testicular Cancer

Tarone RE, Hayes HM, Hoover RN, Rosenthal JF, Brown LM, Pottern LM, Javadpour N, O'Connell KJ, Stutzman RE (Natl Cancer Inst, Bethesda, Md; Westat Inc, Rockville, Md)

J Natl Cancer Inst 83:1497–1499, 1991 1–17

Background.—Military working dogs that served during the period of the Vietnam conflict have been reported to have had a significantly increased risk of testicular tumors, and testicular dysfunction was found in dogs who served and died in Vietnam. Because carcinogenic risk to dogs can be a useful indicator of increased risk to humans, the risk of testicular cancer was assessed in men who served in Vietnam.

Subjects.—Subjects (aged 18–42 years) with testicular cancer newly diagnosed between 1976 and 1981 were matched with controls who had cancers other than cancer of the genital tract. Questionnaires provided information on military service. The analysis was restricted to 137 case subjects and 130 control subjects.

Findings.—A twofold increased risk of testicular cancer was observed in Vietnam veterans, with a greater risk found in younger Vietnam veterans. These 2 findings were also observed in the dog study. Smoking, educational status, and branch of military service had little effect on the odds ratio. A study of Air Force veterans of Operation Ranch Hand, who sprayed the herbicide Agent Orange, reported 3 testicular cancers in 995 veterans, compared with no testicular tumors among 1,299 Air Force veterans who flew air transport in Southeast Asia.

Conclusion.—A twofold increased risk of testicular cancer (with a greater risk for younger veterans) was observed in this study. Further study is warranted on the possible etiologic role of Agent Orange and other risk factors in observed testicular abnormalities in Vietnam veterans.

Case-Control Study of Canine Malignant Lymphoma: Positive Association With Dog Owner's Use of 2,4-Dichlorophenoxyacetic Acid Herbicides

Hayes HM, Tarone RE, Cantor KP, Jessen CR, McCurnin DM, Richardson RC (Natl Cancer Inst, Bethesda, Md; Univ of Minnesota, St Paul; Colorado State Univ, Ft Collins; Purdue Univ, West Lafayette, Ind)

J Natl Cancer Inst 83:1226–1231, 1991 1–18

Background.—Mounting evidence suggests that phenoxyacetic acid herbicides, especially 2,4-dichlorophenoxyacetic acid (2,4-D), are associated with an increased risk of non-Hodgkin's lymphoma in farmers. Potential exposures to animals are substantial, especially because 2,4-D is commonly used by lawn care companies. Although malignant lymphoma, the canine equivalent of non-Hodgkin's lymphoma, has been studied extensively, its cause remains unknown. The relationship of this tumor to chemical exposures,—2,4-D in particular—was investigated in a case-control study.

Methods.—Dogs with confirmed malignant lymphoma were identified from the records of 3 collaborating veterinary medicine teaching hospitals. Two age-matched control groups of animals were also selected—1 from among all other tumor cases and the other from among dogs seen for any other diagnostic reason. The dogs' owners were sent a questionnaire or were interviewed by telephone as to the use of chemicals in and around the home. A total of 491 case households, 466 nontumor control households, and 479 tumor control households responded; the response rates were 84%, 80%, and 82%, respectively.

Results.—The owners of dogs that had malignant lymphoma were significantly more likely to use 2,4-D on their lawn or to use a commercial lawn care company, for an odds ratio of 1.3. Among those households in which the owner 2,4-D 4 times a year or more, the risk of malignant lymphoma increased to a twofold excess. These findings were consistent with studies reporting a modest association between agricultural exposure to 2,4-D and the risk of non-Hodgkin's lymphoma.

Conclusions.—There is an association between the use of 2,4-D herbicide and malignant lymphoma in pet dogs. The risk is even higher when the herbicide is applied several times per year. Further study of the health implications of exposure to 2,4-D is warranted in humans.

▶ These 2 studies (Abstracts 1–17 and 1–18) seem to be reaching for a conclusion that the data do not really support. Extrapolations from dogs to men seem risky. Very few men sit in grass saturated with phenoxyacetic acid herbicides and then lick off the herbicides. The study documenting a twofold risk of testicular cancer (Abstract 1–17) is of marginal statistical significance. The dog study (Abstract 1–18) is curious, but it begs the question of the health of the dog owners themselves. I would argue that the nature of a dog's exposure is likely to be both qualitatively and quantitatively different from that of a man's exposure.

Studies of individuals exposed to phenoxyacetic acid herbicides do not necessarily agree with each other. One study of more than 5,000 individuals working in plants producing such chemicals failed to document any significantly increased risk of cancer, although its power to detect increases in very rare cancers was small (1). Even in studies that conclude that such herbicide exposure is a risk, the risk is small. The development of lymphoma or testicular cancer in a young individual is of serious concern. However, both were known to occur in young men before exposure to herbicides became a veteran's benefits issue. The available data are simply not strong enough to confirm that exposure to herbicides has exerted a major influence on the frequency of these tumors.—D.L. Longo, M.D., F.A.C.P.

Reference

1. Fingerhut MA, et al: *N Engl J Med* 324:212, 1991.

Additional Reading

Henderson BE, Ross RK, Pike MC: Toward the primary prevention of cancer. *Science* 254:1131–1138, 1991.

Weinberg RA: Tumor suppressor genes. *Science* 254:1138–1146, 1991.

Aaronson SA: Growth factors and cancer. *Science* 254:1146–1153, 1991.

Solomon E, Borrow J, Goddard AD: Chromosome aberrations and cancer. *Science* 254:1153–1160, 1991.

Adams JM, Cory S: Transgenic models of tumor development. *Science* 254:1161–1167, 1991.

zur Hausen H: Viruses in human cancers. *Science* 254:1167–1173, 1991.

▶ If you have an hour or 2 to obtain a priceless education in state-of-the-art cancer etiology, check out this issue of *Science*. This wonderful series of articles appeared in the November 22, 1991 issue. All the articles are well written and authoritative. At the very least, a physician should read the article by Henderson et al., which debunks the myths surrounding some of the information concerning diet and environmental factors. If you are a fan of biotechnology, the article by Adams and Cory describes the most powerful new tool yet. Do yourself a favor and at least skim the articles. Also, keep copies in your office for inquisitive patients.

Mickisch GH, Merlino GT, et al: Transgenic mice that express the human multidrug-resistance gene in bone marrow enable a rapid identification of agents that reverse drug resistance. *Proc Natl Acad Sci U S A* 88:547–551, 1991.

▶ Multidrug resistance gene 1-transgenic mice provide a useful system to determine the bioactivity of agents that reverse multidrug resistance.

Haut M, Steeg PS, et al: Induction of nm23 gene expression in human colonic neoplasms and equal expression in colon tumors of high and low metastatic potential. *J Natl Cancer Inst* 83:712–716, 1991.

▶ In contrast to studies in breast cancer, increased expression of the *nm23* gene was not associated with metastatic potential in colorectal tumors. It remains to be established in colon cancer that the *nm23* product is not inactivated by a mutation.

Wunder JS, Czitrom AA, et al: Analysis of alterations in the retinoblastoma gene and tumor grade in bone and soft-tissue sarcomas. *J Natl Cancer Inst* 83:194–200, 1991.

▶ Of the high-grade sarcomas, 40% had detectable alterations in the retinoblastoma-1 gene compared with 9% of the low-grade tumors.

Hollstein M, Sidransky D, et al: *p53* mutations in human cancers. *Science* 253:49–53, 1991.

▶ An excellent review on the role of *p53* mutation in human cancer.

Tanaka K, Oshimura M, Kikuchi R, et al: Suppression of tumorigenicity in human colon carcinoma cells by introduction of normal chromosome 5 or 18. *Nature* 349:340–342, 1991.

▶ Allelic loss of the APC gene on *5q* and the DCC gene on *18q* are associated with colon cancer; experimental replacement of the missing alleles appears to reverse the phenotype to more benign behavior.

Chen P-L, Chen Y, Bookstein R, et al: Genetic mechanisms of tumor suppression by the human *p53* gene. *Science* 250:1576–1580, 1991.

▶ The malignant phenotype of a tumor cell lacking endogenous *p53* could be reversed by giving the cell a single copy of the wild-type *p53* gene; in the presence of both mutant and wild-type *p53,* wild-type was dominant, a finding similar to prior findings with the retinoblastoma gene.

Blot WJ, Devesa SS, Kneller RW, et al: Rising incidence of adenocarcinoma of the esophagus and gastric cardia. *JAMA* 265:1287–1289, 1991.

▶ Although the incidence of gastric cancer is decreasing, adenocarcinoma of the esophagus and gastroesophageal junction is increasing by 4% to 10% per year, mainly in white men.

Davis DL, Ahlbom A, Hoel D, et al: Is brain cancer mortality increasing in industrialized countries? *Am J Indust Med* 19:421–431, 1991.

▶ Brain cancer mortality does appear to be increasing.

Barzilay J, Heatley GJ, Cushing GW: Benign and malignant tumors in patients with acromegaly. *Arch Intern Med* 151:1629–1632, 1991.

▶ Growth hormone may affect a variety of tissues and could act as a mitogenic signal for a tissue that had sustained a prior mutagenic injury; malignant tumors were 2.45 times more common in patients with acromegaly than in patients with other types of pituitary tumors.

Sidransky D, Frost P, Von Eschenbach A, et al: Clonal origin of bladder cancer. *N Engl J Med* 326:737–740, 1992.

▶ Vogelstein lab breakthrough #101: multiple tumors of the bladder appearing at different sites in the bladder at different times all contained evidence of origin from a common clone (based on analysis of allelic loss on autosomes and X-inactivation).

2 Cancer Prevention and Control

Risk Factors

Bone Cancer Incidence Rates in New York State: Time Trends and Fluoridated Drinking Water

Mahoney MC, Nasca PC, Burnett WS, Melius JM (New York State Dept of Health, Albany; State Univ of New York, Albany)

Am J Pub Health 81:475–479, 1991 2–1

Background.—The health effects of artificial fluoridation of drinking water have long been a topic of debate. The finding that rats that ingest a high fluoride diet have an increased incidence of osteosarcoma has raised new questions about the association between fluoridated water and bone cancers. Trends in the incidence of bone cancers were examined, including the incidence of osteosarcoma in areas with and without fluoridated water.

Methods.—The data for the analysis came from the New York State Cancer Registry and included only primary malignancies of the bone occurring in residents of New York State, exclusive of New York City. After comparison of the average annual age-specific rates of bone cancer and osteosarcoma, the incidence of bone cancer and osteosarcoma was evaluated among residents of communities with fluoridated and nonfluoridated water supplies.

Results.—Among male populations younger than 30 years of age, the incidence of bone cancer has increased significantly since 1955; however, there has been no change in the incidence for female populations. For individuals of both sexes who were older than 30 years of age, the incidence of bone cancer decreased significantly during the same time period. Among both sexes and age groups, there was essentially no change in the incidence of osteosarcoma. From 1976 to 1987, the average annual age-adjusted incidence of osteosarcoma in areas with fluoridated water was no different from the incidence in areas without fluoridated water.

Conclusions.—There appears to be no association between fluoridated drinking water and the incidence of bone cancers, including osteosarcoma. An increasing incidence of bone cancers is evident, particularly among younger individuals. The role of fluoride in these cancers might be more thoroughly investigated by using an analytic study design with more careful assessment of residential history and fluoride exposure.

▶ For a variety of reasons, fluoridation of public drinking water has been hotly debated for more than 40 years. Despite its substantial benefit in reducing the incidence of dental caries, periodic waves of concern are expressed both in the media and by various public groups. Most recently, because of the evidence of increased osteosarcoma in rats ingesting high-fluoride diets, there have been concerns about possible increases in osteogenic sarcoma in those populations exposed to fluoridated drinking water. This study looks carefully at fluoride- and nonfluoride-exposed populations in the state of New York. Although a significant increase in bone cancer among males younger than 30 years of age was noted in general, there was no increase in fluoride-exposed populations compared with nonexposed populations. Overall, there was a significant decrease in bone cancer incidence among both males and females older than 30 years of age, and no substantial difference in any subset of patients was related to fluoride exposure. Although the study does not precisely assess the magnitude of fluoride exposure, it is reassuring and suggests that bone cancers are not linked to fluoride in drinking water.—R.C. Young, M.D. F.A.C.P.

Contacts Between Adults as Evidence for an Infective Origin of Childhood Leukaemia: An Explanation for the Excess Near Nuclear Establishments in West Berkshire?

Kinlen LJ, Hudson CM, Stiller CA (Univ of Oxford, Oxford, England)
Br J Cancer 64:549–554, 1991 2–2

Background.—It has been proposed that, in relation to childhood leukemia, a community's response to underlying infection can be disturbed by increases in new social contacts. The social trend for individuals to work outside of their home community could be relevant to this hypothesis. Census data on workplace was used to investigate this possibility.

Methods.—The census data included 28 county boroughs whose boundaries were unchanged by a major reorganization in 1974. This permitted accurate comparisons of workplace data from the 1971 and 1981 censuses. A sum of outward and inward movement of workers was calculated in each borough and then ranked according to the extent of commuting increase. The details of leukemia incidence were drawn from the National Registry of Childhood Tumors.

Results.—A significant trend in leukemia incidence was seen at ages 0–14 years, and a suggestive trend was found at ages 0–4 years. In these age groups (from 1972 to 1985), the only significant increases in leukemia among 10 similar sized groups of county districts ranked by commuting increase were in the highest tenth for commuting increase. Even after exclusion of Reading, which is in an area where an excess of leukemia has been linked to nearby nuclear facilities, these excesses persisted. The entire Reading area showed more commuting increases than 90% of the districts in England and Wales.

Conclusions.—Evidence supports the infection-based hypothesis that contact between adults may affect the incidence of childhood leukemia. Population dynamics are relevant to herd immunity; therefore, they should be considered when an excess of childhood leukemia is seen in a community.

▶ This report reveals another aspect of the infection/immunity theory of childhood leukemia causation. The theory is that the greater the number of outside physical contacts a community has, the greater the likelihood of bringing in an infective and leukemogenic agent. The data in this paper suggest that, insofar as it can be measured, communities with the greatest inward and outward movement of workers ranked highest in the frequency of childhood leukemia. Although they examine only a small part of the infectious etiology hypothesis, studies like this make it possible to begin developing more precise scientific measures. Of course, the goal is to identify the leukemogenic agent or agents so that one may either counsel avoidance or develop immunization procedures.—J.V. Simone, M.D.

Dietary Pesticides (99.99% All Natural)

Ames BN, Profet M, Gold LS (Univ of Calif, Berkeley; Lawrence Berkeley Lab, Berkeley, Calif)

Proc Natl Acad Sci U S A 87:7777–7781, 1990 2–3

Background.—There is an imbalance in data and perceptions about the potential hazards of chemicals to humans, because of the numerous toxicologic examinations of synthetic chemicals and the lack of investigations of natural chemicals. The natural pesticides found in the diet were examined.

Discussion.—By weight, 99.99% of the pesticides found in the American diet are natural chemicals that plants produce to protect themselves. It is estimated that humans consume 1.5 g of natural pesticides per day (with vegetarians consuming greater amounts); it has also been suggested that humans ingest 5,000 to 10,000 different natural pesticides and breakdown products. Few of these toxins have been tested for carcinogenicity. Catechol-type phenolics are more widespread than other natural pesticides, and they may have an antimicrobial role, oxidizing when a plant is wounded. Exposure to natural rodent carcinogens may cast doubt on the relevance of far lower levels of exposure to synthetic carcinogens. The intake of rodent carcinogens from synthetic residues is only approximately .05 mg per day. Cooking produces approximately 2 g of burned material that contains many rodent carcinogens per individual per day. Coffee contains nearly 10 mg per cup, but it cannot be shown to be a risk factor in humans. In high-dose protocols, in vitro studies of natural pesticides are commonly positive. Some carcinogenic plant toxins are clastogenic at far lower levels than their concentrations in food.

Conclusions.—Natural and synthetic chemicals appear equally likely to be positive in animal cancer tests. At the low doses of most human exposures, the comparative hazards of synthetic pesticide residues are insignificant.

▶ More than a decade ago, Doll and Peto suggested that environmental pollution was responsible for less than 2% of all cancers. Nevertheless, there has been major concern about the potential cancer risk associated with environmental pesticides. Several previous publications that were reviewed in the 1991 YEAR BOOK suggested an association between lymphoma and pesticide exposure. This review by Bruce Ames provides a careful analysis of the various natural pesticides and their potential risk. Although many of these compounds are rodent carcinogens, the study illustrates the difficulty in using this information to provide a direct estimate of hazard to humans. The chief exposure is to natural plant pesticides that are present in the environment in 10,000 times the quantity that synthetic pesticide residues are found. What is remarkable about the data is that humans are exposed to a vast array of different pesticides (as many as 5,000–10,000 different types), each with a different spectrum of carcinogenic risk. The extent to which this array of naturally occurring carcinogens plays a role in our background risk of cancer is problematic. As the article emphasizes, although vegetarians are exposed to a significantly larger amount of these natural carcinogens, the cancer risks are actually decreased in individuals who consume large amounts of fruits and vegetables. Presumably, the anticarcinogenic vitamins and anti-oxidants from fruits and vegetables outweigh the carcinogenic risk.—R.C. Young, M.D., F.A.C.P.

Community Lifestyle Characteristics and Risk of Acute Lymphoblastic Leukaemia in Children

Alexander FE, Ricketts TJ, McKinney PA, Cartwright RA (Univ of Leeds, Leeds, England)

Lancet 336:1461–1465, 1990 2–4

Introduction.—Clusters of childhood leukemia have been noted in isolated communities, rapidly growing communities, and dormitory villages. Data on the incidence of acute lymphoblastic leukemia (ALL) were compared at ward level to relate incidence to aspects of community lifestyle.

Methods.—The incidence data came from 2 specialist registries. The data were taken from the Leukemia Research Fund Data Collection Survey, which covers 22 counties in England and Wales. The incidence of ALL reported by this registry was related to community characteristics identified in routine census and Ordnance Survey data. Data from the Yorkshire Region Children's Tumor Registry covered a different time period and were used to test the main findings. The indicators of ward lifestyle included socioeconomic status, commuting distance, urban-rural status, settlement type, distance from a built-up area, and settlement isolation.

Results.—Especially for children aged 1–7 years, the town and village wards had higher risks than built-up wards and other wards. Highly significant increases in risk were seen with distance from a built-up area. A twofold excess (the greatest risk) was seen in wards of higher socioeconomic status and in children aged 1–7 years, which is the childhood peak.

Conclusion.—The lifestyle of isolated communities, particularly those of higher socioeconomic status, may be conducive to some unusual exposure that ultimately increases the risk of childhood leukemia. These results are consistent with the modest effects of area socioeconomic status and the nonsignificant excess in rural (compared with urban) areas.

▶ This is a provocative paper. Basically, it observes that the incidence of childhood leukemia is greatest in higher socioeconomic groups that live in isolated communities away from dense, urban areas. This fits reasonably well with the hypothesis of Greaves (1), who proposed that reduced antigenic challenges in infancy result in more susceptibility to a variety of infectious agents, some of which might provoke leukemogenesis. This paper by no means proves that relationship; however, childhood ALL is a peculiar disease in many respects. The peak incidence between 3 and 6 years of age has led to the belief that a viral agent causes the disease. The unusual susceptibility to a wide variety of chemotherapeutic agents make it 1 of the few disseminated malignancies to be curable with hemotherapy alone. Furthermore, the response to therapy is far better in infants than in teenagers and adults. All these features have encouraged the belief in an infectious agent that causes a malignant aberration in lymphoid development. One hopes that investigations of this type will continue and will be complemented by the new technology in molecular epidemiology that may make it possible to prove appropriate associations.—J.V. Simone, M.D.

Socioeconomic Status and Cancer Survival

Cella DF, for the Cancer and Leukemia Group B (Rush-Presbyterian–St Luke's Med Ctr, Chicago, Ill)

J Clin Oncol 9:1500–1509, 1991 2–5

Background.—Socioeconomic status (SES) is associated with cancer survival. It was investigated whether race, income, or educational level predicts either the initial performance status (IPS) of patients entering a clinical trial or longer survival after adjusting for differences from IPS and other prognostic indicators.

Study Design.—Survival data from 8 Cancer and Leukemia Group B protocols were analyzed for 961 patients with lung cancer, 577 with multiple myeloma, 231 with gastric cancer, 174 with pancreatic cancer, 87 with breast cancer, and 58 with Hodgkin's disease. Adjustments were made for differences in survival rate that were attributable to cancer type, IPS, age, and 14 other protocol-specific prognostic indicators, and the predictive value of SES was determined.

Results.—White or nonwhite race did not significantly predict survival time; however, income and education did. Those patients with lower annual incomes and lower educational levels had significantly shorter survival times than patients with higher incomes or educational levels. Although these survival differences were associated with severity of disease at initial diagnosis, they could not be fully explained by it. Even after controlling for all known prognostic variables, SES exerted a small but significant effect on cancer survival.

Conclusions.—Patients with cancer who are economically and educationally disadvantaged may need treatment programs that include education about treatment and compliance. Such education may be necessary, even after the diagnosis has been made and treatment has begun. Because SES is related to survival independent of all known prognostic variables, it should be included in clinical trial databases to provide more accurate testing of the effectiveness of new treatments.

▶ This study and others suggest that where individuals live, how much money they make, and their level of education play a role in cancer incidence and survival. There are also some racial differences in cancer incidence. For example, Baquet and colleagues (1) found a significantly higher incidence of lung, stomach, cervix, and prostate cancer among blacks than among whites; they also found a significantly higher incidence of rectal and breast cancer among whites. However, when age-adjusted incidence data were correlated with socioeconomic status, whites showed a higher overall cancer risk at all sites combined. It is the disproportionate distribution of blacks in the lower socioeconomic levels that accounts for much (but not all) of the excess cancer burden among blacks.

There is some evidence that blacks do not use the medical care system to the same extent as whites, and that there is an inverse relationship between poverty and the use of preventive medical care, such as screening and early detection services (2). Some of this underutilization is related to an inability to pay for services, and some apparently is related to a fatalistic attitude about the outcome of serious illnesses by individuals of low income or poor education (3). Most of the data would argue that implementation of preventive and/or screening measures for certain cancers in particular high-risk groups would make a significant impact on the dismal statistics. For example, programs designed to stop smoking are needed, and having poor women undergo Papanicolaou testing might significantly lower the incidence of cervical cancer.—D.L. Longo, M.D., F.A.C.P.

References

1. Baquet CR, et al: *J Natl Cancer Inst* 83:551, 1991.
2. Blendon RJ, et al: *JAMA* 261:278, 1989.
3. Freeman HP: *Cancer* 39:266, 1989.

Household Magnetic Fields and Childhood Leukemia: A Critical Analysis

Michaelson SM (Univ of Rochester)

Pediatrics 88:630–635, 1991 2–6

Background.—The past 2 decades have seen an increased interest in the link between the hazards of exposure to the magnetic and electrical fields from high-voltage power lines and household appliances and cancer. Public anxiety over the possibility of such an association has greatly increased. The available human data on this subject were studied to determine whether this anxiety is justified.

Methods.—Residences usually obtain electric power as direct current and/or alternating current of 50 or 60 Hz. Electrical fields form from electric charges around a conductor, whereas magnetic fields form around the area of the flow of AC electric current. The literature shows that approximately 40 studies have researched the association between human cancer frequency and exposure to power frequency.

Results.—Wertheimer and Leeper's early study of 344 children who died before 19 years of age found a higher incidence of cancer in residences near "high-current configurations." It was estimated that children living near these high-current configurations had a 2–3 times greater chance of having cancer than children residing near a low-current configuration. Later studies, using similar measurement parameters, found either no association or weak associations between living near high electric current(s) and the frequency of cancer. Wertheimer and Leeper's later study resulted in an association between the incidence of both childhood and adult cancer and the number of high-current power lines found near the patients' residences. However, systematic current measurements were not obtained at the subjects' homes. A Swedish study also found a weak association between tumor occurrence and residential location near magnetic fields, but the current levels were again based on the kind of wiring configurations used—not on direct measurement. Savitz et al. did a more complete study in Denver, Colorado, by actually measuring current near the homes of 356 patients with childhood cancers. They found only a weak correlation (odds ratio, 1–1.5) between all types of cancers and the presence of magnetic fields in a dose-response manner. A study performed in Seattle, Washington, found no correlation between wire configurations and magnetic fields and the incidence of acute nonlymphocytic leukemia.

Conclusions.—This review and assessment of the available epidemiologic studies found a somewhat weak association between a higher risk of cancer and household exposure to 60-Hz magnetic fields. Animal studies have not linked cancer and current exposure, and scientists have not proposed a cohesive hypothetical mechanism for this association.

▶ There has been a major focus in the media and the lay press about the potential of electromagnetic fields, high voltage transmissions lines, and electrical appliances to increase the risk of cancer. Although several earlier studies have suggested an increased risk, comprehensive analysis of the published literature to date does not support a definite cause-and-effect relationship between such exposures and leukemia. Animal studies have not documented such an increased risk, and no sound biophysical mechanism has yet been proposed for such a risk. Although none of this can be taken to prove that no risk exists, this paper suggests that, at present, there is little scientific evidence for an association between electromagnetic fields and cancer.—R.C. Young, M.D., F.A.C.P.

Cancer in Populations Living Near Nuclear Facilities: A Survey of Mortality Nationwide and Incidence in Two States

Jablon S, Hrubec Z, Boice JD Jr (Natl Cancer Inst, Bethesda, Md)

JAMA 265:1403–1408, 1991 2–7

Objective.—Studies from England, Scotland, and Wales have shown increases in the incidence of leukemia and lymphoma in young individuals living near certain nuclear facilities. Therefore, a mortality survey was done in populations living near nuclear installations in the United States.

Study Design.—Populations in 107 counties with or near nuclear facilities were studied. All the installations studied began operating before 1982. Each county was matched to 3 control counties in the same area.

Observations.—From 1950 to 1984, more than 900,000 cancer deaths occurred in populations near the nuclear facilities. There were 1.8 million deaths from cancer in the 292 control counties. Deaths caused by leukemia and other cancers were not more frequent in the study counties compared with the control counties. Before plant start-up, the relative risk for death from childhood leukemia in the study counties was 1.08 compared with the control counties; after start-up, that risk was 1.03. At all ages, the relative risks of leukemia deaths were 1.02 before start-up and .98 after start-up. Cancer incidence data were also available for the counties in 2 states. After the start-up of 1 facility, the standardized registration ratio for childhood leukemia was significantly increased; however, this increase also predated the start-up of this facility.

Discussion.—These findings do not suggest that nuclear facilities have not caused any cancer deaths in nearby populations. However, if nuclear facilities do pose a risk to individuals living near such facilities, then that risk is too small to be detected by a survey such as this one.

▶ The public and the media continue to be concerned about the potential cancer risks of exposure to low-level radiation associated with nuclear facilities. In the 1991 YEAR BOOK (p 23), we reviewed an article that addressed the definable cancer risks from the Three Mile Island accident and detected no substantial increase in any malignancy. This study looks at the problem from a broad perspective and evaluates populations living near all nuclear facilities in the United States. It examines 900,000 cancer deaths occurring during a 35-year period in 107 counties with or near nuclear installations. The study is reassuring, because the investigators did not detect a significant increase either in specific cancer types or in cancer in general in regions near nuclear facilities.—R.C. Young, M.D., F.A.C.P.

Tobacco Exposure

Passive Smoking and Cancer Risk: The Nature and Uses of Epidemiological Evidence

Woodward A, McMichael AJ (Univ of Adelaide, Adelaide, Australia)

Eur J Cancer 27:1472–1479, 1991 2–8

Background.—Because the risk of cancer in nonsmokers often leads to public social practices (e.g., the restriction of smoking in restaurants or airplanes), the evidence that supports this position was analyzed. The interpretation of results of epidemiologic studies and their use in legal arguments about passive smoking and its relationship to cancer were examined.

Methods.—The epidemiologic research published until this analysis began was studied. The studies that were analyzed in detail included those on lung cancer and passive smoking.

Results.—The relative risk estimates for lung cancer development in smoke-exposed nonsmokers ranged from .75 to 2.55 in the case-controlled epidemiologic studies, with most risk estimates above 1. The 3 cohort studies assessing passive smoking's relationship to lung cancer found relative risks of 1.1 for women in the United States and 1.91 for Japanese women whose husbands smoked. No pattern in the estimation of relative risk associations was found for studies investigating the link between various childhood cancers and passive smoking. No evidence exists that passive smoking causes cancer by a mechanism other than smoke-induced lung cancer. Passive smoking research has been affected by a lack of observational research, although many physicians conclude that no statistically significant data exist to conclude that passive smoking causes lung cancer. However, several research points actually preclude such a conclusion (e.g., the types of statistical analyses performed, the attempt to extrapolate a dose-response association while the specific causal component of lung cancer remains unidentified, the mislabeling of bias and confounding factors, biases occurring at the publication of data, and the use of epidemiologic data for policy making). The legal ramifications of proving cancer risks from passive smoking remain complex and incomplete.

Conclusions.—Although most epidemiologic studies suggest that passive smoking can lead to lung cancer, more questions must be answered before public and legal policy issues on this matter can be settled.

▶ The risks of exposure to passive smoking have dramatically influenced the public's view of smoking. Once content to leave smokers alone, the public has become more activist about exposure to smoking, both at home and in the workplace. The authors of this study have examined the evidence for a relationship between passive smoking and cancer. Although some studies have suggested increases in maxillary sinus, leukemia, and cervix cancers, these authors conclude that persuasive data exist only for an increase in lung cancer risk.—R.C. Young, M.D., F.A.C.P.

Uterine Cervical Cancer Risk in Cigarette Smokers: A Meta-Analytic Study

Licciardone JC, Brownson RC, Chang JC, Wilkins JR III (Texas College of Osteopathic Medicine; Missouri Dept of Health, Columbia; Ohio State Univ, Columbus)

Am J Prev Med 6:274–281, 1990 2–9

Introduction.—A recent study found an increased risk for uterine cervical cancer in smokers but not in former smokers. The probability of detecting a statistically significant risk was also greater in current smokers than in former smokers. To increase the statistical power of analysis when assessing the risk of uterine cervical cancer in current and former smokers, a meta-analysis was performed on the results of studies that examined the role of cigarette smoking in the cause of uterine cervical cancer.

Methods.—A MEDLINE search of 1966–1988 data identified 139 studies that examined cigarette smoking and uterine cervical cancer, but only 5 of these were case-control studies reporting appropriate and complete data for meta-analysis. A recent study by Licciardone et al. also was included.

Results.—Using the graphic approach to meta-analysis (as described by Walker and his colleagues in 1988), all 6 studies demonstrated significantly increased odds ratios for current smokers, ranging from 1.54 to 2.9. However, there was only weak evidence for an excess risk of cervical cancer in former smokers. Meta-analysis further suggested that any excess risk of cervical cancer in former smokers may decline precipitously after discontinuation of smoking.

Conclusion.—Although the rate of cigarette smoking for women in the United States has decreased, this decrease has been most impressive among well-educated women and women in the upper socioeconomic levels. These findings further support the need for aggressive antismoking campaigns among women of lower educational and socioeconomic levels.

▶ Previous studies have suggested an increase in the risk of cervical cancer in cigarette smokers. This meta-analysis of case-controlled studies looked at 5 carefully done earlier studies including more than 1,800 cases and 3,500 controls. Figure 2 in the original article illustrates the odds ratio for cervix cancer in current smokers. This large analysis confirms earlier studies that suggested that the risk of cervical cancer was not increased in former smokers. This finding emphasizes the importance of smoking cessation programs to public health, particularly among women in the lower educational and socioeconomic levels, in whom the risk of cervix cancer is high.—R.C. Young, M.D., F.A.C.P.

A Double-Blind Trial of 16-Hour Transdermal Nicotine Patch in Smoking Cessation

Tønnesen P, Nørregaard J, Simonsen K, Säwe U (Bispebjerg Hosp, Copenhagen; Kabi Pharmacia Therapeutics, Helsingborg, Sweden)

N Engl J Med 325:311–315, 1991 2–10

Background.—The only treatment for quitting smoking that has increased the long-term rates of quitting (compared with placebo) is the use of nicotine chewing gum combined with psychological support. Use of the 24-hour transdermal nicotine patch has increased short-term smoking cessation in 5 to 6 trials. Nicotine gum is usually used when the smoker wishes, and the act of chewing may have therapeutic value. The patch delivers a fixed dose of nicotine with no self-regulation, but it may have improved compliance compared with gum. The efficacy of a 16-hour transdermal nicotine patch in smoking cessation was examined in a double-blind study.

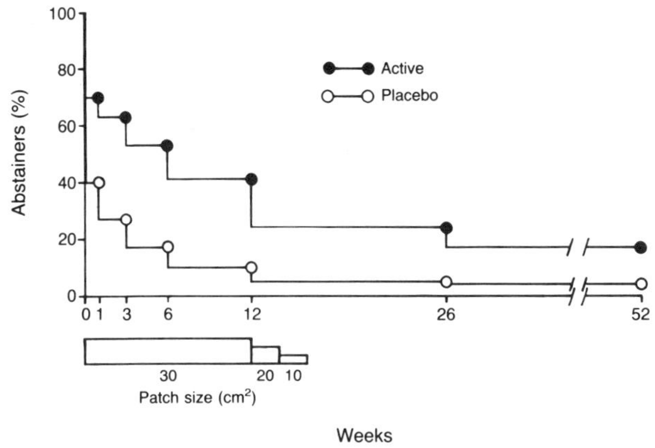

Fig 2–1.—Time to relapse in 289 smokers using nicotine skin patches or placebo patches. (Courtesy of Tønnesen P, Nørregaard J, Simonsen K, et al: *N Engl J Med* 325:311–315, 1991.)

Methods.—The subjects were sequentially and randomly assigned to receive either active treatment or placebo. Of 289 subjects, 145 were given the nicotine patch and 144 were given the placebo patch for 16 weeks. Nicotine substitution attained with the patch was measured by salivary cotinine.

Results.—The active treatment produced sustained abstinence rates of 53% at 6 weeks, 41% at 12 weeks, 24% at 26 weeks, and 17% at 52 weeks. The abstention rates in the group treated with the nicotine patch were significantly better than the abstinence rates of 17%, 10%, 5%, and 4% in those patients in the placebo-patch group at the same intervals (Fig 2–1). Only 2 patients in the nicotine patch group and 1 patient in the placebo group discontinued treatment because of side effects.

Conclusion.—After 12 months, the number of successful abstainers from smoking was higher among subjects who received the nicotine patch compared with those who received the placebo patch. The 17% abstinence rate of abstainers in the nicotine-patch group at the end of 1 year is comparable with the relapse rates and results in treating subjects with alcohol or opiate addiction. The 17% abstinence rate is lower than the rates found in studies that combined the use of nicotine chewing gum with behavioral therapy.

▶ Transdermal nicotine patches have become increasingly popular as an integral part of smoking cessation programs. Because these patches deliver a sustained release of nicotine, they are not in and of themselves a solution; however, they do assist in breaking smoking-related behavioral patterns, and they do not expose the individual to the carcinogenic materials present in incompletely burned tobacco. This double-blind, randomized trial demonstrates improved smoking cessation after 6 and 12 weeks (hardly surprising, because nicotine is simply being supplied by the patch). More importantly, it demonstrates an abstinence rate of 17% at 1-year follow-up. Although this rate was statistically better than that found in the placebo-patch group, the authors emphasize that earlier placebo-controlled trials using nicotine chewing gum and behavioral therapy documented a 49% abstinence rate. Nevertheless, trials with nicotine gum alone often report 1-year abstinence rates of approximately 11%. Although this study illustrates that the nicotine patch is not a panacea for smoking cessation, it does offer an easy and convenient method of initiating an integrated smoking cessation program.—R.C. Young, M.D., F.A.C.P.

Health Effects of Radon Exposure: Report of the Council on Scientific Affairs, American Medical Association

Hendee WR, for the American Medical Association Council on Scientific Affairs (Chicago)

Arch Intern Med 151:674–677, 1991 2–11

Background.—Scientists agree that exposure to randon is a health hazard. However, there is controversy about the risks of lower radon concentrations, including those present in homes. The health risks associated with radon were reviewed, particularly the effects of lower concentrations.

Discussion.—As of October 1989, the United States Environmental Protection Agency (EPA) had reported data on 37,313 homes in 25 states. A total of 74% had radon concentrations below .148 becquerel (Bq)/L; 24% had levels between .148 and .74 Bq/L; and 2% had levels greater than .74 Bq/L. The average level was .148 Bq/L. A review of 38 studies that involved homes in 21 states (3–179 homes per study) concluded that the average level of radon in United States homes was .055 Bq/L. Higher concentrations were found in winter. Most studies of the health effects of radon have been retrospective and have involved underground miners. In general, these studies have suggested that the risk of lung cancer increases in proportion to the intensity and duration of exposure to radon. Some studies of residents living in homes with elevated levels of radon have reported significant associations with lung cancer rates, but others have not. Estimates based on studies of miners are appropriate for estimating residential risks, according to the recent authoritative Biological Effects of Ionizing Radition IV report. This report concluded that cigarette smoking increased the lung cancer risk associated with radon. However, there have been few studies of health outcomes in occupants of homes with high levels of radon. Estimates should consider patterns of occupancy and the age of the occupants, because the induction period for lung cancer is 10–20 years. The most widely used approaches to control of radon exposure are removing the source, preventing or reducing the entry of radon, and increasing the ventilation rate. State radiation control and regional offices of the Environmental Protection Agency are excellent sources of information about these measures.

Conclusion.—In advising patients, physicians should bear in mind the costs and benefits of remedial actions. Patients should be assured that quitting smoking is by far the best way to avoid lung cancer.

▶ Television programs continue to warn us that radon is the second most common cause of lung cancer. However, they neglect to emphasize that it is a very distant second to cigarette smoking. In the 1991 YEAR BOOK (p 21), we reviewed a paper by Henshaw that suggested an association between radon and myeloid leukemia (1). This report of the Council on Scientific Affairs of the American Medical Association presents information on the frequency of elevated levels of radon and the magnitude of those levels. Uranium miners were used as a control population. The council suggests that only 11% of individuals in homes exposed to .70 Bq/L will experience exposure levels above the minimum required to document an increased incidence of lung cancer in miners. The evidence suggests that the risk of lung cancer associated with radon exposure is increased in smokers, and the authors re-emphasize that quitting smoking is by far the best way to avoid lung cancer.—R.C. Young, M.D., F.A.C.P.

Reference

1. Henshaw DL, et al: *Lancet* 335:1008, 1990.

Breast Cancer

Improving Physicians' and Nurses' Clinical Breast Examination: A Randomized Controlled Trial

Campbell HS, Pilgram CA, Fletcher SW, Morgan TM, Lin S (Univ of North Carolina at Chapel Hill; Univ of North Carolina at Wilmington; Bowman-Gray School of Medicine, Winston-Salem, NC)
Am J Prev Med 7:1–8, 1991 2–12

Introduction.—Although clinical breast examination is the major breast cancer screening method practiced, the examination competence of health professionals is not optimal. The changes in health professionals' accuracy in lump detection and examination skills were evaluated after a training program using lifelike silicone breast models.

Methods.—A total of 32 graduate nurses and 64 internal medicine residents participated in the randomized pretest/posttest design. The training emphasized systematic examination and development of tactile skills to detect lumps of varying sizes, degrees of hardness, and depth of placement in the silicone breast models. The experimental group of participants received instruction in lump discrimination and search techniques within 2 weeks of the pretest. All participants were retested 4 months later.

Results.—The mean sensitivity increased in the experimental group but decreased in the control group. Specificity decreased in the experimental group and increased in the control group. The experimental group improved significantly in 5 of 6 techniques, whereas the control group improved in only 1. The duration of the examination was an independent predictor of sensitivity. The medical records of women seen by a subset of the experimental and control groups during the 6 months after training showed no significant differences in the proportion of abnormal breast examinations reported or the number of mammograms ordered between the 2 groups.

Conclusions.—Health professionals who participate in a training program using silicone breast models can develop accuracy in lump detection and tactile skills. In this study, the experimental group that received the training had increased sensitivity but decreased specificity; however, the training program improved the health professionals' accuracy and skill in performing clinical breast examination.

▶ Although physicians rarely receive careful instruction in the technique of breast examination, the public presumes that they have great expertise. This study looked at a randomized controlled trial of health professionals who were given instructions in breast examination in an integrated program developed by the Mammatech Corporation. Using silicone models of lumps of various sizes, hardness, and depth, the sensitivity, specificity, and technique were evaluated both before and 4 months after the training program. Although sensitivity in the experimental group increased from 57% to 63%, specificity in the trained group decreased from 56% to 41%. Interestingly, physicians had higher sensitivity but lower specificity than nurses when doing breast examinations. The training program did seem to increase the accuracy of clinical breast examination; however, the investigators were unable to determine any significant increase in the reporting of abnormal breast examinations or an increase in the number of mammograms ordered by either the trained or the control group of physicians. Clearly, as in most aspects of physical examination, proper instruction and experience is necessary to perfect this important technique. It is difficult to see how physicians could possibly instruct patients in breast self-examination, when they received no formal instruction themselves.—R.C. Young, M.D., F.A.C.P.

Prostate Cancer

The American Cancer Society National Prostate Cancer Detection Project: Findings on the Detection of Early Prostate Cancer in 2425 Men

Mettlin C, Lee F, Drago J, Murphy GP, Investigators of the American Cancer Society National Prostate Cancer Detection Project (Roswell Park Mem Inst, Buffalo; St Joseph Mercy Hosp, Ann Arbor, Mich; The Ohio State Univ, Columbus; American Cancer Society, Atlanta)
Cancer 67:2949–2958, 1991 2–13

Introduction.—In 1987, a multicenter, multidisciplinary study called the American Cancer Society National Prostate Cancer Detection Project was initiated. The study examined 3 procedures for the detection of prostate cancer: the digital rectal examination (DRE), transrectal ultrasound (TRUS), and the prostate specific antigen (PSA) assay. The results of the initial phase of this study were reviewed.

Methods.—By June 1990, 2,425 self-selected men who were not previously suspected of having prostate cancer had been examined. On the basis of TRUS or DRE, biopsy was recommended for 396 (16.3%) men. The results of 330 completed biopsies showed 52 cancers detected by DRE and/or TRUS. The estimated sensitivity of TRUS was significantly greater compared with DRE, but the estimated specificity of DRE was greater. The occurrence of increased PSA levels significantly increased the positive predictive value of both TRUS and DRE.

Conclusion.—The DRE, TRUS, and PSA assays for early detection of prostate cancer can be applied to large numbers of men at risk. Although TRUS is significantly more sensitive to the presence of cancer than DRE, DRE has greater specificity. Increased PSA levels significantly increased the positive predictive value of both TRUS and DRE.

▶ Numerous factors enter into the design of effective screening strategies in cancer, including a demonstration that early detection improves survival, the availability of tests with adequate sensitivity and specificity, patient acceptance of the screening procedure, and cost-effectiveness that is primarily based on the incidence of the disease and the cost of the screening tests. Prostate cancer is common, highly curative in its early stage, and detectable using DRE, TRUS, and serum PSA assays. Consequently, large screening programs for prostate cancer have been developed, including those of the American Cancer Society and the National Cancer Institute.

In this study, men were screened using all 3 procedures: DRE, TRUS, and PSA. The most important finding in this study was that, in men whose PSA levels were normal, a positive TRUS and DRE (alone or in combination) had a low likelihood of predicting that cancer would be detected on biopsy. This suggests that TRUS should not be performed unless the PSA level is elevated. A DRE should remain as part of a routine physical examination and as a screening test because of its ease, cost, and potential for detecting colorectal cancer in addition to prostate cancer. Even though additional studies are still in progress, the case for PSA as a useful screening test is convincing.—R.F. Ozols, M.D., Ph.D.

Routine Screening for Cancer for the Prostate

Gerber GS, Chodak GW (Univ of Chicago Pritzker School of Medicine)

J Natl Cancer Inst 83:329–335, 1991 2–14

Introduction.—Mortality from prostatic cancer has changed little in the past 3 decades, in part because of the large number of men with advanced disease at the time of diagnosis. A national survey suggests that only approximately 60% of patients have clinically localized disease when their tumors are initially diagnosed.

Problems in Screening.—Randomized studies of screening are necessary to avoid lead-time bias and length-time bias. Tumors found when screening asymptomatic patients tend to be less aggressive than those diagnosed by usual methods in symptomatic men. Overdetection is also a problem; a large majority of men who are found at autopsy to have prostatic cancer never have clinical manifestations.

Methods.—Digital rectal examination may have a limited ability to detect small tumors confined to the prostate. In addition, it has a low positive predictive value. The estimation of prostatic acid phosphatase is also limited. The role of prostate-specific antigen in screening for prostatic cancer remains uncertain. Transrectal ultrasonography appears to detect more cancers than digital rectal examination, but its positive and negative predictive values are low, and clinically insignificant tumors may be detected.

The Patient With Symptomatic BPH.—Prostatic cancer may be seen in as many as 20% of men who undergo surgery for benign prostatic hyperplasia. Fine-needle aspiration is a simple means of detecting clinically significant tumors in men scheduled for prostatectomy, and it is safer than transperineal or transrectal core biopsy. The role of random biopsy before prostatectomy in men with benign prostatic hyperplasia remains to be established.

▶ Prostate cancer is now 1 of the most common cancers diagnosed in American men. Although a variety of screening tools exist, including digital rectal examination, transrectal ultrasound, and determination of serum prostatic specific antigen levels, there has been little change in the mortality rate from prostate cancer in the past 30 years. Despite existing screening techniques, approximately 40% of patients are seen with either distant metastases or extracapsular tumor spread. These authors review the current approaches to prostate cancer screening and emphasize the lack of evidence, documenting decreased mortality from such screenings. They emphasize the lead-time and length-time bias associated with screening asymptomatic patients. That, coupled with the common finding of asymptomatic prostate cancer in autopsy series of elderly males, makes the significance of screening data difficult to interpret. After a comprehensive review of existing information, the authors concluded that a large randomized trial of prostate cancer screening is required to document survival benefit, and until such a trial is completed, prostate cancer screening by any modality must be considered experimental.—R.C. Young, M.D., F.A.C.P.

Colon Cancer

Nutritional Factors in Colorectal Cancer Risk: A Case-Control Study in Majorca

Benito E, Stiggelbout A, Bosch FX, Obrador A, Kaldor J, Mulet M, Muñoz N (Unitat d'Epidemiologia i Registre de Càncer de Mallorca, Mallorca, Spain; The Netherlands Cancer Inst, Amsterdam; Internatl Agency for Research on Cancer, Lyon, France; Hosp "Son Dureta," Mallorca, Spain)

Int J Cancer 49:161–167, 1991 2–15

Background.—A previous population-based study of colorectal cancer suggested that cruciferous vegetables had a protective effect, that meat consumption increased risk of colon cancer, and that consumption of dairy products increased the risk of rectal cancer. Further analysis of this study, concentrating on the effect of specific nutrients on colorectal cancer risk, was done.

Methods.—The study took place in the Spanish Mediterranean island of Majorca and included 286 patients with cancer, representing all patients with confirmed colon and rectal cancers seen during a 4-year period; 295 population controls; and 203 hospital controls. Intake of 29 nutrients and of total calories was estimated by use of food composition tables and ad hoc estimates of portion sizes. For each nutrient, after adjustment for total calorie intake, the relative risks for quartiles of nutrient consumption were calculated.

Results.—The dietary intake of total calories in the middle quartiles carried a 1.6 relative risk (RR) of having colorectal cancer. The highest quartile of calorie intake was associated with an RR of 2.6. For cholesterol consumption, the RRs were .9, 1.7, and 1.7, for the 2nd, 3rd, and 4th quartiles, respectively. The intake of fiber from legumes and folic acid appeared to have a protective effect. All of these associations and trends attained statistical significance. Of the main energy-supplying nutrients, protein—especially animal protein, carried RRs of 1, 1.1, 1.7, and 2.5, and carbohydrates carried RRs of 1, 1.5, 1.4, and 2.2. An increased intake of lipids or saturated fats had no effects.

Conclusion.—Total energy intake, probably as a reflection of nonexpended energy, appears to be an important risk factor for colorectal cancer. Vegetables, or the nutrients commonly found in them, may have a protective effect. Public health programs to prevent colorectal cancer should recommend a moderate calorie intake in relation to physical activity level and high consumption of vegetables.

▶ This well-performed epidemiologic study places more emphasis on total calorie intake than on total fat intake as a risk factor for colorectal cancer. In most Western diets, high fat consumption is associated with high calorie consumption. Thus, the relative contribution of fat vs. calories is difficult to discern. When experimental carcinogenesis studies vary the fat content in isocaloric diets, it is difficult to see a contribution from fat. Additional support for the role of calories comes from experiments at the other end of the caloric intake spectrum. In animal studies, low-calorie diets dramatically reduce the incidence of neoplasms, whether the carcinogenic insult is chemical or viral. The protective effect of vegetables is consistent with a contribution from fat. It is believed that fat is converted into carcinogenic moieties by bile acids, and that diets high in vegetable fiber clear the carcinogenic materials from the colon in a more timely fashion. There is a lot more to learn about the contribution to colon cancer.

In what must be his 100th amazing and important contribution to our understanding of cancer, Bert Vogelstein and his group have found a way to detect mutant *ras* proteins in stool samples (1). Because *ras* mutations are noted in approximately 50% of colon tumors, the detection of *ras* will not necessarily detect all colon tumors. However, it is likely that if a mutant *ras* protein is detectable, then the other classes of genetic change that Vogelstein and his colleagues have noted in colon cancer may also be detectable. Thus, it becomes conceivable that patients could be screened for colon cancer by the performance of a test on a stool sample, and that unpleasant and expensive colonoscopy procedures could be reserved for patients with detectable abnormal stool proteins or genes.—D.L. Longo, M.D., F.A.C.P.

Reference

1. Sidransky D, et al: *Science* 256:102, 1992.

3 Pediatric Oncology

Introduction

There is little question that the most successful cancer treatment regimens have been realized in pediatric oncology. Cure rates in excess of 80% are now realized in Wilms' tumor and lymphomas, and cure rates of 70% or more are now anticipated in acute lymphoblastic leukemia. With some notable exceptions, there has been gradual progress in most of the solid tumors. In the recent past, this has meant relatively few *major* advances in therapy, so the panorama of interesting literature has changed in composition. There is now a growing interest in etiology and pathogenesis—both with respect to environmental factors—as well as in the increasingly exciting genetic research. In the past several years, leukemia therapy has been undergoing a process of fine tuning in an attempt to squeeze out a few more cures and reduce the late effects. There has also been increasing interest in biological therapies, both in leukemias and solid tumors, as is reflected in several papers in this section.

Success in brain tumor therapy continues to lag behind the other forms of childhood cancer. In a sense, the status of brain tumor therapy is where the status of leukemia and Wilms' tumor therapy was some 25 years ago. Another important aspect of today's literature is the evolution of reportage on late effects. Although there is still retrospective observational literature, there is a growing amount of interest in early detection and intervention as means of avoiding any catastrophic consequences of therapy. All in all, there appears to be a slow but steady progress in the improvement of treatment regimens, and increasing excitement for the future of diagnosis and therapy that the new biological research tools will provide.

Joseph V. Simone, M.D.

Leukemia and Lymphoma

▶ ↓ The treatment of childhood lymphoblastic leukemia is 1 of the success stories in cancer therapy. The papers in this section include those that demonstrate principles of therapy that have been partially responsible for that advance; those that demonstrate attempts at fine tuning therapy; and, finally, those that use the newer biological approaches.—J.V. Simone, M.D.

Improved Outcome in Childhood Acute Lymphoblastic Leukaemia With Reinforced Early Treatment and Rotational Combination Chemotherapy

Rivera GK, Raimondi SC, Hancock ML, Behm FG, Pui C-H, Abromowitch M, Mirro J Jr, Ochs JS, Look AT, Williams DL, Murphy SB, Dahl GV, Kalwinsky DK, Evans WE, Kun LE, Simone JV, Crist WM (St Jude Children's Research Hosp, Memphis; Univ of Tennessee, Memphis)
Lancet 337:61–66, 1991 3–1

Introduction.—The results from several clinical trials suggest that the intensification of early treatment may help to prevent treatment failure in childhood acute lymphoblastic leukemia (ALL). Most of these strategies have been used for patients with poor prognosis. Patients with a more favorable prognosis were evaluated in a more recent study.

Methods.—A total of 358 consecutive untreated patients with a median age of 5 years was assessed. A 4-agent remission-induction therapy was reinforced with teniposide plus cytarabine and high-dose methotrexate with leucovorin rescue, followed by rotational combination chemotherapy. Those patients who had complete remission were randomized (according to prognosis) to conventional continuation treatment or to

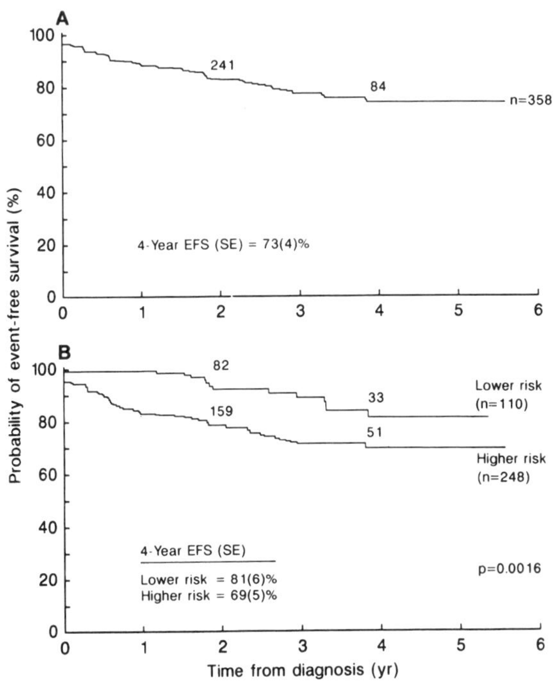

Fig 3–1.—Kaplan-Meier estimates of event-free survival for all patients in study (**A**) and lower risk and higher risk groups (**B**). *Numbers on curves* indicate patients still at risk of relapse; the *P* value was determined by log-rank test. (Courtesy of Rivera GK, Raimondi SC, Hancock ML, et al: *Lancet* 337:61–66, 1991.)

treatment with 4 pairs of drugs rotated either weekly or every 6 weeks. In addition to intrathecal therapy that was given to all patients, those patients with higher risk also received 1,800-cGy cranial irradiation after 1 year of remission.

Results.—Complete remission was achieved in 99% of the lower risk group and in 95% of the higher risk group. At a median follow-up of 40 months, the 4-year event-free survival estimates were 73% for the group as a whole, 81% for lower risk patients, and 69% for higher risk patients (Fig 3–1). During the 6-year study period, there were 62 relapses, most of which occurred in the bone marrow. Secondary acute myeloid leukemia developed in 8 children with a poorer prognosis. Multivariate analysis showed that a leukocyte count greater than 50×10^9/L, common lymphocytic leukemia antigen (CALLA)-negative blasts, and a pseudodiploid or hypodiploid karyotype independently predicted an unfavorable outcome. Treatment was generally well tolerated, and the children received most courses as outpatients.

Conclusion.—This regimen may cure 69% to 77% of patients younger than 18 years who have ALL. In lower risk patients, the high 4-year event-free survival rate suggests that intensive early therapy and conventional postremission treatment may often be adequate to secure durable remissions.

▶ This rather large series of patients from a single institution (my own) has had a gratifying result. It is yet another example of the importance of early aggressive therapy in childhood ALL. It has become clear over the years that one must provide very strong therapy as early as possible in the treatment of these patients if one hopes to have a significantly large percentage of good results. This study also tested another issue, i.e., whether the rapid rotation of different pairs of agents would reduce the likelihood of resistant leukemia cell clones emerging, thus improving the long-term results. This facet of the study showed no difference between patients who received agents rotated weekly vs. those who had agents rotated every sixth week. So, at least within the framework of this study as designed, giving the maximum-tolerated dosages of multiple agents was more important than the time sequence of exposure.

As results in ALL studies improve to—perhaps—a 70% to 80% cure rate, it becomes increasingly difficult to make major changes in subsequent studies for fear of jeopardizing those patients that might be cured with the existing approaches. Nonetheless, some modifications are possible, and it is important to continue testing those modifications in an attempt to further improve the outcome and reduce toxicity.—J.V. Simone, M.D.

Monthly Pulses of Vincristine and Prednisone Prevent Bone Marrow and Testicular Relapse in Low-Risk Childhood Acute Lymphoblastic Leukemia: A Report of the CCG-161 Study by the Childrens Cancer Study Group

Bleyer WA, Sather HN, Nickerson HJ, Coccia PF, Finklestein JZ, Miller DR, Littman PS, Lukens JN, Siegel SE, Hammond GD (Children's Hosp and Med Ctr, Seattle; Univ of Southern California, Los Angeles; Children's Hosp of Los Angeles; Children's Hosp, Long Beach, Calif; Marshfield Clinic, Marshfield, Wis, et al)

J Clin Oncol 9:1012–1021, 1991 3–2

Introduction.—Methotrexate (MTX) and mercaptopurine (6MP) are the drugs of choice for the eradication phase of acute lymphoblastic leukemia (ALL), also known as maintenance therapy. The addition of other drugs to MTX and 6MP has not been shown to increase the cure rate. However, the findings of 1 study showed that children at low risk for relapse appeared to benefit from the later addition of monthly pulses of vincristine and prednisone (VCR-PDN) during maintenance therapy.

Patients.—Included in the study were 698 previously untreated children with ALL, aged 3–6 years, with an initial white blood cell count less than 10,000/μL and fewer than 25% L2 cells in the bone marrow. At the end of induction therapy with VCR, PDN, L-asparaginase, and intrathecal MTX (IT MTX), 631 children were randomized to receive monthly pulses of VCR-PDN during maintenance therapy. This was given in addition to standard therapy with 6MP and MTX, and either cranial irradiation administered during consolidation or IT MTX given every 3 months. All patients received 6 doses of IT MTX during induction and consolidation. The minimum follow-up was 4.25 years.

Results.—Life-table analysis revealed that 76.7% of the children who received VCR-PDN in addition to standard therapy with 6MP and MTX had a 5-year disease-freee survival (DFS), regardless of whether they received cranial irradiation. In contrast, only 63.9% of the children who received standard 6MP-MTX therapy without the monthly VCR-PDN pulses had a 5-year DFS. The difference in relapse-free survival was primarily the result of bone marrow relapse; in boys, it was also the result of testicular relapse. Among nonirradiated children, the 5-year DFS rate was 79% for those treated with 6MP-MTX and VCR-PDN pulses, and 61.2% for those treated with 6MP-MTX alone. There was no significant difference in the 5-year DFS among irradiated children.

Conclusion.—In view of the potential deleterious effects of cranial irradiation, a maintenance therapy regimen of 6MP-MTX supplemented with monthly VCR-PDN pulses and maintenance IT MTX appears to be the best of the 4 regimens studied in patients with acute ALL who are initially at low risk for relapse.

▶ This large study from the Children's Cancer Study Group, which opened in 1978 and closed to new entries in 1983, includes an evaluation of the best prognostic group that could be identified. All patients received 6MP and MTX maintenance therapy and were randomized either to receive or not receive monthly VCR-PDN pulses. The study demonstrated, not surprisingly, that those patients who received VCR-PDN pulses had a better outcome. The reason this result is not surprising is that it has long been demonstrated that a combination of 6MP and MTX given alone in conventional dosage was inferior maintenance therapy to any regimen that included more agents. The premise of this study was that one might identify a group of patients with very low risk who were exceptions and needed less therapy. Instead, it demonstrated that there are still no exceptions to the rule. However, when this study was designed in the mid-1970s, that fact might not have been as clear.

An editorial comment: the use of "low risk" as a definition of any form of disseminated cancer rankles the bones. Even at best, 20% of the patients in this selected group died of their disease. Is there any disease with a 20% mortality that we are willing to call low risk? I suggest the use of relative terms such as "better" risk or "worse" risk so that we don't fool ourselves into thinking that leukemia, even in highly selected subpopulations, may be viewed in the same way as nonmalignant diseases.—J.V. Simone, M.D.

Improved Treatment Results in Boys With Overt Testicular Relapse During or Shortly After Initial Therapy for Acute Lymphoblastic Leukemia: A Pediatric Oncology Group Study

Buchanan GR, Boyett JM, Pollock BH, Smith SD, Yanofsky RA, Ghim T, Wharam MD, Crist WM, Vietti TJ, Johnson W, Rivera GK (Univ of Texas Southwestern Med Ctr at Dallas; Cleveland Clinic Foundation; Univ of Florida, Gainesville; Stanford Univ School of Medicine, Stanford, Calif; Cross Cancer Ctr, Edmonton, Alberta, Canada, et al)

Cancer 68:48–55, 1991 3–3

Background.—In boys with acute lymphoblastic leukemia (ALL) the testis is the second most common site of extramedullary relapse. Previously, patients with overt testicular relapse during or shortly after initial chemotherapy nearly always had bone marrow relapse later and died of disease.

Study Design.—An intensive protocol [Pediatric Oncology Group (POG) 8303] was evaluated in 38 boys who had ALL and overt testicular relapse between 1983 and 1987. All had relapsed within 6 months of the end of initial continuation chemotherapy. Systemic reinduction therapy included prednisone, vincristine, daunorubicin, and asparaginase. A brief intensive consolidation phase of teniposide and cytarabine doses followed. The patients then received weekly rotating treatment with vincristine/cyclophosphamide and teniposide/cytarabine for 2 years, with or without 4-drug reinforcement pulses given at 16-week intervals. Testicular irradiation was given during reinduction therapy. In addition, the patients received intrathecal chemoprophylaxis with 3 drugs every 4–6 weeks.

Results.—All 38 patients had clinical remission after reinduction. Thirteen remained in complete remission for 34+ to 74+ months (Fig 3–2). Three patients withdrew while in remission, whereas 22 had further re-

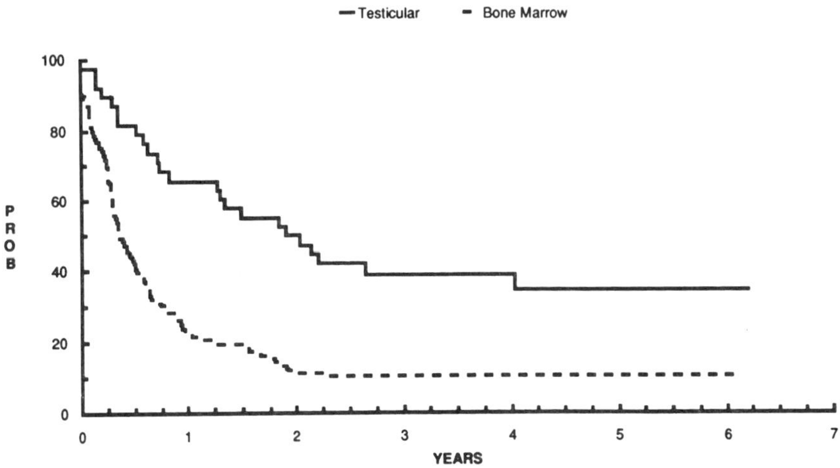

INTERVAL	Testicular Prob(SE)	Fail	N	Bone Marrow Prob(SE)	Fail	N
0- 6 Mos	81.6(6.3)	7	38	42.3(4.1)	87	153
6-12 Mos	65.8(7.7)	6	31	22.2(3.4)	30	63
12-18 Mos	55.3(8.1)	4	25	19.5(3.3)	4	33
18-24 Mos	50.0(8.1)	2	21	11.1(2.6)	12	28
24-30 Mos	42.1(8.9)	3	19	10.4(2.6)	1	16
30-36 Mos	38.9(9.2)	1	13	10.4(2.6)	0	15
36-42 Mos	38.9(9.2)	0	11	10.4(2.7)	0	14
42-48 Mos	38.9(10.1)	0	11	10.4(3.0)	0	13
48-54 Mos	34.5(10.6)	1	9	10.4(3.5)	0	11
54-60 Mos	34.5(16.1)	0	7	10.4(4.0)	0	8
60-66 Mos	34.5(19.8)	0	3	10.4(5.7)	0	6
66-72 Mos	34.5(28.0)	0	2	10.4(7.0)	0	3
72-78 Mos		0	1		0	2

Fig 3–2.—Comparison of the probability of event-free survival for the 38 patients with overt testicular relapse (OTR) *(solid line)* with 153 patients with first bone marrow relapse *(dashed line)* who were treated on the same protocol. The horizontal axis begins on the date of the second complete remission. An abridged life table is also shown. The OTR patients had a statistically significant disease-free survival advantage over those with first relapse in the bone marrow (number of observed to expected failures was 24:49.9 for OTR vs. 134:108.1 for bone marrow relapse patients, $P = .0001$). (Courtesy of Buchanan GR, Boyett JM, Pollock BH, et al: *Cancer* 68:48–55, 1991.)

lapse, 2 at the testicular site. Five of 18 patients who electively discontinued treatment relapsed. Severe toxicity was infrequent, and continuation treatment was well tolerated.

Conclusion.—Approximately one third of boys with ALL who have testicular relapse do well when treated with POG protocol 8303, exhibiting a prolonged second remission with the possibility of cure.

▶ Although the results of this study of testicular relapse are better than those of earlier studies, only 13 of 38 patients remained in complete remission at the time of this report. This underscores the dictum that any relapse is bad for the patient. However, it also demonstrates support for the hypothesis that testicular relapse may reflect an early systemic relapse that is more easily detected in the testes because of the site and obvious nature of testicular swelling. Because one has an opportunity to detect relapse sooner, aggressive systemic therapy can be initiated earlier, providing a greater chance of obtaining a good result. This reinforces a general principle of cancer therapy in pediatric patients: the sooner one can apply aggressive therapy to any tumor, the better the result.—J.V. Simone, M.D.

Survival of Children and Adolescents With Acute Lymphoid Leukemia: A Study of American Indians and Hispanic and Non-Hispanic Whites Treated in New Mexico (1969 to 1986)

Foucar K, Duncan MH, Stidley CA, Wiggins CL, Hunt WC, Key CR (Univ of New Mexico, Albuquerque)

Cancer 67:2125–2130, 1991 3–4

Introduction.—Advances in the treatment of childhood acute lymphoid leukemia (ALL) during the past 30 years have yielded dramatic improvements in survival. However, preliminary data from the New Mexico Tumor Registry has suggested that American Indians have worse survival than Hispanic and non-Hispanic whites. The clinical and pathologic features of children with ALL were reviewed to identify the factors that might explain this difference.

Methods.—During an 18-year period, 196 American Indian, Hispanic white, and non-Hispanic white children were treated for ALL; 14% were American Indians, 46% were Hispanic whites, and 39% were non-Hispanic whites. The treatment regimens varied during the study period, but patients from the various ethnic groups received similar treatment based on their standard risk factor assessment; most received multidrug chemotherapy and CNS prophylaxis. The factors affecting survival were assessed using multivariate statistical analysis.

Results.—For those patients who received antileukemic therapy, the median survivals ranged widely according to sex and ethnicity (Figs 3–3 and 3–4). Non-Hispanic white girls survived 140 months, compared with 8 months for American Indian boys. The highest initial median leukocyte count, 23.8 × 10^9/L, was found in American Indian boys. Com-

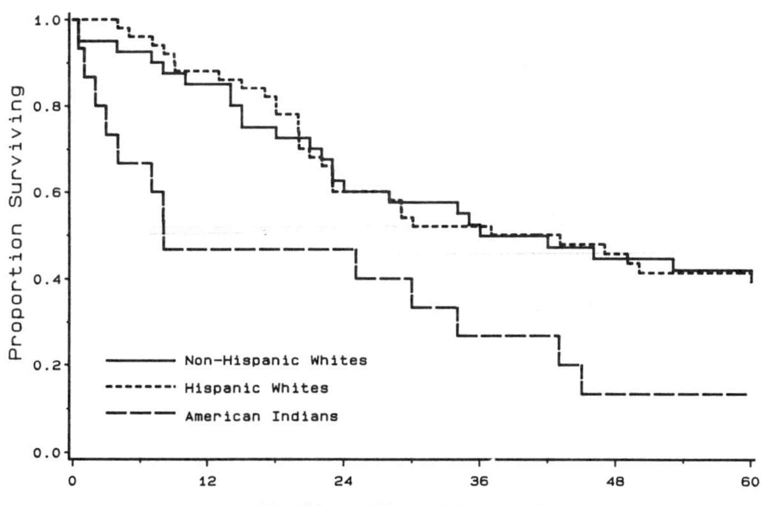

Fig 3–3.—Survival for treated boys by ethnic group. (Courtesy of Foucar K, Duncan MH, Stidley CA, et al: *Cancer* 67:2125–2130, 1991.)

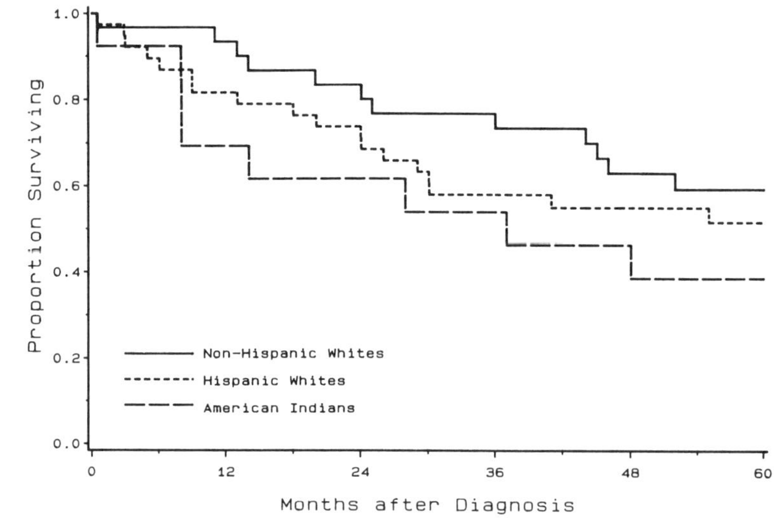

Fig 3–4.—Survival for treated girls by ethnic group. (Courtesy of Foucar K, Duncan MH, Stidley CA, et al: *Cancer* 67:2125–2130, 1991.)

pliance problems, including treatment delays and stopping maintenance treatment, were most common in American Indian children. All other clinical and pathologic features evaluated were distributed similarly among the ethnic and gender groups. Initial white blood cell count, age, and gender were the independent prognostic variables for survival. Possible (but confounded) variables included ethnicity and compliance problems.

Conclusion.—American Indian children with ALL have reduced survival compared with other ethnic groups. Ethnicity and compliance problems may influence outcome, but these are confounded variables. Studies are under way to seek biological differences in the types of leukemia found in these 3 ethnic populations. A higher initial white blood cell count may be found in American Indian patients.

▶ This important paper from New Mexico gives us sad news. American Indian children with ALL fared much worse than their white or Hispanic counterparts. The authors suggest that, because of the geographic distances and social conditions, treatment compliance with protocol therapy was more difficult for the American Indian population and may have been a major factor in the poor outcome. However, as has been discovered among black children, there may be biological factors that explain the poor outcome, e.g., a subtype of leukemia with a poorer prognosis may be more prevalent in certain populations. One hopes the authors will pursue these studies to try to identify the reason for these differences. This may help us understand how to better treat all children, and, in particular, how we might help those unfortunate children who have a terrible outcome that is not acceptable in the 1990s.—J.V. Simone, M.D.

Childhood Cancer and Ethnic Group in Britain: A United Kingdom Children's Cancer Study Group (UKCCSG) Study

Stiller CA, McKinney PA, Bunch KJ, Bailey CC, Lewis IJ (Univ of Oxford, Oxford, England; Univ of Leeds; Seacroft Hosp, Leeds, England)

Br J Cancer 64:543–548, 1991 3–5

Background.—There have been few reports of the patterns of cancer incidence in children of various ethnic groups in Britain. The observation of a high frequency of Hodgkin's disease in Asian children prompted an analysis of ethnic variations in the occurrence of childhood cancer.

Methods.—The analysis included data from the United Kingdom Children's Cancer Group, which registers more than two thirds of all childhood cancer in Britain. Since 1981, when information on ethnic groups was first recorded, 7,658 children with cancer have been treated at pediatric oncology centers. A case-control approach was used to analyze the relative frequency of cancer diagnostic groups between ethnic groups by the log-linear method of Kaldor et al. The method allowed for regional variations in the ages and diagnostic groups of the children studied.

Results.—The patterns of incidence of acute lymphoblastic leukemia (ALL) were similar in white children and children of Asian (or Indian subcontinent) origin and in those of West Indian origin. Compared with white children, Asian children had an estimated relative risk of acquiring Hodgkin's disease of 2.09. For children age 4 years and younger, this risk increased to 6.67. Asian children had approximately half the incidence of Wilms' tumor and rhabdomyosarcoma, but West Indians had a significant excess of Wilms' tumor (relative risk, 2.55). There was a higher incidence of unilateral retinoblastoma in Asian and West Indian children, but this was not significant.

Conclusions.—Environmental determinants in the country of residence, which are probably related to lifestyle factors, appear to affect the incidence of childhood ALL. In contrast, retinoblastoma, Wilms' tumor, the Hodgkin's disease in early childhood appear to be related more to ethnicity than geographic location. The excesses described may represent genetic or environmental factors.

▶ It has long been known in the United States that there is a difference in the incidence of certain malignancies in different racial groups, as well as a difference in the response to therapy. The most striking example is that the incidence of ALL in black children is approximately one half of that found in white children. However, as a group, black children respond less well to therapy than do white children. Also, Ewing's sarcoma of bone is almost unknown in the black population of the United States.

The ethnic differences reported in this paper are of sufficient magnitude to be important, but the cause of these differences in unknown. It is very likely that environmental factors (if one includes ambient viruses and other infectious agents) must play a role in some of these tumors. Because it is well known that retinoblastoma and Wilms' tumor, for example, have strong genetic correlations, the prevalence of these predisposing genetic factors could easily be different in the various ethnic populations. This is a useful type of investigation, because it tells us where to apply the new molecular tools when trying to understand the etiology and pathogenesis of cancer.—J.V. Simone, M.D.

Importance of 6-Mercaptopurine Dose in Lymphoblastic Leukemia

Hale JP, Lilleyman JS (Children's Hosp, Sheffield, England)

Arch Dis Child 66:462–466, 1991 3–6

Introduction.—The long-term survival of children with lymphoblastic leukemia has improved strikingly in the United Kingdom during the past decade. Since 1980, long-term survival has improved 20%, but morbidity and mortality from treatment also increased when a policy of physician compliance to a much more strict regimen of permitted modifications in doses was instituted.

Methods.—The possibility that higher maintenance doses of 6-mercaptopurine (6MP) contributed to the improved outcome was investigated. Data on 30 children in whom lymphoblastic leukemia was diagnosed before 1980 were compared with those of 55 in whom it was diagnosed after this time.

Results.—The median total dose of 6MP increased 22% after 1980. According to the protocol, the dose should have increased by an average of 9%. At the same time, the relapse-survival at 5 years improved 18%. After 1980, boys were prescribed significantly more 6MP than girls. Dose reductions for myelosuppression were less frequent in boys.

Conclusion.—A change in the amount of 6MP prescribed during maintenance treatment apparently resulted from altered criteria for dose reduction rather than a change in the recommended maximum dosage. In the future the 6MP dosage will be titrated to myelotoxicity in all children. In this way, it may be possible to prevent children with higher tolerance from being inadvertently undertreated.

▶ This paper is included as a reminder of an important principle in leukemia therapy: children have widely different tolerances of chemotherapy, and the dosage of therapy should be adjusted to the maximum tolerated. Physicians may become slaves to a dosage prescribed by a protocol and, as long as no problems develop, they may believe that they are giving optimal therapy. This is not necessarily true. It is important to increase the dosage in patients who are extremely tolerant, because it clearly makes a difference in the outcome.—J.V. Simone, M.D.

Recombinant Interferon Alfa Given Before and in Combination With Standard Chemotherapy in Children With Acute Lymphoblastic Leukemia in First Marrow Relapse: A Pediatric Oncology Group Pilot Study

Ochs J, Brecher ML, Mahoney D, Vega R, Pollock BH, Buchanan GR, Whitehead VM, Ravindranath Y, Freeman AI (Univ of Tennessee, Memphis; Roswell

Park Mem Inst, Buffalo, NY; Baylor College of Medicine, Houston, Univ of Texas Southwestern Med Ctr, Dallas; Emory Univ School of Medicine, Atlanta; et al)
J Clin Oncol 9:777–782, 1991 3–7

Objective.—As many as one third of children with acute lymphoblastic leukemia (ALL) have relapse, most often in the bone marrow. A pilot study was designed to evaluate high-dose recombinant interferon alfa (rIFN-α) given as a single agent before standard reinduction treatment for ALL in relapse.

Study.—Thirty-one children with ALL in first-treatment marrow relapse received rIFN-α, 30 megaunits/m^2/day intravenously for 10 days. Standard reinduction therapy with 4 drugs and multidrug continuation therapy ensued. At this stage, rINF-α was given subcutaneously 3 days a week at 3-week intervals.

Results.—Two patients had partial remission after the initial course of rIFN-α therapy. Two others had progressive disease. Three patients had dose-limiting toxicity. Eventually, almost three fourths of the children had marrow remission. All but 1 tolerated continuation therapy well. One child required a lower dose of rINF-α because of CNS toxicity. Five patients remained in remission after 26–36 months. In no case was it necessary to lower the dose of standard chemotherapeutic agents.

Conclusions.—Therapy with high-dose rIFN-α alone had a modest antileukemic effect in children with marrow relapse of ALL. In contrast to experience in adults, pulse rINF-α therapy did not compromise the intensity of standard continuation chemotherapy.

▶ Interferon has had a long run in our consciousness since it was touted as a wonder drug on the cover of *Time* some years ago. However, it has failed to live up to its promise as a cure-all, and it certainly is not very effective in childhood leukemia. As with most new anticancer agents, introducing the agent is only half the battle; finding the right application for it is the other half. It is unlikely that interferon will be a significant factor in *acute* leukemias in children, but read on.—J.V. Simone, M.D.

Response to Alpha-Interferon In Children With Philadelphia Chromosome-Positive Chronic Myelocytic Leukemia

Dow LW, Raimondi SC, Culbert SJ, Ochs J, Kennedy W, Pinkel DP (St Jude Children's Research Hosp, Memphis; Univ of Texas; MD Anderson Cancer Ctr, Houston; Univ of Tennessee, Memphis)
Cancer 68:1678–1684, 1991 3–8

Introduction.—Recombinant α-interferon (α-INF) induces hematologic remissions in adult patients with Philadelphia chromosome-positive chronic myelocytic leukemia (Ph$^+$ CML) and suppresses the Ph$^+$ clone in some patients. The therapeutic efficacy and toxicity of long-term daily administration of α-IFN were studied in children with Ph$^+$ CML.

Patients/Treatment.—Fifteen children (aged 2.5–20 years) with Ph$^+$ CML were treated with a daily dose of α-IFN, 5 × 10^6 units/m^2, given intramuscularly. The daily dose was increased to 10 × 10^6 units of α-INF per m^2 if the leukemia was inadequately controlled. Before α-IFN therapy, all patients received an initial cytoreductive therapy with either hydroxyurea or busulfan for a median of 7 months (range, 6 weeks–46 months). At the beginning of α-IFN therapy, the leukocyte counts ranged from 5 to 101 × 10^9/L, and the marrow myeloid to erythroid ratios decreased to a median 4.9:1 in 10 patients.

Outcome.—Ten children had an initial hematologic response, and 9 showed a reduction in the percentage of Ph$^+$ marrow cells. At 48–204 weeks after initiation of therapy, 4 patients had no detectable Ph$^+$ cells, including 2 patients who remained free of Ph$^+$ cells and another patient in whom the p210 *bcr-abl* protein in marrow cells and the *bcr-abl* gene rearrangements in the blood cell were not detected. Therapy was discontinued before week 104 because of early hematologic responses without a decrease in Ph$^+$ cells in 3 patients, early resistant disease in 1, blast crisis in 1, progressive disease in 2, seizure attributed to a high-dose α-IFN in 1, and inadequate trial of α-IFN resulting from aseptic necrosis or poor compliance in 2. Recombinant α-IFN therapy was well tolerated, and the most common side effects included fever, malaise, myalgia, fatigue, and pain at the injection site. Three patients had skin lesions that resolved with cessation of therapy. Therapy was discontinued because of seizures, aseptic necrosis, and myelofibrosis.

Conclusion.—Long-term daily administration of α-IFN, in combination with an effective cytoreductive agent, can suppress and possibly eliminate Ph$^+$ cells in approximately 33% of children with Ph$^+$ CML, which is similar to the percentage previously reported in adults. Therapy is well tolerated in children. The optimal duration of α-IFN therapy is unknown.

▶ Unlike its results in acute leukemia in children, interferon appears to have some efficacy in chronic leukemia in children (as it does in chronic leukemia in adults.) Because bone marrow transplantation is currently the only curative regimen for chronic myelocytic leukemia, and because a majority of patients will not be eligible for transplantation as a result of the lack of a matched donor or some other problem, it is gratifying to see even the modest response obtained with this newer agent. Clearly, a combination of cytoreductive therapy and biological therapy is warranted.—J.V. Simone, M.D.

Autologous Bone Marrow Transplantation in High Risk Remission T-Lineage Acute Lymphoblastic Leukemia Using Immunotoxins Plus 4-Hydroperoxycyclophosphamide for Marrow Purging

Uckun FM, Kersey JH, Vallera DA, Ledbetter JA, Weisdorf D, Myers DE, Haake R, Ramsay NKC (Univ of Minnesota Health Sciences Ctr, Minneapolis; Oncogen Corp, Seattle)

Blood 76:1723–1733, 1990 3–9

Introduction.—Some patients with acute lymphoblastic leukemia (ALL) are at high risk of relapsing after receiving current first-line chemotherapy. Those patients who have a medullary relapse during or shortly after first-line treatment have a poor outlook.

Methods.—Autologous marrow transplantation was performed in 14 consecutive patients with T-lineage ALL in complete remission to eradicate residual disease. Immunotoxins directed against the CD5/Tp67 and CD7/Tp41 T-lineage differentiation antigens were used to purge the autografts in conjunction with the cyclophosphamide congener 4-hydroperoxycyclophosphamide (4-HC). High-dose radiotherapy and chemotherapy were administered before marrow transplantation.

Results.—Of the 14 patients, 9 relapsed a median of 2.5 months after marrow transplantation. Relapse was likely when a new quantitative minimal residual disease assay, which combines fluorescence-activated flow cytometry with cell sorting by leukemic progenitor-cell assays, demonstrated high numbers of residual progenitor cells before marrow transplantation.

Conclusion.—Recurrent leukemia in these patients reflects inefficient pretransplant radiochemotherapy, not inadequate purging of marrow autografts. The minimal residual disease detection assay may help in timing marrow transplantation properly and in determining whether further treatment is necessary.

▶ This paper confirms the suspicion that many clinicians have had concerning autologous marrow transplantation. Getting rid of the leukemia in the patient was at least as great a problem as getting rid of the residual leukemia cells in the marrow to be returned to the patient. The authors used a sensitive technique for detecting minimal residual disease, and they demonstrated that, after therapy, patients still harbored large numbers of leukemia cells before the transplant. The bad news is that the treatment is not as successful as one might have hoped. The good news is that the technology is improving to the point where one might be much more specific and effective in clearing the leukemia from the patient and cleansing autologous marrow of residual leukemia cells. There is a silver lining in this cloud.—J.V. Simone, M.D.

Arthritic Presentation of Childhood Leukaemia

Bradlow A, Barton C (Royal Berkshire Hosp Battle Hosps, Reading, England)

Postgrad Med J 67:562–564, 1991 3–10

Introduction.—As many as one third of children with leukemia have bone or back pain or joint swelling, and more than half have bony abnormalities on roentgenograms at the time of presentation. Data on 3 children with leukemia who were initially thought to have juvenile chronic arthritis were reviewed.

Features.—All of the patients were symptomatic for at least 4 months before leukemia was diagnosed. One patient was thought to have systemic juvenile chronic arthritis, or Still's disease, but a low white blood cell count should have cast doubt on this impression. In 1 patient, the presence of lymphadenopathy and hepatosplenomegaly promoted marrow aspiration after attempted treatment with prednisolone. The third patient had no signs of leukemia until the white blood cell count decreased during treatment with sulfasalazine. Examination of synovium from the affected knee joint was not helpful.

Recommendation.—Children with arthritis of recent onset should undergo radiographs. Marrow aspiration should be considered, especially if there is adenopathy, hepatosplenomegaly, or neutropenia. Repeated marrow aspirations may be necessary to detect leukemia.

▶ I include this paper for a personal reason. Having been at a large referral center for many years, I have been distressed once or twice each year to see a patient who has been given an incorrect diagnosis of rheumatoid arthritis, has undergone steroid therapy with transient improvement, and has subsequently been given a diagnosis of acute lymphoblastic leukemia. This is not simply a matter of delaying the diagnosis, but a question of compromising the opportunity for a cure by giving inadequate therapy for the leukemia and allowing resistant disease to develop. As the authors point out, the patients had symptoms for an extended period of time, and the physician should have been tipped off by the persistence of a low leukocyte count. Therefore, I offer a strong reminder: a bone marrow aspiration should be considered in a child who is seen with symptoms of arthritis and also happens to have a low leukocyte count. In addition, a high degree of suspicion will alert radiologists to look for typical changes in radiographs of the ends of bones.—J.V. Simone, M.D.

Acute Myeloid Leukaemia in Childhood: The Costs and Benefits of Intensive Treatment

Phillips M, Richards S, Chessells J (Hosp for Sick Children, London; Inst of Child Health, London; Clinical Trials Service Unit, Oxford, England)

Br J Haematol 77:473–477, 1991 3–11

Introduction.—Treatment for acute myeloid leukemia (AML) has become increasingly intensive in recent years. Treatment responses and resource use were compared in 2 groups of children with AML: 99 treated in 1972–1982 (group A), and 53 treated in 1983–1987 (group B).

Management.—The children in group A usually received cytarabine, daunorubicin, and various other drugs at the outset. Most treatment was given on an outpatient basis. Those who entered remission received intrathecal chemotherapy and late cranial irradiation. Children in group B received thioguanine in addition to cytarabine and daunorubicin and were given a second course of the same drugs. The third course included amsacrine, 5-azacytidine, and etoposide. Intrathecal therapy was given with cytarabine, methotrexate, and hydrocortisone. Marrow transplantation was much more frequent in group B cases.

Results.—The remission rates were 67% for children in group A and 87% for those in group B. Thirteen early deaths occurred in group A and 4 occurred in group B. The overall event-free survival was 12% at 5

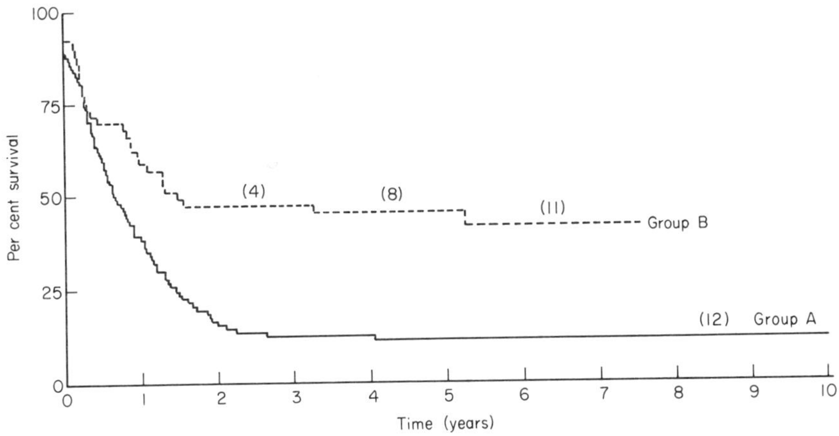

Fig 3–5.—Event-free survival in the 2 series of patients. The *numbers in parentheses* refer to the numbers of children still alive and in remission at specific time periods. (Courtesy of Phillips M, Richards S, Chessells J: *Br J Haematol* 77:473–477, 1991.)

years in group A and 45% in group B (Fig 3–5). Survival was highest in patients in group B who underwent marrow transplantation in first remission (Fig 3–6).

Discussion.—A real improvement in outlook is evident for children with AML, but this is achieved at the cost of hospitalization and intensive medical and nursing care. There remains much room for improvement.

▶ This analysis of the results of treatment of AML in children is a sad reminder that we have improved the outcome at considerable cost. Much more aggres-

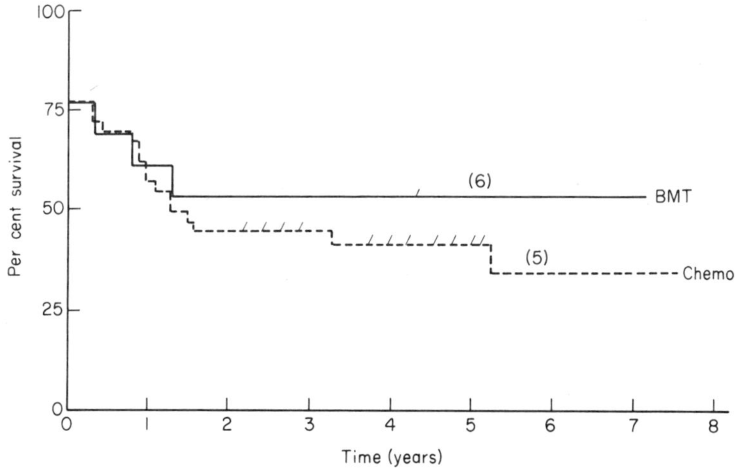

Fig. 3–6.—A comparison of event-free survival in patients who received allogeneic marrow transplantation and those who received chemotherapy. All deaths before 15 weeks have been counted a death at week 1. The *marks on the graph* indicate patients alive in remission, whereas the *numbers in parentheses* refer to children alive and in remission after 5-year follow-up. (Courtesy of Phillips M, Richards S, Chessells J: *Br J Haematol* 77:473–477, 1991.)

sive therapy, including bone marrow transplantation, has been necessary to improve the long-term survival. The costs are enormous in terms of hospitalization time, antibiotics, and nursing care. No one is happy with what is necessary to obtain these results; however, it is the best we have at the present time. The reason that progress has been far less spectacular in myeloid leukemia than in ALL is unknown. The self-evident explanation is that we simply don't have as many effective agents for AML. One hopes that the increasing body of knowledge on myeloid growth factors may provide alternative therapeutic strategies.—J.V. Simone, M.D.

Leukaemia and Paternal Radiation Exposure

Watson GM (Australian Atomic Energy Commission Research Establishment, Lucas Heights, NSW)

Med J Aust 154:483–487, 1991 3–12

Introduction.—In a previously published report, it was inferred that a father's exposure to ionizing radiation increases the risk of leukemia in his children. A critical comment on this conjecture is provided, and more substantial confirmation is advised before the dissemination of such alarming suggestions.

Data Analysis.—This previously published article is statistically weak, because the leukemia cluster near the town of Sellafield could have been a chance finding, and the number of cases was not statistically significant compared with previous reports of clusters of patients with leukemia. Genetically, leukemia is not recognized to be transmitted as a Mendelian trait in the manner required by the previous study. The children of the Japanese who were exposed to nuclear explosions have not manifested genetic effects or increases in leukemia or other cancers and they have been observed on a large scale. This contradicts the supposition that the Sellafield children were affected by paternal radiation exposure.

Conclusions.—The premature release of such alarming information is likely to cause a rash of lawsuits by patients with cancer against British Nuclear Fuels Limited, which operates in Sellafield, and against other nuclear facilities. Claimants may be disappointed because the study's disturbing conclusion was not well substantiated.

▶ This paper was written to urge caution readers about the results of an earlier study that was reported in the 1991 YEAR BOOK (1). That study, by Gardner et al., suggested that paternal exposure to radiation increased the incidence of leukemia in subsequent offspring, thereby implying that gonadal exposure was responsible. This paper raises some objection to the conclusions of that study, urging caution in stretching that conclusion too far. However, one might be forgiven for viewing this attempted rebuttal with a jaundiced eye, because of the organization at which the author is employed. One should interpret these data with interest but with a healthy dose of skepticism, waiting for convincing confirmation from either side.—J.V. Simone, M.D.

Reference

1. Gardner MJ, et al: *Br Med J* 300:423, 1990.

Pediatric Solid Tumors

Improved Survival at 2 and 5 Years in the LMCE1 Unselected Group of 72 Children With Stage IV Neuroblastoma Older Than 1 Year of Age at Diagnosis: Is Cure Possible in a Small Subgroup?

Philip T, Zucker JM, Bernard JL, Lutz P, Bordigoni P, Plouvier E, Robert A, Roché H, Souillet G, Bouffet E, Michon J, Lopez M, Vilcoq JM, Gentet JC, Philip I, Landenstein R, Favrot M, Chauvin F (Hôpital Debrousse, Lyon; Institut Curie, Paris; Hôp Nord/Hôp de la Timone, Marseille; Centre Hospitalier Régional, Strasbourg; Centre Hospitalier Universitaire, Vandoeuvre les Nancy, France; et al)

J Clin Oncol 9:1037–1044, 1991 3–13

Introduction.—Several phase II studies have shown promising response rates among patients with metastatic neuroblastoma who were treated with high-dose chemotherapy and autologous bone marrow transplantation (BMT). However, it is still not clear whether the improved outcomes were the result of changes in the induction regimen or consolidation with BMT. The prognostic factors of disease-free survival were identified in a group of unselected patients treated for stage IV neuroblastoma.

Patients.—In 1982–1987, 72 children with stage IV neuroblastoma, aged 1–14.5 years, were entered into the study. After induction therapy, 18 patients were in complete remission, 8 were in very good partial remission, 42 were in partial remission, and 4 had disease progression. In 62 patients, treatment consisted of vincristine, high-dose melphalan, and fractionated total-body irradiation. Thereafter, 57 patients received purged autologous BMT, and 5 received histocompatible allogeneic BMT; 10 patients did not undergo BMT. The median observation time was 59 months.

Results.—Progression-free survival (PFS) for the 10 patients who did not undergo BMT was 20% at 2 years and 0% at 4 years. The PFS for the 62 patients who underwent BMT was 40% at 2 years, 20% at 4 years, and 13% at 7 years. After 4–7 years of follow-up, 6 of the 72 patients were still free of disease, and 6 were still alive with disease but without progression. In a historic control group of 56 patients, only 12% achieved PFS at 2 years. Age, gender, the type of induction regimen, and the quality of excision did not contribute to outcome, nor did they influence whether the children receiving BMT were in complete remission/very good partial remission or in partial remission. A negative bone scan after induction was the only factor that was strongly predictive of survival.

Conclusion.—Among children with stage IV neuroblastoma who are older than 1 year of age at the time of diagnosis, normalization of bone metastasis before autologous BMT appears to be the major prognostic factor of relapse-free survival and survival at 2 years. The effect at 5 years is less clear.

▶ Neuroblastoma is a tantalizing tumor. Biologically, it is the most interesting of pediatric solid tumors. For example, spontaneous regression during the first year of life is not unusual. On the other hand, once neuroblastoma is disseminated in patients older than 1 year, it is extremely difficult to cure, despite transient responses to many forms of therapy. Only a small proportion of these patients is ever cured with current forms of treatment, despite very aggressive chemotherapy and BMT regimens. In this paper, Dr. Philip and his colleagues report the result in a sizeable treatment series using autologous BMT. Although the initial response rates were encouraging and the progression-free survival was superior in this study compared with older studies, the overall results are nothing to crow about. The slope of the progression-free survival curve was better in the more recent study, mainly because of an improved outcome in the first 6 months; this suggests that better supportive care avoided early deaths. Nonetheless, because the study group continued to fail relentlessly throughout the course of follow-up, the final outcome was not significantly different from the older study.

We saw the same kind of modest improvement in the early studies of childhood leukemia in the 1960s, i.e., improved remissions and median durations of remission without improvements in the cure rate. This led to a progressive improvement in the durations of remission until a cure frequency was achieved. There has been a gradual increase in the cure rate in childhood leukemia in subsequent years. An optimist would say that this result bodes well for the future of neuroblastoma therapy because of the similarity of improvement to the early studies of childhood leukemia; however, there is a major difference. For childhood leukemia, there had been several very effective individual chemotherapeutic agents, and some of the success was a result of the appropriate organization of the regimen for the optimal use of those agents. The modest improvement demonstrated in this study is the result of a very aggressive regimen that uses all effective agents and BMT. It is not easy to see what modifications in this regimen might be made to push the curve higher. One suspects that new effective agents or biological regimens would be required to make a substantial difference in the cure rate.—J.V. Simone, M.D.

Low-Dose Interferon Gamma Renders Neuroblastoma More Susceptible to Interleukin-2 Immunotherapy

Sigal RK, Lieberman MD, Reynolds JV, Shou J, Ziegler MM, Daly JM (Univ of Pennsylvania School of Medicine, Philadelphia; Children's Hosp of Philadelphia)
J Pediatr Surg 26:389–396, 1991 3–14

Background.—Neuroblastoma (NB) remains a deadly childhood tumor. Although surgery alone may achieve a cure in as many as 90% of the children who are seen with localized disease, regionally advanced and metastatic NB remain generally resistant to multimodal treatment. Nevertheless, occasional cases of spontaneous regression of widespread disease suggest that immunotherapy might prove effective.

Study Design.—Mice bearing subcutaneous C1300 NB were randomized to receive daily injections of 25,000, 50,000, or 100,000 units of recombinant interferon-γ intraperitoneally for 6 days. Splenocytes taken at the time of sacrifice were tested for natural killer (NK) activity toward YAC, an NK-sensitive lymphoma, and toward C1300-NB.

Observations.—Treatment with interferon initially increased class I MHC antigen expression and then reduced it in a dose-dependent manner. The higher doses of interferon augmented the NK cytotoxic activity of splenocytes. No regimen had much impact on the development of immunity toward C1300-NB. Interferon administration prolonged survival slightly. Recombinant interleukin-2 had a somewhat more pronounced effect; the greatest prolongation of survival occurred when both interferon and interleukin-2 were given.

Discussion.—These findings warrant clinical trials of sequential immunotherapy (using interferon-gamma and recombinant interleukin-2) in patients with advanced NB. Future studies might profitably focus on regimens for optimally generating effector cells rather than on tumor modification.

▶ This study in mice is included in the belief that new approaches are required to make any substantial progress in disseminated neuroblastoma. If biologic therapy is to work in any pediatric tumor, neuroblastoma should be a prime candidate. It was inevitable that modest results obtained with individual biologicals might be improved by the combination of 2 or more such agents. This study demonstrates that the sequence of interferon and interleukin-2 was important in prolonging survival in these animals. It also provides some insight into how one might best administer these biologicals to patients.—J.V. Simone, M.D.

Enhanced Resection and Improved Survival in Murine Neuroblastoma (C1300-NB) After Preoperative Immunotherapy

Fowler CL, Brooks SP, Squire R, Rich GA, Rossman JE, Finegold MJ, Allen JE, Cooney DR (State Univ of New York and the Children's Hosp, Buffalo; Texas Children's Hosp, Houston)

J Pediatr Surg 26:381–388, 1991 3–15

Background.—Survival rates have not increased for children with advanced neuroblastoma (NB) in several decades. Because NB appears to be an immunogenic tumor, immunotherapy has been proposed as an alternative or adjunctive measure.

Study Design.—Three immunomodulating agents were tested for efficacy when given preoperatively to mice with C1300-NB. The agents used included low-dose cyclophosphamide, interleukin-2 (IL-2), and retinyl palmitate (RP). The effects of these agents on expression by tumor of class I major histocompatibility complex (MHC) antigens were examined.

Observations.—Combination immunotherapy with low-dose cyclophosphamide, IL-2, and RP increased the survival of mice bearing C1300-NB and inhibited tumor growth to a significant degree. Surgical resection was aided by immunotherapy. Also, the expression of class I MHC antigens was enhanced.

Discussion.—A combination of biological response modifiers, given in nontoxic doses, may be an effective part of multimodal treatment for neuroblastoma. This approach could be used preoperatively without suppressing immune defenses.

▶ Another mouse study is included to suggest another potential use of immunotherapy in children with neuroblastoma. Conventional wisdom states that immunotherapy will be the most effective when the patient's tumor has been reduced to the minimal residual size possible. This study provides an interesting reversal of that wisdom, giving biologicals in combination with other agents before an attempted surgical resection. The 1 caution in interpretation of this study is that the preoperative treatment included cyclophosphamide as well as IL-2 and RP. Although the cyclophosphamide was administered as an immunomodulating agent in low dosage, it is also an effective antitumor agent. This approach needs much further study.—J.V. Simone, M.D.

Multimodal Therapy for the Management of Localized Ewing's Sarcoma of Pelvic and Sacral Bones: A Report From the Second Intergroup Study

Evans RG, Nesbit ME, Gehan EA, Garnsey LA, Burgert O Jr, Vietti TJ, Cangir A, Tefft M, Thomas P, Askin FB, Kissane JM, Pritchard DJ, Neff J, Makley JT, Gilula L (Mayo CLinic, Rochester, Minn; Univ of Minnesota Med School, Minneapolis; Univ of Texas MD Anderson Cancer Ctr, Houston; Washington Univ School of Medicine, St Louis; Rhode Island Hosp, Providence; et al)

J Clin Oncol 9:1173–1180, 1991 3–16

Background.—Early results from the first Intergroup Ewing's Sarcoma Study (IESS-I) (1973–1978) suggested that doxorubicin or pulmonary irradiation is helpful when added to vincristine, dactinomycin, and cyclophosphamide (VAC) therapy in patients with primary nonpelvic lesions but not in those with a primary pelvic lesions. This prompted the development of a protocol in IESS-II for patients with Ewing's sarcoma localized to the pelvis and sacrum.

Study Design.—Fifty-nine patients in IESS-III (1978–1982) with disease in the pelvic and sacral bones were compared with 68 who were previously entered in IESS-I. The patients received high-dose intermittent treatment with vincristine, cyclophosphamide, doxorubicin, and dactinomycin for 6 weeks before and 70 weeks after local treatment. Those who did not have complete resection were given a dose of 55 Gy to the tumor bed.

Outcome.—A significant advantage was apparent for the IESS-II patients. The survival at 5 years was 63%, compared with 35% for those in IESS-I. The respective rates of complete remission were 68% and 13%. Local recurrences were more than twice as frequent in the IESS-I group.

Intensified therapy appeared to control lung metastasis more effectively than the IESS-I protocol, and bone metastases were also less frequent. More than 60% of the patients had severe toxicity, and 1 died of congestive failure secondary to Adriamycin toxicity. Three patients had life-threatening cardiotoxicity.

Conclusion.—High-dose chemotherapy and radiotherapy have improved the survival of patients with Ewing's sarcoma of the pelvic and sacral bones to the level reported for those with disease in nonpelvic sites.

▶ Bone tumors involving the flat bones of the body present a special problem to the therapist. Clean resections are usually impossible, which leaves one wondering what to do at the local site in addition to giving systemic combination chemotherapy. This report from the IESS group affirms what has been believed for some time: intensive chemotherapy is superior to lung irradiation in controlling lung metastases, and aggressive radiation therapy to the local site decreased the frequency of local recurrence. Ewing's sarcoma is 1 of the success stories in pediatric oncology, because it has been treated as a systemic disease rather than a localized disease. Thus, although aggressive combination chemotherapy is the first line of treatment, the bony nature of the primary tumors makes localized treatment necessary. Radiation therapy has been the most effective form of local therapy, and it must be appropriately sequenced with chemotherapy.—J.V. Simone, M.D.

Long-Term Follow-Up of Ewing's Sarcoma of Bone Treated With Combined Modality Therapy

Kinsella TJ, Miser JS, Waller B, Venzon D, Glatstein E, Weaver-McClure L, Horowitz ME (Natl Cancer Inst; Univ of Wisconsin, Madison)

Int J Radiat Oncol Biol Phys 20:389–395, 1991 3–17

Introduction.—Initial studies of combined modality treatment for Ewing's sarcoma of bone showed significant improvements in the 2–3-year disease-free survival rate during radiation therapy or surgery alone; however, there have been no long-term follow-up studies.

Methods.—Data on 107 patients with Ewing's sarcoma of bone who were entered into the 3 trials during a 12-year period were reviewed. The patients had a median age of 15 years; only 10 patients were older than 25 years. The patients received 4 cycles of either a 2-drug regimen (cyclophosphamide [CTX] and vincristine [VCR]) or a 3-drug regimen (CTX, VCR, and either actinomycin-D or doxorubicin). They also received 50 Gy of local irradiation to the involved bone. At presentation, 80 patients had localized and 27 had metastatic disease. There was more than 1 site of metastasis in 11 patients. The median potential follow-up was greater than 15 years.

Results.—Of the patients, 27% remained alive. The quickest declines in disease-free (DFS) and overall survival (OS) appeared in the first 5 years of follow-up: DFS was 29% and OS was 39%. Of the patients with metastases, only 2 survived longer than 5 years. The DFS was 52% at 2

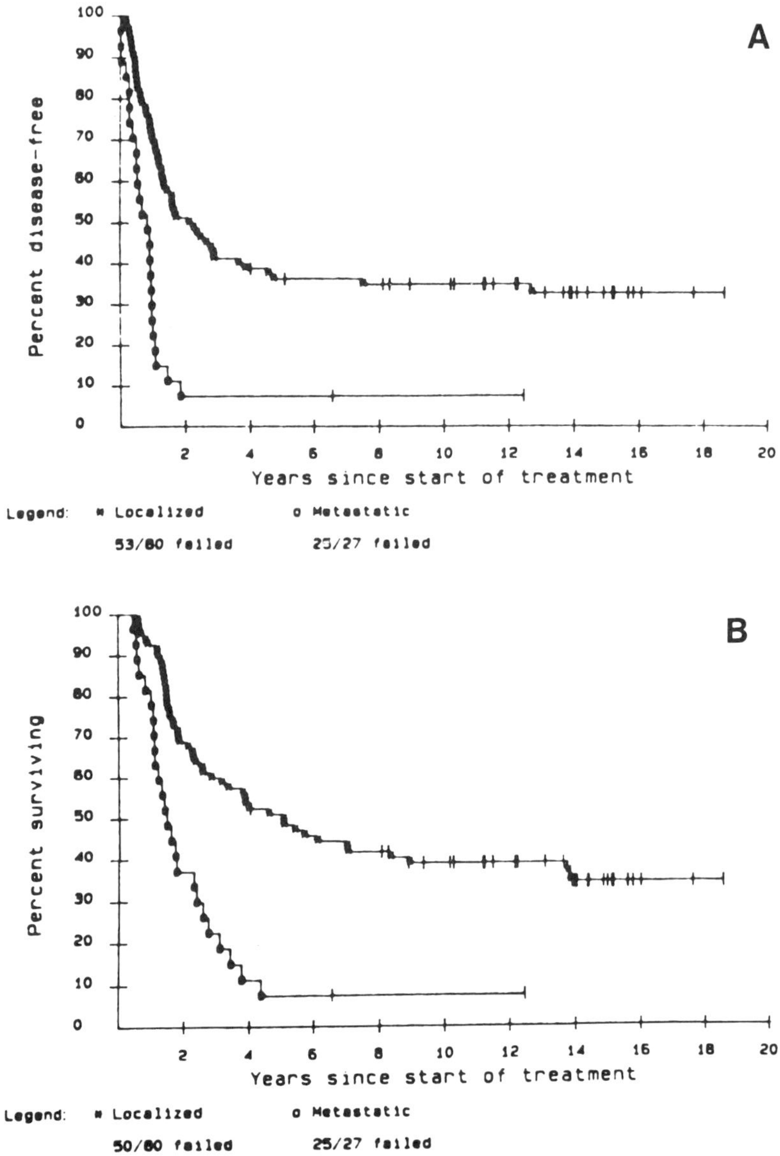

Fig 3–7.—Disease-free (**A**) and overall survival (**B**) curves for Ewing's sarcoma in patients with localized disease *(exes)* or metastatic disease *(circles)*. (Courtesy of Kinsella TJ, Miser JS, Waller B, et al: *Int J Radiat Oncol Biol Phys* 20:389–395, 1991.)

years, 37% at 5 years, 35% at 10 years, and 33% at 15 years for patients with localized disease. The OS was 68% at 2 years, 51% at 5 years, 39% at 10 years, and 34% at 15 years (Fig 3–7). The first site of failure was local relapse in 11 patients. The variable with the most significant effect on DFS and OS was metastatic disease, followed by age older

Relative Risk Estimates for Disease-Free and Overall Survival Using Cox Proportional Hazard Model

	Disease-free interval		Overall survival	
	Relative risk	Confidence interval (95%)	Relative risk	Confidence interval (95%)
Metastatic disease	6.6	(3.3, 13)	5.8	(2.9, 12)
Age >25	4.1	(1.9, 8.9)	3.7	(1.7, 8.2)
High LDH in localized disease patients	3.7	(1.7, 8.3)	3.3	(1.5, 7.2)
Central sites in localized disease patients	2.5	(1.2, 5.2)	2.5	(1.2, 5.0)

(Courtesy of Kinsella TJ, Miser JS, Waller B, et al: *Int J Radiat Oncol Biol Phys* 20:389–395, 1991.)

than 25 years, high lactate dehydrogenase levels in localized disease, and central primary tumor in localized disease (table).

Conclusion.—Most patients with Ewing's sarcoma of the bone who are treated with combined-modality therapy appear to relapse within 5 years; however, relapse may occur as late as 15 years. Local failure is not uncommon, but it does not appear to affect overall survival.

▶ This paper is important because it gives the long-term follow-up that is so frequently missing. These studies were completed years ago, and they represent nothing new. On the other hand, it is important to see that the long-term follow-up does not reveal any major proportion of late failures after 5 years. The reader must appreciate that, 20 years ago, 5-year data meant *actual* 5-year data, where the minimum period of follow-up was 5 years for every patient. Today's 5-year data represent actuarial projections, with a median period of follow-up that is maybe only 2.5 years—and sometimes even less. For this reason, today's 5-year data are not as reliable as they once were. Indeed, comparable data to the 5-year figures of the 1960s and 1970s would represent 10-year data today. Because actuarial projections have become the standard in oncology today, there is an increasing need for authors who show significant differences among different treatments to publish the long-term follow-up data that confirm their initial conclusions which, even with 5-year actuarial data, must be considered only preliminary today.—E. Glatstein, M.D.

The Contribution of Salvage Surgery to the Management of Childhood Osteosarcoma

Pastorino U, Gasparini M, Tavecchio L, Azzarelli A, Mapelli S, Zucchi V, Morondi F, Bellani FF, Valente M, Ravasi G (Instituto Nazionale Tumori; Instituto Gaetano Pini, Milan, Italy)

J Clin Oncol 9:1357–1362, 1991 3–18

Introduction.—The long-term survival for children with osteosarcoma has increased from 20% to 60% during the past 2 decades as a result of effective multimodality therapies. Salvage surgery has made a major contribution to this positive change. The real benefit of salvage surgery was assessed in a consecutive series of patients with childhood osteosarcoma.

Methods.—A total of 210 consecutive patients (20 years of age or younger) with primary osteosarcoma was treated between January 1970 and December 1988. Of these, 174 had a complete surgical resection of the primary tumor. Of the 174 patients, 72 (mean age, 12.8 years) were treated between 1970 and 1981 with surgery and chemotherapy, whereas 102 (mean age, 13.2 years) were treated between 1982 and 1988 with surgery plus neoadjuvant chemotherapy.

Findings.—Of the 174 patients, isolated lung metastases developed in 91, 42 in the first period and 49 in the second period. Extrapulmonary metastases occurred as the initial sign of relapse in 7% of both patient groups. The preoperative clinical staging accuracy improved significantly during the time periods, with chest CT becoming the standard staging procedure. The overall cancer-free 5-year survival increased significantly, from 35% to 58% during the second time period. At 5 years, the disease-free survival increased from 38% to 45%; whereas isolated lung metastases decreased from 58% to 48%. Macroscopic complete resection of the lung metastases was performed in 17% of the patients in the first time period and in 55% of those in the second time period. The overall survival from the detection of lung metastases increased significantly, from 0% to 28% at 5 years.

Conclusions.—These results indicate that systemic salvage surgery for lung metastases after chemotherapy increases the overall cure rate in these young patients with osteosarcoma. Salvage surgery should be considered the gold standard for management of limited metastatic disease.

▶ So the reader is not misled, you must start with a caveat in the first sentence of the abstract. The long-term survival (and even cure) for children with osteosarcoma has increased to approximately 60%, but only for those patients who have apparent localized disease in an extremity at the time of diagnosis. Those patients with flat bone tumors or metastatic disease at diagnosis do not have nearly that good a result. This paper points to an unusually successful approach for patients with osteosarcoma in whom metastases to the lung develop. The authors report a large series of patients in whom isolated lung metastases developed after surgical removal of the primary tumor plus adjuvant or neoadjuvant chemotherapy. As the investigators became more aggressive in removing isolated lung metastases in recent years, this resulted in an improvement in survival. The overall survival from the detection of lung metastases increased from 0% to 28% at 5 years. This mimics the experience of other centers.

It is a mystery why aggressive removal of lung metastases salvages a significant minority of patients with this tumor. In virtually every malignant tumor, pulmonary metastases after definitive surgery and multiagent chemotherapy signal certain death. What is it about osteosarcoma that makes it possible to salvage some of these patients? Does the early and complete resection of the primary tumor remove some influence? Does the chemotherapy somehow modify the metastatic cells? Is the lung a basically hostile environment for osteosarcoma? Surely, some metastatic cells fail to grow in the lung and do not develop into metastatic nodules. Until the answers to some of these questions provide further leads in therapy, we must be grateful that we can salvage even a small percentage of patients in whom lung metastases develop.—J.V. Simone, M.D.

The Effect of Preoperative Therapy on the Histologic Features of Wilms' Tumor: An Analysis of Cases From the Third National Wilms' Tumor Study

Zuppan CW, Beckwith JB, Weeks DA, Luckey DW, Pringle KC (Loma Linda Univ, Calif)

Cancer 68:385–394, 1991 3–19

Introduction.—Although preoperative chemotherapy has become a common treatment for Wilm's tumor in the United States, it is not common in Europe, where clinicians are concerned about the histologic compromise from the anticancer agents. Study results from 140 young patients with Wilms' tumor who underwent preoperative chemotherapy were evaluated.

Methods.—A total of 140 patients who had received chemotherapy were selected from the Third National Wilms' Tumor Study (NWTS-3), and biopsy material was obtained to determine the predominant histologic pattern. Tumor area, mitotic criteria, other tumor factors, and disease-free survival were also assessed.

Findings.—The 140 children represented 5.6% of the 2,489 children registered in the NWTS-3. After the initial analysis, post-therapy resection material was available for 83 cases: 48% had had stage IV disease; 43%, stage III; 5%, stage II; and 4%, stage I. The favorable histology type Wilms' tumor with distant metastases at diagnosis (stage IV) demonstrated poorer disease-free survival when compared with tumors without distant metastases. In the subset of 108 patients with favorable histology Wilms' tumor, 79% were alive and disease free at the last follow-up visit. Those tumors that had responded well to therapy appeared decimated at resection and had broad expanses of bland connective tissue. They also had proliferative fibrohistiocytic nodules, hemosiderin-carrying macrophages, and evidence of recent hemorrhages. The patient outcome correlated with the proportion of differentiated elements after therapy and lower mitotic activity. Nine of the 83 resection samples had anaplasia (11%).

Conclusions.—These findings, although limited by the absence of a standardized preoperative therapy protocol and by the relatively intense therapy all patients received, point to the potentially important criteria for future controlled studies. The possible benefits of preoperative tumor reduction must be balanced against the risk of either overtreatment or undertreatment because of the lack of knowledge regarding tumor stage.

▶ Even though 80% to 90% of children with Wilms' tumor can be cured, investigators continue to search for ways of curing the remaining 10% or 15%. This paper addresses, but unfortunately does not completely resolve, a question that has concerned Wilms' tumor for many years: Is there any advantage to giving preoperative chemotherapy to patients with large or metastatic Wilms' tumor rather than definitive surgery followed by chemotherapy? The authors found an association between the degree of tumor destruction by preoperative chemotherapy and the outcome, which should surprise no one. But one must wonder whether the results justify the modification of histology that chemotherapy must induce, with the loss of important landmarks that help to identify and treat the small percentage of patients who fail to respond to modern therapy. Thus, one cannot recommend preoperative chemotherapy or radiotherapy, except in rare circumstances in which the size or location of the tumor is an immediate threat to life or normal renal function.—J.V. Simone, M.D.

Extended Followup of Bilateral Wilms Tumor: Results of the National Wilms Tumor Study

Montgomery BT, Kelalis PP, Blute ML, Bergstralh EJ, Beckwith JB, Norkool P, Green DM, D'Angio GJ (Mayo Clin and Foundation, Rochester, Minn; Children's Hosp, Denver; Natl Wilms Tumor Data and Statistical Ctr, Seattle; Roswell Park Cancer Inst, Buffalo, NY; Children's Hosp of Philadelphia)

J Urol 146:514–518, 1991 3–20

Background.—Over the past 2 decades, considerable literature about Wilms' tumor has been produced, attesting to the dramatic improvement in the survival of children with this disease as noted in the third National Wilms' Tumor Study (NWTS). One aspect of the long-term survival of the NWTS patients not fully explained relates to renal function and late relapse. An attempt was made to establish the long-term survival for those NWTS patients with synchronous bilateral disease.

Methods.—Patients in the NWTS-2 and NWTS-3 were registered between January 1974 and July 1986. A total of 209 children registered with synchronous bilateral disease. After applying exclusion criteria, 140 patients remained for restrospective review and 45 new patients were added, providing 185 patients for analysis. Treatment changed during the study period, with 109 (59%) patients undergoing surgical resection, whereas 65 (35%) of the patients had tumor biopsy only, followed by chemotherapy with or without radiotherapy and subsequent surgery.

Results.—The overall survival for patients with synchronous bilateral Wilms' tumor was 83%, 73%, and 70% at 2, 5, and 10 years, respectively (Fig 3–8). At follow-up, 133 of the 185 patients remained free of disease. Of the 18 patients demonstrating evidence of unfavorable histology, 14 died of tumor progression, for a 5-year survival of 20%. Diagnosis at a younger age and a lower tumor substatge significantly improved the prognosis of the patients. Renal failure occurred in 10 patients as-

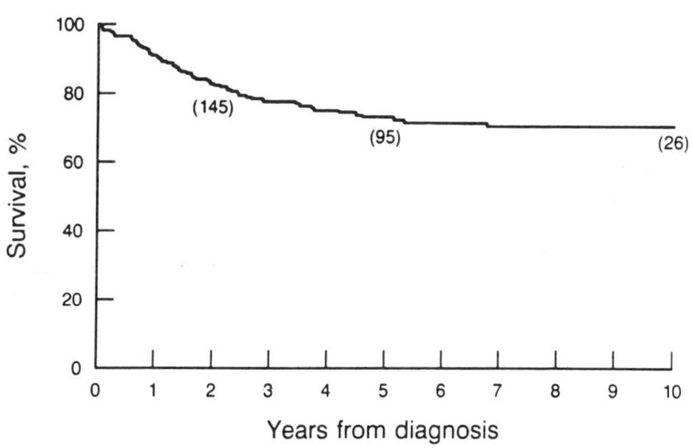

Fig 3–8.—The overall survival curve for children with synchronous bilateral Wilms' tumor registered with NWTS. The number of patients under observation at 2, 5, and 10 years of follow-up is shown in parentheses. (Courtesy of Montgomery BT, Kelalis PP, Blute ML et al: *J Urol* 146:514–518, 1991.)

sessed at follow-up. Those patients requiring hepatic and pulmonary resections of the metastatic tumor had poor outcomes.

Implications.—These findings showed that children with Wilms' tumor do well if they do not undergo immediate resection of the primary tumor. One advantage of delaying the tumor resection is that the renal-sparing tumor removal can follow the chemotherapy.

▶ This report of a large number of children with bilateral Wilms' tumor provides very important follow-up information. First, a majority of these children can be cured, despite the surgical, chemotherapeutic, or radiation effects on the residual normal kidney tissue. The study also provides the very useful information that preoperative chemotherapy can reduce the loss of normal renal tissue. This is an excellent example of cooperative group studies at their best. The authors gathered the results in a rare form of tumor during an extended period of time, and they were able to develop some clear guidelines for the therapeutic approach. We are fortunate that Wilms' tumor is so responsive to multiple forms of therapy. There are few malignancies seen with multiple involved sites that are curable in more than half of the patients.—J.V. Simone, M.D.

Intensive Chemotherapy and Low-Dose Radiotherapy for the Treatment of Advanced-Stage Hodgkin's Disease in Pediatric Patients: A Pediatric Oncology Group Study

Weiner MA, Leventhal BG, Marcus R, Brecher M, Ternberg J, Behm FG, Cantor A, Wharam M, Chauvenet A (Hackensack Med Ctr, Hackensack, NJ; Johns Hopkins Univ, Baltimore; Univ of Florida, Gainesville; Roswell Park Mem Inst, Buffalo, New York; Washington Univ School of Medicine, St Louis; et al)
J Clin Oncol 9:1591–1598, 1991 3–21

Introduction.—In 1984, the Pediatric Oncology Group began a pilot study using 8 cycles of alternating mechlorethamine, vincristine, procarbazine, prednisone/doxorubicin, vinblastine, bleomycin, dacarbazine (MOPP/ABVD) therapy plus low-dose radiotherapy to treat 62 patients with advanced-stage Hodgkin's disease.

Methods.—The patients (mean age, 12 years) received 4 cycles of MOPP alternating with 4 cycles of ABVD. Low-dose radiotherapy was given at the end of chemotherapy to those patients who achieved complete remission. The dose to lymphoid tissue and bone lesions was 2,100 cGy, and that to nonlymphoid organs was limited to 1,050 cGy.

Results.—Complete remission was achieved in 87% of patients at the end of chemotherapy. Survival after a median follow-up of nearly 3 years was 91%, and the actuarial 3-year event-free survival rate was 77%. Females did better than males, and those with stage IV disease had a relatively poor outlook. Of the 6 deaths, 3 were caused by progressive Hodgkin's disease. Treatment was well tolerated; the major problem was neutropenia.

Conclusion.—This combined chemotherapy/radiotherapy regimen for advanced-stage Hodgkin's disease is safe in the short term. Further study will clarify the role of radiotherapy and delineate the long-term toxic effects of this treatment.

▶ With such a high cure rate in pediatric Hodgkin's disease, there have been major efforts to reduce the potential for late effects that result from therapy. These efforts include attempts to eliminate or reduce the dosage of nitrogen mustard and other alkylating agents; to reduce the frequency of splenectomy used in staging procedures; and to reduce the amount of radiation given. In this study, the amount of radiotherapy was reduced by approximately one third, and the middle-term outcome was acceptable. However, because of their age, irradiation of the vertebral column in pediatric patients is likely to impair growth—even when the dose is reduced to 2,100 cGy. Furthermore, the likelihood of secondary acute myeloid leukemia developing is compounded when alkylating agents are given in addition to radiation therapy. It remains to be seen, therefore, whether reductions in the dosage of radiation therapy will have any significant effect on the frequency of serious late complications.—J.V. Simone, M.D.

Additional Reading

Bowman LC, Hancock MD, Santana VM, et al: Impact of intensified therapy on clinical outcome in infants and children with neuroblastoma: The St. Jude Children's Research Hospital experience. *J Clin Oncol* 9:1599–1608, 1991.

▶ This is an optimistic report of a large series of patients with neuroblastoma. The outcome of all patients with all stages of disease was better than expected—57% 4-year survival. Of course, patients older than 1 year of age with disseminated disease did poorly; however, a 20% long-term survival is projected for those treated in the modern era compared with the small percentage of survival achieved in earlier studies. Progress may be slow, but even in this difficult disease, there is some light.

Chan HSL, Haddad G, Thorner PS, et al: P-glycoprotein expression as a predictor of the outcome of therapy for neuroblastoma. *N Engl J Med* 325:1608–1614, 1991.

▶ This is an interesting report that could be useful if confirmed. Although I'm not a fan of "prognostic factors," this report is intriguing because p-glycoprotein is related to multiple drug resistance. Thus, this prognostic factor could directly guide therapeutic intervention.

Uckun FM, Ramsey NK, Waddick KG, et al: In vitro and in vivo radiation resistance associated with CD3 surface antigen expression in T-lineage acute lymphoblastic leukemia. *Blood* 78:2945–2955.

Niemeyer CM, Gelber RD, Tarbell NJ, et al: Low-dose versus high-dose methotrexate during remission induction in childhood acute lymphoblastic leukemia (Protocol 81-01 Update). *Blood* 78:2514–2519.

Henze G, Fengler R, Hartmann R, et al: Six-year experience with a comprehensive approach to the treatment of recurrent childhood acute lymphoblastic leukemia (ALL-REZ BFM 85). A relapse study of the BFM group. *Blood* 78:1166–1172.

Neglia JP, Meadows AT, Robison LG, et al: Second neoplasms after acute lymphoblastic leukemia in childhood. *N Engl J Med* 325:1330–1336, 1991.

Rubin CM, Arthur DC, Woods WG, et al: Therapy-related myelodysplastic syndrome and acute myeloid leukemia in children: Correlation between chromosomal abnormalities and prior therapy. *Blood* 78:2982–2988, 1991.

Berman E, Little C, Gee T, et al: Reasons that patients with acute myelogenous leukemia do not undergo allogeneic bone marrow transplantation. *N Engl J Med* 326:156–160, 1992.

Eguiguren JM, Riberio RC, Pui CH, et al: Secondary non-Hodgkin's lymphoma after treatment for childhood cancer. *Leukemia* 5:908–911, 1991.

4 Hematologic Malignancies

Introduction

I think that most physicians who treat patients with Hodgkin's disease and non-Hodgkin's lymphoma believe that they are able to effectively treat most patients. The improvements in the treatment of Hodgkin's disease have been readily reflected in the declining mortality of the disease (1). However, there has not been a comparable decline in mortality from non-Hodgkin's lymphoma in population-based cancer registries. This could be a result of a number of factors: the therapies may not be as good as we think they are; the therapies may not be used in the community in the way that they were reported; only a fraction of patients are actually getting the newer therapies; or there may be other explanations. Nevertheless, more progress is required to achieve the same results that have been seen with Hodgkin's disease therapy in other hematologic malignancies.

Dan L. Longo, M.D., F.A.C.P.

Reference

1. Feuer EJ, et al: *J Clin Epidemiol* 44:141, 1991.

Hodgkin's Disease

Lymphography: Current Role in Oncology
Moskovic E, Fernando I, Blake P, Parsons C (Royal Marsden Hosp, London)
Br J Radiol 64:422–427, 1991 4–1

Introduction.—Because the number of lymphograms performed at oncology centers has decreased since the introduction of techniques such as CT, the 1980–1989 data from a major oncology center were reviewed to determine whether there is still a role for lymphography in oncology.

Results.—In 1980, 536 lymphograms were performed; in 1989, 101 were performed. Nearly 40% of the total number of lymphograms in 1980 were performed on patients with lymphoma, whereas in 1989, only 4% were performed on these patients. Instead, 90% of the lymphograms were performed on patients with gynecologic malignancies, especially carcinoma of the cervix. Data analysis suggested that only in carcinoma of the cervix can a lymphogram provide useful information on gynecologic malignancy.

Conclusion.—The decrease in the use of lymphography is, for the most part, justified. However, when CT is negative for nodal disease in patients with stage IB carcinoma of the cervix and in the staging of some Hodgkin's lymphomas, a lymphogram is still useful.

▶ This particular subject is near and dear to my heart. Current imaging techniques have gradually resulted in more and more staging that is dependent on CT or MRI. The only criterion they have for neoplasm is size. Although MRI has the potential to give more than a size criterion, this has not been commonly used thus far. The lymphogram still allows one to assess the internal architecture of the nodes, which is frequently the only site of abnormality when the node is of normal size. Using some arbitrary cut-off (e.g., 1.5 cm) is obviously capricious at best. Does anyone seriously believe that sizing the node at 1.5 cm can reliably distinguish neoplasm within a 1.4 cm node?

The main problem is that, because few lymphograms are being done these days, most of the diagnostic radiologists are uncomfortable with the interpretation. Thus, the usual interpretation is "of concern," or "suspicious," or "worrisome." These descriptions do not help much in terms of interpretation. Although they may make the diagnostician feel better, they really don't help the oncologist. The simple fact is that the lymphogram is a relatively gross tool; therefore, one has to be very careful about *not* overinterpreting the lymphogam. In the hands of those who really know how to interpret them (as does this group from the Royal Marsden) lymphograms still have an important role to play in oncology. It is my strong belief that they still play a major role in the staging of lymphomas, despite the disagreement of many of my colleagues. Approximately 10% of the time—when the CT or MRI is normal—the lymphogram is abnormal. Most of the time, we have confirmed this histologically.

In addition to the enormous amount of information on staging, there is also the value of having the nodes imaged for setting treatment portals, as well as for following the nodes during and after treatment with simple flat plates of the abdomen. This latter use of the lymphogram is remarkably unappreciated by many oncologists, despite its economy in terms of assessing intra-abdominal nodes that respond to treatment.—E. Glatstein, M.D.

Radiation Therapy Versus Combination Chemotherapy in the Treatment of Early-Stage Hodgkin's Disease: Seven-Year Results of a Prospective Randomized Trial

Longo DL, Glatstein E, Duffey PL, Young RC, Hubbard SM, Urba WJ, Wesley MN, Raubitschek A, Jaffe ES, Wiernik PH, DeVita VT Jr (Natl Cancer Inst, Bethesda, Md)

J Clin Oncol 9:906–917, 1991 4–2

Objective.—Radiation therapy results in the cure of approximately 75% of patients with early-stage Hodgkin's disease. Some investigators have recommended adding chemotherapy to radiation therapy in an effort to improve upon these results. However, rather than accept combined modality related toxicities, it is reasonable to evaluate the effects of chemotherapy alone in these patients. A prospective trial comparing radiotherapy with mechlorethamine, vincristine, procarbazine, and prednisone (MOPP) chemotherapy was begun in 1978, enrolling patients with laparotomy-staged early Hodgkin's disease.

Study Design.—A total of 136 patients with stage IA to $IIIA_1$ disease was entered into the trial and followed for a median of 7½ years. All patients were untreated. The extent of megavoltage radiotherapy depended on the stage of disease.

Results.—Overall, survival at 10 years was projected as 81%, and disease-free survival was projected as 74%. All 30 patients with peripheral stage IA disease had a complete remission with radiotherapy, and none have relapsed. Those patients with more advanced-stage disease relapsed less frequently when given MOPP chemotherapy. The projected 10-year survival for patients given chemotherapy is 92%, compared with 76% for those given radiotherapy. Patients who relapsed after chemotherapy were not more resistant to salvage treatment than were those who relapsed from radiotherapy-induced remission. Acute hematologic toxicity was more evident with chemotherapy, but there were no treatment-related deaths in either group.

Discussion.—The final choice between these treatment options will depend in large part on long-term survival and the frequency of treatment-related complications. It is evident that MOPP chemotherapy is at least as effective as radiotherapy in early-stage Hodgkin's disease.

▶ This National Cancer Institute study demonstrated that MOPP chemotherapy was significantly better than radiation therapy in the treatment of patients with central stage IA, IB, IIA, IIB, and $IIIA_1$ disease who were randomized in this study. If one excludes the patients with stage $IIIA_1$ and massive mediastinal disease (who are now believed to be better treated with chemotherapy), the significance between the 2 arms disappears. However, it is possible to conclude from this study that 1 option for patients with clinical early-stage Hodgkin's disease is to forego the staging laparotomy and receive combination chemotherapy on the basis of clinical staging.

A second similar study by Cimino and colleagues (1) obtained similar results with either MOPP chemotherapy or radiation therapy after laparotomy staging in patients with stage IA and IIA Hodgkin's disease. However, a recent update (2) of this 1989 study reversed its conclusions based on the differences in salvageability of relapsed patients. Twelve patients treated with MOPP and 12 patients treated with radiation therapy relapsed. Ten of the 12 relapsed patients who were initially treated with radiation therapy were successfully salvaged with chemotherapy, and 10 of the 12 relapsed patients treated with chemotherapy died. The updated survival data showed that the MOPP-treated patients with stage IA and IIA disease had only a 56% overall survival at 8 years. This is significantly lower than every other report of patients with early-stage disease treated with chemotherapy alone, and it is lower than would be expected even in asymptomatic advanced-stage patients. It is very important to sort out whether patients with early-stage disease who are treated with chemotherapy have a different prognosis than patients with early-stage disease who are treated with radiation therapy. However, the equation for dealing with the choice of therapy will also need to balance the very high rate of late morbidity and mortality related to the use of chemotherapy.—D.L. Longo, M.D., F.A.C.P.

References

1. Cimino G, et al: *J Clin Oncol* 7:732, 1989.
2. Biti GP, et al: *J Clin Oncol* 10:378, 1992.

Treatment of Advanced-Stage Massive Mediastinal Hodgkin's Disease: The Case for Combined Modality Treatment

Longo DL, Russo A, Duffey PL, Hubbard SM, Glatstein E, Hill JB, Jaffe ES, Young RC, DeVita VT Jr (Natl Cancer Inst, Bethesda, Md)

J Clin Oncol 9:227–235, 1991 4–3

Background.—In some patients with massive mediastinal Hodgkin's disease, the addition of radiation therapy to chemotherapy can improve outcome. Toxicity is high, and it is best to ensure that each modality is not optimally effective when used alone. The outcomes of 49 patients with massive mediastinal Hodgkin's disease treated by chemotherapy alone were evaluated.

Patients.—Presenting radiographs of 192 patients treated with mechlorethamine, vincristine, procarbazine, and prednisone (MOPP) chemotherapy were examined. A total of 49 patients had mediastinal masses measuring greater than one third of the greatest posteroanterior chest diameter. There were 29 males and 20 females (median age, 22 years). Disease stage was IIB in 5 patients and III or IV in 44.

Outcome.—A total of 71% of the patients achieved complete remission. The relapse rate among these patients was 40%, although 4 patients achieved lasting remissions with subsequent therapy. The overall survival was 39% at a median follow-up of 20 years, and disease-free survival for patients who achieved a complete response was 60%. Of the 9 patients who received mantle therapy after a maximal response to MOPP, only 1 relapsed, compared with 50% of the patients who achieved a complete response to MOPP alone. Disease-free survival was plotted as a function of treatment (Fig 4–1). There was a near-significant difference in tumor mortality between patients treated with MOPP and combined modality, but overall, the survival difference was not significantly different because of the late complications of combined therapy.

Conclusions.—Retrospective analysis suggests that combined radiation therapy and chemotherapy in patients with advanced Hodgkin's disease and massive mediastinal involvement may result in improved control of disease. Additional chemotherapy regimens with mantle radiation therapy may improve on the results that were found. A complete remission rate of 85% has been reported in a preliminary study.

▶ Chemotherapy alone is associated with an approximately 50% probability of relapse in patients with advanced-stage Hodgkin's disease who also have large

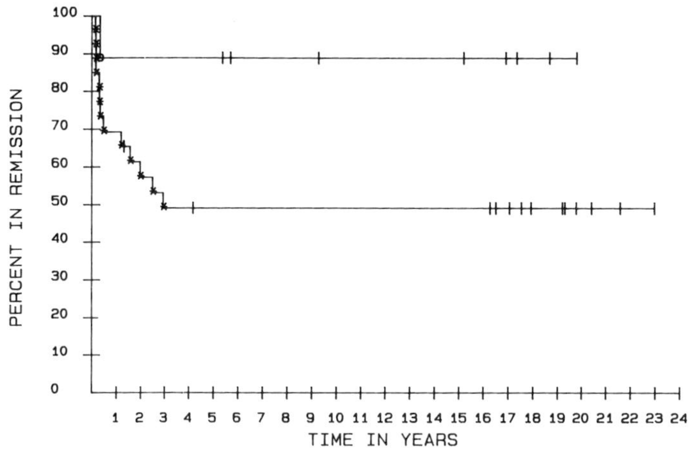

Fig 4–1.—Kaplan-Meier plot of disease-free survival of complete responders as a function of treatment. *Asterisk* = patients treated with MOPP alone, 13/26 failed. *Open circle* = patients treated with MOPP followed by mantle-field irradiation, 1/9 failed. The plateau of the curve of patients treated with MOPP is at 49%; for the patients treated with combined modality, the plateau is at 89% (P_2 = 0.53). (Courtesy of Longo DL, Russo A, Duffey PL, et al: *J Clin Oncol* 9:227–235, 1991.)

mediastinal masses. The late toxicities associated with MOPP plus radiation therapy have made us interested in evaluating MOPP/ABVD (Adriamycin, bleomycin, vinblastine, and dacarbazine) plus radiation therapy in these patients who seem to require both modalities to achieve disease eradication. Massive mediastinal disease is the only form of Hodgkin's disease in which primary combined-modality therapy appears to be indicated.

Several treatment experiences that used combined-modality therapy in patients with advanced-stage disease have been reported (1–4). The results are quite good when low-dose radiation to the involved nodes is added as an adjunct to combination chemotherapy. However, the only randomized trials to specifically address the role of radiation therapy in patients with advanced-stage disease have gotten either equivocal (5) or negative results (6,7). There may be important advantages to adding radiation therapy in those subsets of patients that have been demonstrated to have higher relapse rates, such as patients with massive mediastinal disease. However, on the basis of currently available data, the toxicities that are associated with combined-modality therapy and the efficacy of well-delivered combination chemotherapy make it difficult to see a routine role for radiation therapy in the treatment of all patients with an advanced stage of disease.—D.L. Longo, M.D., F.A.C.P.

References

1. Brizel DM, et al: *Int J Radiat Oncol Biol Phys* 19:535, 1990.
2. Connors JM, Klimo P: *Semin Hematol* 24(suppl 1):35, 1987.
3. Vose JM, et al: *J Clin Oncol* 9:1421, 1991.
4. Yahalom J, et al: *J Clin Oncol* 9:2193, 1991.
5. Yelle L, et al: *J Clin Oncol* 9:1983, 1991.
6. Glick J, et al: *Blood* 76(suppl 1):350A, 1990.
7. Crowther D, et al: *J Clin Oncol* 2:892, 1984.

Outcome of Treatment of First Relapse of Hodgkin's Disease After Primary Chemotherapy: Identification of Risk Factors From the British Columbia Experience 1970 to 1988

Lohri A, Barnett M, Fairey RN, O'Reilly SE, Phillips GL, Reece D, Voss N, Connors JM (British Columbia Cancer Agency, Vancouver, BC, Canada)

Blood 77:2292–2298, 1991 4–4

Background.—Less than 30% of patients remain free of disease after salvage therapy for patients with Hodgkin's disease who relapse after multiagent chemotherapy. To identify factors that may influence the outcome of salvage strategies, the records of 80 patients who had relapses after potentially curative primary chemotherapy for Hodgkin's disease were examined. Freedom from second failure (FF2F) was considered as the major end point.

Patients.—The patients were divided into 4 groups based on primary chemotherapy: 24 were initially treated with 3 cycles of mechlorethamine, vincristine, prednisone, and procarbazine (MOPP) and wide-field radiation therapy (group 1); 25 had 6 cycles of MOPP (group 2); 15 were treated initially with MOPP plus doxorubicin, bleomycin, vinblastine, and dacarbazine, and received conventional salvage regimens (group 3); and 16 received similar primary therapy as group 3 but received high-dose chemotherapy and autologous bone marrow transplantation as salvage therapy (group 4).

Findings.—The actuarial FF2F for all patients was 38% after a median follow-up of 75 months for patients who were alive. Three risk factors had significant impact on the outcome of treatment: stage IV disease at primary diagnosis, B symptoms at relapse, and time from primary treatment to relapse of less than 1 year. Actuarial FF2F at 5 years was 17% when 1 or more of these risk factors were present which was significantly less than the FF2F of 82% when none of these factors was present. The impact of these factors was independent of the type of primary chemotherapy as well as salvage strategies including high-dose chemotherapy and autologous bone marrow transplantation. Interestingly, those patients with none of these risk factors at relapse who were treated with doxorubicin-based chemotherapy or extended-field irradiation, or both had excellent outcome.

Summary.—The outcome of salvage treatment for patients with Hodgkin's disease in first relapse after primary chemotherapy depends on the presence or absence of 3 risk factors: initial stage IV disease, B symptoms at relapse, and time to relapse of less than 1 year.

Conventional-Dose Salvage Combination Chemotherapy in Patients Relapsing With Hodgkin's Disease After Combination Chemotherapy: The Low Probability for Cure

Longo DL, Duffey PL, Young RC, Hubbard SM, Ihde DC, Glatstein E, Phares JC, Jaffe ES, Urba WJ, DeVita VT Jr (Natl Cancer Inst, Bethesda and Frederick, Md)

J Clin Oncol 10:210–218, 1992 4–5

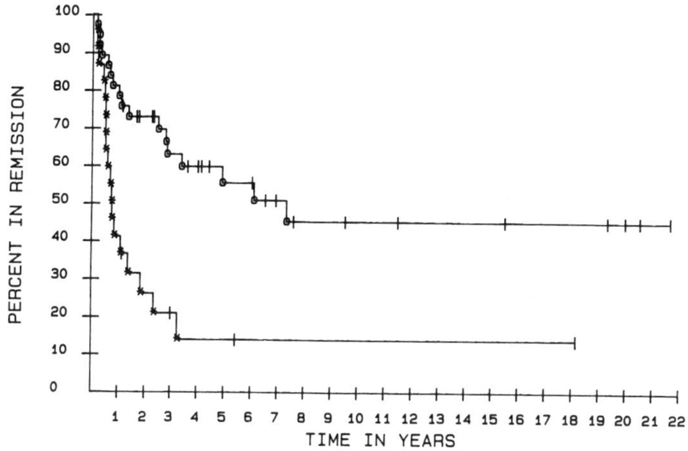

Fig 4–2.—A Kaplan-Meier plot of the disease-free survival of patients obtaining a second complete remission as a function of the length of initial remission. Those patients with a short initial remission (<1 year, *; 18 of 23 failed) had significantly less durable second remissions (14% at 4 years) than patients with long (>1 year, *open circles;* 17 of 37 failed) initial remissions (45% at 21 years) (P_2 = .0003). (Courtesy of Longo DL, Duffey PL, Young RC, et al: *J Clin Oncol* 10:210–218, 1992.)

Introduction.—Salvage treatment was evaluated in 107 patients with Hodgkin's disease who had relapsed after combination chemotherapy had induced a complete remission. They represented 28% of all patients who had a complete response to treatment in 1964–1990.

Management.—A large majority of patients seen before 1979 received mechlorethamine, vincristine, procarbazine, prednisone (MOPP) therapy, with or without MOPP or carmustine for maintenance. Only those patients with systemic involvement at the time of relapse received chemotherapy as the initial salvage treatment.

Outcome.—Half the relapses occurred within a year of complete remission. Overall survival is projected to be 17% at 20 years. The only significant factors in survival were age at diagnosis and the length of initial remission. Patients older than 30 years of age at the time of initial treatment had a poorer outlook, as did those who were in remission for less than a year (Fig 4–2). A large majority of patients with a longer initial remission responded well to MOPP therapy for relapse, but acute leukemia and other complications reduced their long-term survival.

Conclusions.—Salvage treatment in conventional doses often cannot sustain complete remission in patients who have relapsed after initial chemotherapy for Hodgkin's disease. Patients who achieve a second remission might do better with high-dose treatment and hematopoietic support.

▶ These studies clearly define the prognosis of patients with advanced-stage disease in whom primary combination chemotherapy does not result in cure. In the experience of Lohri and colleagues (Abstract 4–4), relapsed patients without poor prognostic factors had an 80% probability of long-term survival with conventional-dose salvage chemotherapy that included doxorubicin. The data on salvage of relapses with good prognosis from the National Cancer Institute (Abstract 4–5) are not quite as optimistic, but there is sufficient data for optimism that conventional-dose salvage may be successful. On the other hand, the sobering data from the Vancouver experience reveals that the use of high-dose therapy with bone marrow transplantation in 12 relapsed patients with poor-prognosis characteristics (i.e., short initial remission, initial stage IV disease, or B symptoms at relapse) did not seem to improve their poor prognosis. This is a very small experience; however, other transplant experiences have not analyzed their results based on these prognostic factors.

Indeed, a multicenter experience with high-dose salvage therapy (cyclophosphamide, carmustine, and etoposide) in Vancouver from patients reported a 53% 5-year survival in 56 relapsed patients (1). The Nebraska group reported a 37% 3-year event-free survival in 56 patients who received peripheral blood stem cells rather than autologous bone marrow (2). Are these series starting with patients of similar prognosis? Probably not. Older patients often do not make it to high-dose therapy programs. In addition, patients with marrow disease, either at diagnosis or at relapse, may be excluded. It may be time for a prospective randomized trial comparing conventional-dose chemotherapy alone and the same therapy followed by high-dose therapy with bone marrow transplantation in patients whose initial remission was short, who were seen with stage IV disease, or who relapsed with B symptoms.—D.L. Longo, M.D., F.A.C.P.

References

1. Reece DE, et al: *J Clin Oncol* 9:1871, 1991.
2. Kessinger A, et al: *Blood* 77:2322, 1991.

Life-Threatening Airway Obstruction at the Presentation of Hodgkin's Disease

Jeffrey GM, Mead GM, Whitehouse JMA (Southampton Gen Hosp, Southhampton, England)
Cancer 67:506–510, 1991 4–6

Introduction.—Although Hodgkin's disease often involves the mediastinum, significant mediastinal symptoms are less frequent and severe airway obstruction is rare. Data on 6 patients (aged 19–42 years) with life-threatening airway obstruction during the early clinical course of Hodgkin's disease were reviewed.

Patients.—All patients had life-threatening airway obstruction during an 11-year period. All were in either stage IIA or IIB of the disease; 5 patients had the nodular sclerosing type of Hodgkin's disease, which has a propensity for the mediastinum. Airway obstruction developed during general anesthesia in 3 patients, and another patient showed rapid deterioration after diagnostic bronchoscopy. Respiratory arrest developed in 1 patient after admission, and another had mediastinal adenopathy with invasive disease of the trachea. The maximal diameter of the masses was 9–15 cm. All patients received combined treatment.

Results.—The results of treatment were excellent; all patients were alive at follow-up, with no relapses; 1 patient was alive at more than 90 months.

Conclusion.—Mediastinal Hodgkin's disease may rarely be complicated by life-threatening airway obstruction. General anesthesia with endotracheal intubation should be avoided if possible. Peripheral lymph nodes that could be removed using local anesthetic can be sought, or CT-guided biopsy may provide adequate histologic findings when the mediastinum is the only site of involvement.

▶ Life-threatening airway obstruction, or superior vena cava syndrome, is a well-described clinical presentation of mediastinal (usually nodular sclerosis subtype) Hodgkin's disease. This report adds 6 cases to the previously published reports of patients with severe airway obstruction when initially seen with Hodgkin's disease. The low incidence (2% to 4%) of this complication is of note in light of the frequent presentation of massive mediastinal involvement. The airway obstruction usually becomes apparent as a result of anesthesia or bronchoscopy. However, in these patients there is little—if anything—to be gained by a procedure that requires anesthesia or bronchoscopy. The diagnosis can virtually always be made by a relatively noninvasive procedure (e.g., peripheral lymph node biopsy, bone marrow aspirate, or mediastinal/retroperitoneal fine-needle aspiration). Because massive mediastinal Hodgkin's disease requires combined modality treatment, there is no need for laparotomy, and treatment should be initiated as rapidly as possible.—R.F. Ozols, M.D., Ph.D.

Non-Hodgkin's Lymphoma

Multivariate Analysis of Prognostic Factors in Stage IV Follicular Low-Grade Lymphoma: A Risk Model

Romaguera JE, McLaughlin P, North L, Dixon D, Silvermintz KB, Garnsey LA, Velasquez WS, Hagemeister FB, Cabanillas F (Univ of Texas MD Anderson Cancer Ctr, Houston)

J Clin Oncol 9:762–769, 1991 4–7

Objective.—The records of 96 previously untreated patients with stage IV follicular low-grade lymphoma were reviewed to identify the pretreatment variables influencing outcome. The patients were treated uniformly with cyclophosphamide, doxorubicin, vincristine, prednisone, and bleomycin (CHOP-Bleo) chemotherapy in 1972–1982.

Results.—After a median observation time of 11½ years, the 10-year survival rate was 42%. The overall rate of complete remission was 77%. A total of 15% of the patients lived 10 years without relapsing, and the median failure-free survival time was 30 months.

Prognostic Factors.—Multivariate analysis showed that lymph node size, the degree of marrow involvement, and female sex influenced failure-free survival. The number of extranodal sites of disease was a factor in cause-specific survival. Gender was a very powerful variable. Females with a low tumor burden had the best outlook, whereas males with a high burden did the worst.

Discussion.—Intensive treatment measures (such as marrow transplantation) might be reserved for those patients with stage IV follicular low-grade lymphoma who are most likely to fail. Nevertheless, a sizeable proportion of even low-risk patients are at risk of relapsing at some stage.

▶ The major difficulty with the nihilistic approach to the management of patients with advanced-stage indolent lymphoma is that it fails to take into account the subsets of patients who do very well with currently available therapy and also those subsets of patients whose prognosis is sufficiently poor that a more aggressive approach may be worth considering. Ann Arbor staging is poorly suited to the task of separating patients with indolent lymphoma who have different prognoses. This paper discusses the specific clinical features used to distinguish the subgroups.

An even more intriguing report from this same group of investigators (on a somewhat different group of patients) found that the serum level of β2-microglobulin identified patients of distinct prognosis (1). Those patients with indolent lymphoma who were seen with serum β2-microglobulin levels greater than 3 mg/L had a 36% complete response rate to chemotherapy, and all had relapsed by 42 months. On the other hand, when the serum β2-microglobulin level was below 3 mg/L, the complete response rate was 71%; 85% of the complete responders were in their initial remission at 42 months. The capacity to identify prospectively those patients who have prolonged disease-free survival after conventional-dose chemotherapy would be an important breakthrough in this puzzling group of patients.—D.L. Longo, M.D., F.A.C.P.

Reference

1. Litam P, et al: *Ann Intern Med* 114:855, 1991.

Radiation Sensitivity of Human B-Lineage Lymphoid Precursor Cells

Uckun FM, Mitchell JB, Obuz V, Park CH, Waddick K, Friedman N, Oubaha L, Min WS, Song CW (Univ of Minnesota, Natl Cancer Inst, Bethesda, Md)

Int J Radiat Oncol Biol Phys 21:1553–1560, 1991 4–8

Background.—Although much information is available on the radiobiologic features of human and murine myeloid/erythroid precursor cell populations, little is known about the radiation sensitivity of human B-lineage lymphoid precursor cells (LPCs). The radiation sensitivity of human B-lineage LPC was studied at various developmental stages.

Methods and Findings.—The radiation sensitivity of 8 immunophenotypically distinct B-lineage LPC lines of acute lymphoblastic leukemia or fetal liver origin corresponding to discrete developmental stages of human B-cell ontogeny was analyzed. The B-lineage LPC radiation sensitivity showed a temporal correlation with the distinct stages of develop-

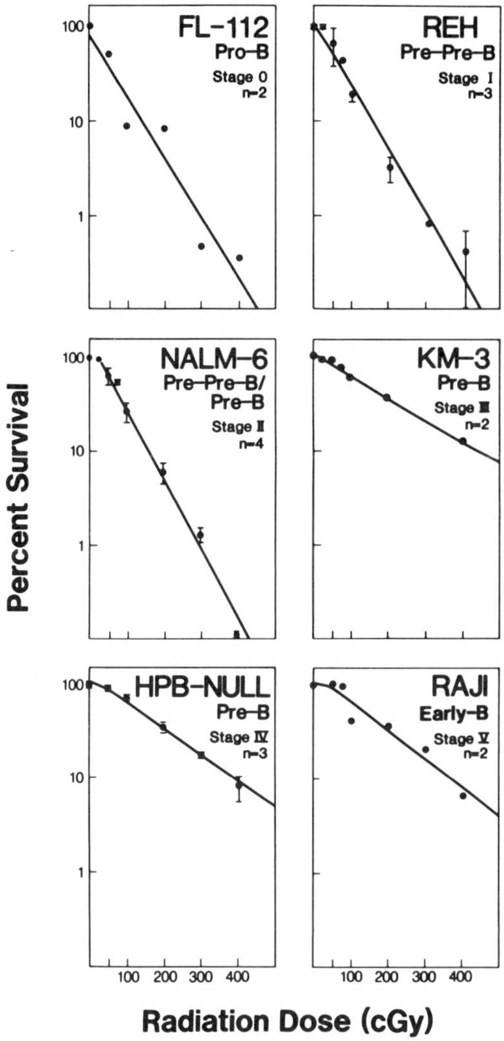

Fig 4–3.—Radiation sensitivity of B-lineage lymphoid precursor cell at discrete developmental stages. The graphs represent the composite radiation survival curves of B-lineage lymphoid precursor cells showing survival of the cells as a function of the radiation dose. The cells were irradiated and assayed for clonogenic growth, and the radiation survival curves were generated by linear regression analysis. See table for details. Bars represent SE. (Courtesy of Uckun FM, Mitchell JB, Obuz V, et al: *Int J Radiat Oncol Biol Phys* 21:1553–1560, 1991.)

ity showed a temporal correlation with the distinct stages of development. The most radiation-sensitive B-lineage LPC populations were the FL112 and FL114 fetal liver pro-B cells with germline immunoglobulin heavy chain genes but rearranged T-cell receptor γ genes, REH acute lymphoblastic leukemia pre-pre-B cells with rearranged IgH and T-cell receptor γ genes, and NALM-6 acute lymphoblastic leukemia pre-pre-B/ pre-B cells corresponding to the earliest 3 stages of human B-lymphocyte

Multiparameter Characterization of Human B-Lineage Lymphoid Precursor Cell Lines

Cell line	Maturational stage	Immunophenotype											Genotype		
		CD7	CD10	CD19	CD24	CD72	CD74	CD75	CD76	Cμ	IgM	IgD	Tγ	Tβ	Cμ
FL112	Pro-B	−	+	+	−	±	−	−	−	−	−	−	RR	GG	GG
FL114	Pro-B	−	+	+	−	±	−	−	−	−	−	−	RR	GG	GR
REH	Pre-Pre-B	−	+	+	+	+	−	−	−	−	−	−	RR	RG	RR
NALM-6	Pre-Pre-B/ Pre-B	−	+	+	+	+	−	±	−	±	−	−	GG	GG	RR
KM-3	Pre-B	−	±	+	+	+	±	+	+	+	−	−	DD	GG	RR
HPB-NULL	Pre-B	−	−	±	+	+	±	±	±	+	±	−	GG	GG	RG
NAMALWA	Early B	−	±	+	+	+	+	+	+	−	+	−	GG	GG	DG
RAJI	Early B	−	±	+	+	+	+	+	+	−	±	+	GG	GG	DG
Controls															
CEM	Pre-T	+	+	−	−	−	−	−	−	−	−	−	RR	RR	GG
MOLT-3	Pre-T	+	−	−	−	−	−	−	−	−	−	−	RR	RR	GG

		Proliferative activity				Biochemical features				
		$\%G_{0/1}$	%S	$\%G_2M$	Proliferation index %	Protein (mg/10^7 cells)	GHS level (μ/mg)	GST activity (nmol/min/mg)	$[pH]_i$	$[Ca^{2+}]i$ (Indo-1 Ratio)
FL112	Pro-B	49.1	28.9	22.0	50.9	1.4	2.1	126.3	7.24	1.39
FL114	Pro-B	65.0	29.7	13.3	43.0	0.5	8.5	N.D	N.D	1.97
REH	Pre-Pre-B	57.5	28.5	17.0	45.5	0.4	0.2	118.7	6.93	2.33
NALM-6	Pre-Pre-B/ Pre-B	51.8	33.0	15.2	48.2	0.3	5.3	58.7	6.91	1.91
KM-3	Pre-B	52.1	32.6	15.3	47.9	0.4	5.8	112.4	7.13	1.88
HPB-NULL	Pre-B	52.0	24.0	24.0	48.0	0.1	8.3	55.3	7.17	1.83
NAMALWA	Early B	48.8	36.2	15.0	51.2	0.5	1.6	94.8	7.05	1.98
RAJI	Early B	49.2	31.1	19.7	50.8	0.3	12.7	3.2	7.05	1.98
Controls										
CEM	Pre-T	65.5	31.0	3.5	34.5	0.1	5.3	180.4	7.10	N.D
MOLT-3	Pre-T	73.7	23.7	2.6	26.3	0.4	2.2	N.D	7.40	N.D

Abbreviations: ND, not determined; *RR*, both alleles rearranged; *GG*, both alleles in germline configuration; *RG*, are allele rearranged, are allele in germline configuration; *DG*, 1 allele deleted is allele in germline configuration; *DD*, both alleles deleted.

The multiparameter characterization of human B-lineage lymphoid precursor cell lines was performed. The biochemical parameters, except for the glutathione-S-transferase (GST) activity are shown as the mean values of multiple (3–4) measurements. The standard errors did not exceed 10% of the mean values. Glutathione-S-transferase activity data were obtained by a single measurement.

(Courtesy of Uckun FM, Mitchell JB, Obuz V, et al: *Int J Radiat Oncol Biol Phys* 21:1553–1560, 1991.)

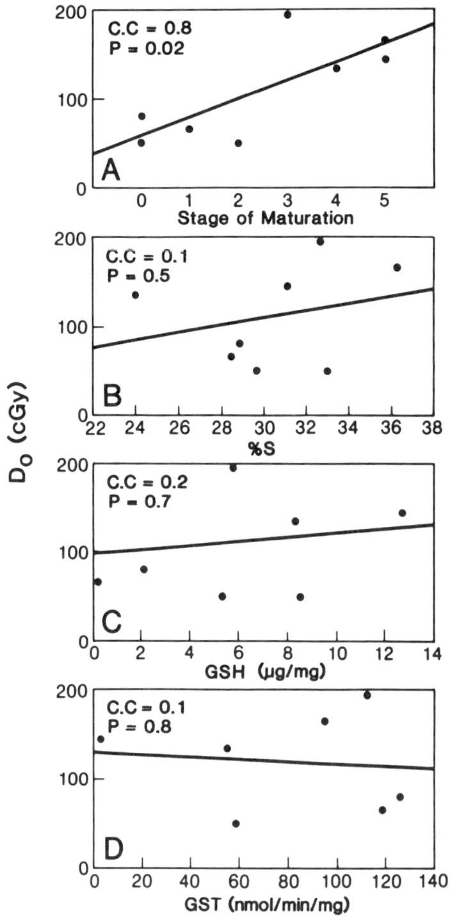

Fig 4–4.—Correlation of cellular radiation sensitivity with stage of maturation. The radiation sensitivity of (e.g., D_o value of the single-dose radiation survival curves) of the B-lineage lymphoid precursor cells was correlated on a continuous scale with stage of maturation, %S, intracellular glutathione content, and glutathione-S-transferase activity by single regression. *Abbreviation: CC,* coefficient of correlation. *P* = *P* value (i.e., statistical significance) of the correlation. (Courtesy of Uckun FM, Mitchell JB, Obuz V, et al: *Int J Radiat Oncol Biol Phys* 21:1553–1560, 1991.)

development. Much more radiation resistant were KM-3 acute lymphoblastic leukemia pre-B, HPB-NULL acute lymphoblastic leukemia pre-B, and sIgM$^+$ RAJI/NAMALWA early B-cell lines corresponding to the later stages of human B-lymphocyte development (table, Figs 4–3 and 4–4).

Conclusion.—The radiation sensitivity of B-lineage LPC decreases during maturation in the B-lineage lymphoid precursor pathway. However, the S-phase index, proliferation index, cellular protein content, intracellular glutathione level, glutathione-S-transferase activity, intracellular pH, and free cytoplasmic calcium concentration were not correlated with B-lineage LPC radiation sensitivity.

▶ The relative radiation sensitivity of B-lineage LPCs is a complicated subject. This paper demonstrates nicely that the radiation sensitivity of B-lineage LPCs varies during maturation. Thus, it is important to know the stage of differentiation of the cells before assuming anything about radiation sensitivity. It is also interesting to note that intracellular chemical composition and S-phase indices do not appear to correlate with radiation sensitivity.—E. Glatstein, M.D.

Immunologic Purging of Marrow Assessed by PCR Before Autologous Bone Marrow Transplantation for B-Cell Lymphoma

Gribben JG, Freedman AS, Neuberg D, Roy DC, Blake KW, Woo SD, Grossbard ML, Rabinowe SN, Coral F, Freeman GJ, Ritz J, Nadler LM (Dana-Farber Cancer Inst, Boston; Harvard Med School)

N Engl J Med 325:1525–1533, 1991 4–9

Background.—Autologous bone marrow transplantation has become a commonly used treatment for advanced cancers. There have been many attempts at purging the bone marrow of residual tumor cells to reduce the chance of relapse; however, the effectiveness of purging has not been proven. To ascertain the efficacy of immunologic purging, clonogenic assays were performed in a tumor cell line in culture.

Methods.—Bone marrow samples were taken from 114 patients with B-cell non-Hodgkin's lymphoma. All had responded to aggressive induction or salvage chemotherapy. Bone marrow was purged with the use of anti–B-cell monoclonal antibodies and rabbit complement before reinfusion. Polymerase chain reaction amplification was used to detect residual lymphoma cells before and after purging. All patients had a transloca-

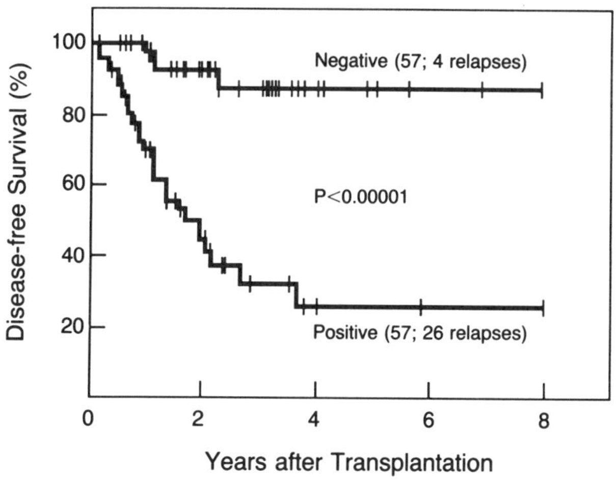

Fig 4–5.—Actuarial probability of disease-free survival after autologous bone marrow transplantation in 114 patients with B-cell non-Hodgkin's lymphoma. "Negative" denotes the patients in whom polymerase chain reaction did not detect residual lymphoma cells after purging, and "positive" denotes the patients in whom polymerase chain reaction did detect residual disease. (Courtesy of Gribben JG, Freedman AS, Neuberg D, et al: *N Engl J Med* 325:1525–1533, 1991.)

tion, t(14;18), that could be amplified by polymerase chain reaction at the time of their initial evaluation.

Results.—A 3- to 6-log destruction of cells in the tumor cell line resulted from immunologic purging in vitro. Polymerase chain reaction detected residual lymphoma cells before purging in all patients. After purging, the bone marrow was completely free of lymphoma cells in 57 patients. These patients had increased disease-free survival compared with those who had detectable residual lymphoma cells (Fig 4–5). Only 4 of these patients had a relapse. The degree of bone marrow involvement and previous response to therapy were unassociated with the ability to purge residual lymphoma cells.

Conclusions.—In patients with lymphoma, ex vivo purging of autologous bone marrow is a clinically useful technique. Reinfusion of bone marrow that contains malignant cells appears to contribute to relapse. The most important predictor of relapse appears to be an inability to purge residual lymphoma cells.

▶ This study reports truly remarkable results. Its first important lesson is that patients with follicular lymphoma who appear to be in complete remission after conventional-dose chemotherapy—in this case CHOP—always have abnormal cells bearing the detectable t(14;18) translocation in the marrow. The second important lesson is that it is possible to use a mixture of monoclonal antibodies and complement to purge those abnormal cells down to a level that, in this study, was not detectable by PCR amplification in half the patients. The third remarkable finding is that the ability to purge the marrow is associated with durable clinical remissions. The corollary of this finding is that the failure to render the marrow PCR negative is associated with a 46% relapse rate. Using actuarial methods, the projected disease-free survival of patients with residual tumor contamination of the marrow is only 25% at 4 years. The fourth surprise is that patients who relapse do so in previously involved nodal sites of disease, just as would be expected in patients relapsing after chemotherapy. This might not be expected if the source of the growing cells is the tumor contaminating the marrow graft. Marrow relapses or extranodal relapses including the lung might have been expected. Either the tumor cells can only grow in nodes that have been conditioned by their prior growth, or the homing capacity of the tumor cells is highly developed, or perhaps the inability to purge the marrow is a surrogate marker for resistance to therapy. Any of these possibilities would be interesting. This is the first study to suggest that marrow purging may play a therapeutic role, and it is 1 of the first studies to show prolonged disease-free survival from aggressive therapy in indolent lymphoma.—D.L. Longo, M.D., F.A.C.P.

The Significance of Circulating Cells Carrying t(14;18) in Long Remission From Follicular Lymphoma

Price CGA, Meerabux J, Murtagh S, Cotter FE, Rohatiner AZS, Young BD, Lister TA (St. Bartholomew's Hosp, London)

J Clin Oncol 9:1527–1532, 1991 4–10

Background.—The t(14;18)(q32;q21) translocation is found in more than 80% of follicular lymphomas. Polymerase chain reaction (PCR) may demonstrate small numbers of t(14;18)-bearing cells—even after the patient is in clinical remission. The presence of this translocation was studied in healthy patients who had achieved clinical remission many years before.

Methods.—The study sample comprised patients who had been in clinical remission from follicular lymphoma for at least 10 years. There were 10 men and 5 women, with age at presentation ranging from 31 to 73 years. One patient was in remission for 23 years. Eight were seen with stage III or IV disease, and 7 were seen with stage I or II disease. The peripheral blood mononuclear cell fractions from these patients were examined with PCR to find cells carrying the t(14;18) translocation. The assay was sensitive enough to find 1 positive cell in approximately 5×10^5 cells.

Results.—Polymerase chain reaction detected t(14;18)-positive cells in 6 patients, all of whom initially were seen with stage III or IV disease. No patient who was seen with stage I or II disease had a positive PCR. All 6 PCR-positive patients remained in clinical remission 1 year later. Amplification of the 14q+ junction regions from formalin-fixed biopsy specimens was successful in 2 cases. According to sequence analysis, the cells circulating when the patient was in remission belonged to the original clone in both cases.

Conclusions.—In patients who have achieved long-term clinical remission from advanced follicular lymphoma, t(14;18)-bearing cells may persist in the circulation for a decade or more. At least some cells that carry the t(14;18) translocation have very low malignant potential. The reliability of these cells in predicting relapse was questioned.

▶ Not everyone agrees that finding cells bearing the t(14;18) translocation is clinically meaningful. In this small series of patients, 6 of 8 patients who were in long-term remission and had originally had advanced-stage disease had detectable abnormal cells in their peripheral blood by PCR; however, the presence of these cells did not appear to be a harbinger of relapse. It is possible that the remaining abnormal cells are incapable of division. It also is possible that they are in some sort of dynamic equilibrium with the host, kept under control by immune mechanisms. The meaning of these persistent cells is contentious—as are many aspects of lymphoma treatment.—D.L. Longo, M.D., F.A.C.P.

The Role of Gene Rearrangements for Antigen Receptors in the Diagnosis of Lymphoma Obtained by Fine-Needle Aspiration: A Study of 63 Cases With Concomitant Immunophenotyping

Katz RL, Hirsch-Ginsberg C, Childs C, Dekmezian R, Fanning T, Ordóñez N, Cabanillas F, Sneige N (Univ of Texas MD Anderson Cancer Ctr, Houston)

Am J Clin Pathol 96:479–490, 1991 4–11

Background.—The use of immunophenotypic markers in addition to cytomorphologic procedures has improved the diagnostic accuracy of

Results of Immunophenotyping and Immunoglobulin and T-Cell Receptor Gene Rearrangements in 63 Patients With Lymphoproliferative Disorders

		Immunocytochemistry on Cell Suspension				***Rearranged***				
Cytologic Diagnosis	***No.***	*Monoclonal (K or λ)*	*T-Cell Phenotype*	***FNA Cell Suspension Polyclonal***	***Other***	*IgH*	*IgL Kappa or Lambda*	*TCRβ Only*	*IgH + TCRβ*	*Germline*
Reactive hyperplasia Cases 1–5	5	0	0	5	0	0	0	1	0	4
Atypical lymphoid proliferation Cases 6–11	6	1	1	4	0	4	3	2	0	0
Small lymphocytic lymphoma Cases 12–19	8	7	1	0	0	7	7	1	0	0
Small cleaved cell Cases 20–34	15	15	0	0	0	14	15	0	1	0
Mixed cell lymphoma Cases 35–41	7	5	2	0	0	5	4	2	0	0

Large cell lymphoma										
Cases 42–55	14	11	0	0	3*	13	13	0	0	1
Small noncleaved cell										
Cases 56–57	2	1	0	0	1†	2	0	0	0	0
Lymphoblastic lymphoma/leukemia										
Cases 58–61	4	0	3++	1	0	1	1	1	2	0
Hodgkin's disease										
Cases 62–63	2	0	0	0	0	0	0	0	0	2
Total	63	40	7	10	4	46	43	7	3	7

Abbreviations: FNA, fine-needle aspiration; *TCRβ,* T-cell receptor β chain gene.

*The only markers expressed were Bl(1), Ki-l(1) or markers were unsatisfactory; + = no markers expressed-"null cell"; ++ = includes 1 case with biphenotypic expression of myelomonocytic markers (My-9) and T-cell phenotype.

(Courtesy of Katz RL, Hirsch-Ginsberg C, Childs C, et al: *Am J Clin Pathol* 96:479–490, 1991.)

lymphoma in fine-needle aspirates of B-cell and T-cell non-Hodgkin's lymphoma. The efficacy of performing genotyping in addition to immunophenotyping as an adjunct to cytologic diagnosis was assessed.

Methods and Findings.—Sixty-three consecutive patients with fine-needle aspirates of lymphoproliferative lesions and concurrent immunophenotyping and genotyping of fine-needle aspirate cell suspensions were studied. A total of 62% of the specimens that appeared to contain non-Hodgkin's lymphoma and were proved to be of B-cell lineage by genotyping were phenotyped accurately and shown to be monotypic for immunoglobulin light chains by cell suspension immunocytochemistry. Genotyping facilitated lineage assignment and/or confirmed clonality in 27% of the specimens that were difficult to establish on the basis of morphologic data. This group included 6 cases of atypical lymphoid proliferations with polyclonal or inconclusive markers, 3 of peripheral T-cell lymphoma, 1 of extracutaneous mycosis fungoides, 4 of lymphoblastic lymphoma, 1 of null cell lymphoma, and 2 specimens with equivocal or technically unsatisfactory markers (table).

Conclusions.—Genotyping for lineage assignment and/or clonality should be done to include cases of atypical lymphoid proliferations, T-cell malignant neoplasms, lymphoid malignant neoplasms with equivocal markers, and differentiation of lymphoid neoplasms from nonlymphoid ones. Genotyping by antigen-receptor gene rearrangement seems redundant when mature B-cell phenotypes demonstrate monoclonality by immunophenotyping.

▶ We have been assessing patients with lymphoma based on morphologic diagnosis for decades; however, the "new biology" ushered in with molecular probes is in the process of changing all that. Clearly, we're in a transition period in terms of the diagnosis of lymphoma. Ultimately, sometime in this next century, a diagnosis will be based on molecular criteria such as these gene rearrangements.

This paper is provocative because of the way these studies have been derived. Fine-needle aspiration represents a simple technology for obtaining additional tissue for the processing and interpretation of these gene rearrangements. This type of procedure is bound to gain favor in the coming years, because it is based on a criterion that is far more specific than that associated with light microscopy. Although, there are still potential problems with the interpretation of some of these studies, this report is a simple indication of the power of such technology. It is almost certainly going to increase during the next few years.—E. Glatstein, M.D.

Similar Outcome of Treatment of B-Cell and T-Cell Diffuse Large-Cell Lymphomas: The Stanford Experience

Kwak LW, Wilson M, Weiss LM, Doggett R, Dorfman RF, Warnke RA, Horning SJ (Stanford Univ Med School, Stanford, Calif)

J Clin Oncol 9:1426–1431, 1991 4–12

Background.—Previous research has suggested that some patients with peripheral T-cell lymphoma have a relatively poor prognosis; however, the clinical significance of immunologic phenotype in diffuse large-cell-lymphoma (DLCL) is debatable. The results of a retrospective analysis of the prognostic significance of immunologic phenotype in 101 previously untreated patients with DLCL were reviewed. All were treated with 3 generations of modern combination-chemotherapy–based protocols.

Methods.—The patients were treated at 1 center between 1975 and 1986 with cyclophosphamide, doxorubicin (Adriamycin), vincristine, and prednisone (CHOP); with methotrexate, bleomycin, doxorubicin, cyclophosphamide, vincristine, and dexamethasone ([M]BACOD); or with methotrexate, doxorubicin, cyclophosphamide, vincristine, prednisone, and bleomycin (MACOP-B). Immunologic phenotype was determined in each patient.

Results.—Immunologic analysis identified 77 cases of B-cell origin, 21 cases of T-cell origin, and 3 cases that lacked B- or T-cell markers. The prognosis for those with B- and T-cell disease did not differ significantly. Those patients with B-cell markers had a complete remission rate of 84%, a 5-year actuarial freedom from disease progression of 38%, and a 5-year actuarial overall survival of 52%. The percentages among those with T-cell markers were 95%, 53%, and 79%, respectively. Five-year actuarial survival rates of patients with stage IV disease also did not differ between the B- and T-cell groups (36% and 56%, respectively).

Conclusion.—Not all patients with peripheral T-cell lymphomas have a poor prognosis. In fact, immunologic phenotype appears to have little prognostic significance for patients with DLCL who are treated with current aggressive chemotherapy regimens. Treatment selection should not be based on immunologic criteria alone.

▶ Another contentious area in lymphoma treatment is the role of cell-surface phenotype in predicting outcome. A number of groups have suggested that cell-surface phenotype affects the prognosis in patients with aggressive histology lymphoma. Most of these claims have been made on patient groups treated either heterogeneously or with combination chemotherapy programs that are not the most effective available. However, there are believable exceptions to this statement. For example, Coiffier and colleagues (1) have reported that patients whose tumors were of T-cell origin did more poorly on the LNH-84 regimen than did those with B-cell tumors. Armitage and colleagues (2) also reported that their 8 patients with stage IV disease and T-cell markers did more poorly after CAP-BOP therapy than those with stage IV disease and B-cell markers; however, there were no differences in outcome for T-cell vs. B-cell lymphomas of other stages. Although it would seem that there are some lymphoma regimens that may be more active against B-cell tumors than T-cell tumors, most of the second and third generation aggressive lymphoma regimens do not have clearly different results based on immunologic phenotype.

The group at the University of Arizona has suggested that tumors failing to express HLA-DR antigens are more aggressive (3). At the National Cancer Institute, we have not seen enough DR-negative cases of lymphoma to meaningfully detect differences in outcome if they existed. An Eastern Cooperative Oncology Group study failed to show significant differences in prognosis based on HLA-DR expression (4). In general, it would appear that the immunologic features of disease are not more important than the clinical prognostic factors. At present, there are not sufficient data to base treatment decisions on immunophenotype.—D.L. Longo, M.D., F.A.C.P.

References

1. Coiffier B, et al: *Ann Oncol* 1:45, 1990.
2. Armitage JO, et al: *J Clin Oncol* 7:1783, 1989.
3. Slymen DJ, et al: *J Clin Oncol* 8:986, 1990.
4. O'Keane JC, et al: *Cancer* 66:1147, 1990.

Value of Follow-Up Procedures in Patients With Large-Cell Lymphoma Who Achieve a Complete Remission

Weeks JC, Yeap BY, Canellos GP, Shipp MA (Dana-Farber Cancer Inst, Boston)
J Clin Oncol 9:1196–1203, 1991 4–13

Objective.—Although approximately two thirds of patients with large-cell lymphoma (LCL) achieve complete remission with initial combination chemotherapy, recurrent disease will develop in many of them. Salvage treatment appears to be most effective in those with minimal disease. Patterns of relapse were examined in 139 patients with LCL who achieved a complete remission on high- to moderate-dose combination (M/m-BACOD) chemotherapy.

Observations.—Thirty-six patients relapsed from complete remission and were compared with 46 others who remained in remission. Only 2 relapses were detected at a presymptomatic stage. Two thirds of the patients relapsed at new sites. Gallium scans detected 90% of the relapses, whereas physical examination detected 80%. The lactate dehydrogenase (LDH) test was 65% sensitive and frequently predicted impending symptomatic relapse. The specificity of LDH estimation was a function of time after completion of treatment.

Recommendations.—It might be best to use the LDH estimate—and perhaps the gallium scan—at frequent intervals to screen for recurrent lymphoma, reserving directed radiography for those with positive screening findings. Aggressive screening might be reserved for those patients who are eligible to receive potentially curative salvage treatment.

▶ This paper reports a finding that I believe to be true because the data are quite clear and convincing. I also know it to be true from my own experience. But, gosh, it's tough to change compulsive behavior that gets rare, intermittent positive reinforcement! I have enormous difficulty with the notion that I should stop doing chest x-rays as a means of following my patients with lymphoma. I have even more trouble with the concept of using a gallium scan as an effective follow-up tool. I see it, but I don't believe it. Nevertheless, this sort of study is bound to be used to formulate reimbursement policies as medical care becomes increasingly managed by cost-effectiveness principles.—D.L. Longo, M.D., F.A.C.P.

Effective Treatment of Small-Noncleaved-Cell Lymphoma With High-Intensity, Brief-Duration Chemotherapy

McMaster ML, Greer JP, Greco FA, Johnson DH, Wolff SN, Hainsworth JD (Vanderbilt Univ, Nashville)

J Clin Oncol 9:941–946, 1991 4–14

Introduction.—The small-noncleaved-cell (SNC) form of lymphoma is recognized as a high-grade, biologically aggressive neoplasm. It is 1 of the least common subtypes of non-Hodgkin's lymphoma. Its response to treatment is poor, and the neoplasm frequently relapses; the long-term survival is less than 20%.

Study Design.—Twenty patients with histologic evidence of SNC non-Hodgkin's lymphoma received intensive chemotherapy in an inpatient setting. Most of the patients had stage IV disease as well as other features associated with a poor prognosis. Two 4-week induction courses were given, the first of which included cyclophosphamide, etoposide, vincristine, bleomycin, and methotrexate. The second course included cyclophosphamide, etoposide, and doxorubicin. Meningeal disease was treated with intrathecal methotrexate.

Outcome.—Complete remission was achieved in 85% of the patients. Two of 3 patients with initial CNS disease and 3 of 6 with marrow involvement entered complete remission. Three fourths of the patients who responded remain in continuous remission a median of 29 months after diagnosis. Two who relapsed died of lymphoma, and 2 other patients died of treatment-related toxicity. Hematologic toxicity was severe.

Conclusions.—Brief, dose-intensive chemotherapy has allowed a majority of patients with SNC lymphoma to survive without disease. Patients must be followed closely for complications of severe myelosuppression.

▶ This is an impressive little study. Three patients with AIDS-related lymphomas were included in this series, and all 3 had a complete response to therapy. The morphologic distinction between diffuse SNC lymphoma of Burkitt's variety and diffuse SNC lymphoma of non-Burkitt's variety can be subtle. In general, there is more heterogeneity in nuclear size in the non-Burkitt's variety. However, the subtle morphologic differences belie more distinctive molecular differences. In 1 recent study of 29 cases of SNC lymphoma, 17 of the 18 Burkitt's variety lymphomas contained *c-myc* rearrangements; none of the 11 non-Burkitt's variety had *c-myc* rearrangements (1). On the other hand, 3 of the non-Burkitt's had *bcl*-2 rearrangements, suggesting a relationship to follicular-center-cell lymphomas. Indeed, in our clinical experience, we have generally treated the rare non-Burkitt's lymphomas similarly to diffuse large-cell lymphomas with similar results. It is possible that diffuse SNC lymphoma of the non-Burkitt's type is another category of lymphoma that the Working Formulation has categorized incorrectly, because it may respond well to regimens used in patients with intermediate grade lymphomas.—D.L. Longo, M.D., F.A.C.P.

Reference

1. Yano T, et al: *Blood* 79:1282, 1992.

Epstein-Barr Virus in AIDS-Related Primary Central Nervous System Lymphoma

MacMahon EME, Glass JD, Hayward SD, Mann RB, Becker PS, Charache P, McArthur JC, Ambinder RF (Johns Hopkins School of Medicine)

Lancet 338:969–973, 1991 4–15

Background.—Human immunodeficiency virus-associated lymphomas originating in the CNS are increasing in frequency, perhaps as a result of increased survival of HIV-infected individuals. Although Epstein-Barr virus (EBV) has been detected in these tumors, the extent of the association has not been determined because of the highly restricted expression of EBV in malignant tissue and the lack of a reliable technique for detection. A new technique for the detection of latent EBV uses short nonprotein coding EBV transcripts (EBERs), which are expressed in much higher quantity than other EBV-latency transcripts.

Methods.—Necropsy material from 18 cases of AIDS-related primary CNS lymphoma and 3 additional brain biopsy specimens were studied. The abundant expression and the characteristic subcellular distribution of EBV-EBER RNAs make them a useful target for EBV detection.

Findings.—The 100% association of AIDS-related primary CNS lymphoma with EBV is significant because EBV is rarely found in most cases of primary CNS lymphoma in nonimmunocompromised individuals, and also because it is absent from a large number of systemic lymphomas in patients with AIDS. This finding suggests that the pathogenesis of AIDS-related primary CNS lymphomas may be distinct from the systemic disease in which only 30% to 50% of the tumors are associated with EBV. The pathogenetic role of EBV is supported by the detection of the latent membrane protein that is implicated as an effector for EBV-associated lymphomagenesis.

Conclusion.—A technique using EBERs RNAs to detect latent EBV found a 100% association between AIDS-related primary CNS lymphoma and EBV. Epstein-Barr virus has a potential role as a tumor marker that may aid in the diagnosis of primary CNS lymphoma in patients with AIDS.

▶ This paper would suggest that the primary CNS lymphoma that occurs in patients with AIDS is similar in its pathogenesis to the primary CNS lymphoma that occurs in the setting of other immunodeficiency states. One might extrapolate from these results that therapy directed at restoring immune function might prevent CNS lymphoma. It is somewhat surprising that, with a fair measure of success deriving from efforts to develop effective antiviral therapies and effective treatments or preventive measures for opportunistic infections, there has been relatively modest or even no success at restoring the immune dysfunction in patients with AIDS. If EBV is the etiologic agent of the CNS lymphomas, then what accounts for the pathogenesis of the peripheral lymphomas in patients with AIDS?—D.L. Longo, M.D., F.A.C.P.

Projections of the Incidence of Non-Hodgkin's Lymphoma Related to Acquired Immunodeficiency Syndrome

Gail MH, Pluda JM, Rabkin CS, Biggar RJ, Goedert JJ, Horm JW, Sondik EJ, Yarchoan R, Broder S (Natl Cancer Inst, Bethesda, Md)

J Natl Cancer Inst 83:695–701, 1991 4–16

Objective.—An increased risk of aggressive non-Hodgkin's lymphoma (NHL) has been described in association with AIDS. This may be of increasing import as advances in antiretroviral treatment and the prevention of opportunistic infection prolong the survival of AIDS patients. This association was examined by reviewing data from the Surveillance, Epidemiology, and End Results (SEER) program of the National Cancer Institute.

Findings.—The number of excess cases of NHL increased substantially in men aged 20–49 years in the period 1983–1987. There was no clear excess of cases of NHL either in women of this age or in men or women older than 49 years of age. Survival after the diagnosis of AIDS increased over time. The projections of current data suggested that, in 1992, from 8% to 27% of all cases of NHL in the United States will be associated with HIV infection.

Discussion.—A considerable increase in AIDS-related NHL is anticipated in the coming years. Therefore, experimental protocols for new AIDS treatments must include long-term follow-up for NHL. The risk of NHL also is increased in several inherited immunodeficiency syndromes and in drug-induced immunodeficiency states.

▶ The risk of NHL has been estimated to be nearly 10% per year for patients with full-blown AIDS in a small cohort of patients on experimental antiviral therapies (1) and approximately 3% of patients who are HIV positive and have full-blown AIDS develop often have lymphoma as their presenting diagnostic finding for AIDS. However, data from a large multisite 2-year prospective observational study of 1,030 patients with AIDS who were being treated with zidovudine suggest that the risk may be lower. Lymphoma developed in 24 (2.3%) of the patients who received zidovudine during 1,463 person-years of follow-up, for a rate of 1.6 cases per 100 person-years of therapy. The lymphoma that develops is usually a highly aggressive one (e.g., small-noncleaved-cell lymphoma of Burkitt's or non-Burkitt's variety). Approximately half of the patients are seen with primary CNS lymphoma. The non-CNS lymphomas generally have gene rearrangements that involve activation of the c-myc gene most often t(8;14)—

and they usually do not show evidence of Epstein-Barr virus involvement in the lymphomagenesis. However, it is a different story for the primary CNS lymphomas.—D.L. Longo, M.D., F.A.C.P.

References

1. Pluda JM, et al: *Ann Intern Med* 113:276, 1990.
2. Moore RD, et al: *JAMA* 265:2208, 1991.

Acute Leukemia

Results of a Randomized Trial Comparing Idarubicin and Cytosine Arabinoside With Daunorubicin and Cytosine Arabinoside in Adult Patients With Newly Diagnosed Acute Myelogenous Leukemia

Berman E, Heller G, Santorsa J, McKenzie S, Gee T, Kempin S, Gulati S, Andreeff M, Kolitz J, Gabrilove J, Reich L, Mayer K, Keefe D, Trainor K, Schluger A, Penenberg D, Raymond V, O'Reilly R, Jhanwar S, Young C, Clarkson B (Mem Sloan Kettering Cancer Ctr, New York)

Blood 77:1666–1674, 1991 4–17

Background.—Idarubicin (IDR), or 4'-demethoxydaunorubicin, is a new anthracycline that is more lipophilic than the parent compound and has a long-lived metabolite. A prospective trial was carried out in 130 adult patients with newly diagnosed acute myelogenous leukemia.

Study Design.—The patients were randomized to receive either IDR combined with cytosine arabinoside (Ara-C), or standard treatment with

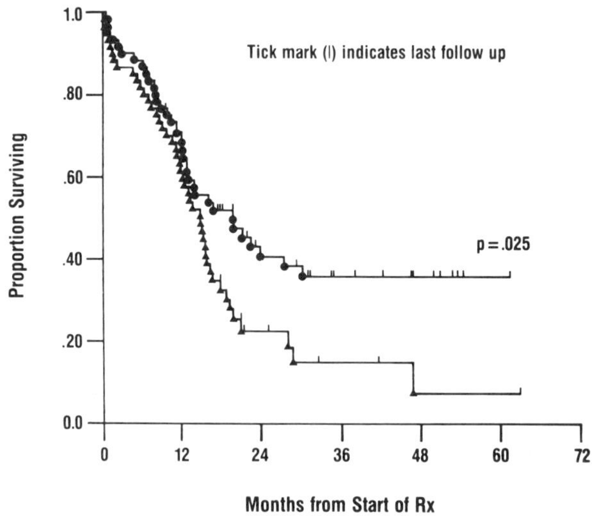

Fig 4–6.—The L-19/L-22 protocols: survival by treatment arm. *Closed circles* indicate IDR/Ara-C treatment (60 patients/25 censored); *closed triangles* indicate DNR/Ara-C treatment (60 patients/15 censored). (Courtesy of Berman E, Heller G, Santorsa J, et al: *Blood* 77:1666–1674, 1991.)

daunorubicin (DNR) and Ara-C. The dose of IDR was 12 mg/m^2/day, given for 3 days, and DNR, 50 mg/m^2/day, was given for 3 days.

Results.—When 60 patients had been assigned to each arm of the study, those given IDR and Ara-C exhibited a better response than those given standard treatment. The respective rates of complete remission were 80% and 58%. The IDR/Ara-C regimen was especially useful to patients with a high initial white cell count. The overall survival was 19.5 months, compared with 13.5 months for patients given standard treatment after a median follow-up of 2½ years (Fig 4–6). Nonhematologic toxicity was comparable in the 2 treatment groups.

Conclusions.—Treatment with IDR/Ara-C can replace DNR/Ara-C therapy for adults with newly diagnosed acute myelogenous leukemia. Both IDR and DNR appear to have equivalent cardiotoxic effects.

Cytarabine Plus Idarubicin or Daunorubicin as Induction and Consolidation Therapy for Previously Untreated Adult Patients With Acute Myeloid Leukemia

Wiernik PH, Banks PLC, Case DC Jr, Arlin ZA, Periman PO, Todd MB, Ritch PS, Enck RE, Weitberg AB (Albert Einstein Cancer Ctr, New York; Adria Labs, Columbus, Ohio; Maine Med Ctr, Portland; New York Med College, Valhalla; Harrington Cancer Ctr, Amarillo, Tex; Yale Univ, New Haven, Conn; Med College of Wisconsin, Milwaukee; Riverside Cancer Inst, Columbus, Ohio; Roger Williams Hosp, Providence, RI)

Blood 79:313–319, 1992 4–18

Background.—The synthetic daunorubicin idarubicin has been shown to be significantly more effective than daunorubicin or doxorubicin against certain leukemias in mice. Idarubicin was compared with daunorubicin in the treatment of acute myeloid leukemia (AML).

Methods.—The study included 214 adults from 32 centers during a 3-year period. For induction therapy, all patients received cytarabine, 100 mg/m^2, as a 7-day continuous infusion. They also received either daunorubicin, 45 mg/m^2/day (A+D), or idarubicin, 13 mg/m^2/day (A+I), on the first 3 treatment days. After they achieved complete remission (CR), patients received 2 courses of the induction regimen, with anthracycline given for 2 days and cytarabine for 5.

Results.—There were 97 evaluable patients in the A+I group and 111 in the A+D group. The complete remission rates were 70% for A+I and 59% for A+D (P = .08). For patients aged 18–50 years, the difference in CR was significant—88% for A+I vs. 70% for A+D. Resistance to induction therapy was significantly more frequent with A+D than with A+I. Achievement of CR was unfavorably affected by hyperleukocytosis in the A+D but not the A+I group. The A+I group had a significantly greater duration of CR and better survival—median survival, 12.9 months vs. 8.7 months for A+D. The A+I group had more prolonged myelosuppression during consolidation therapy and more frequent mild chemical hepatitis.

Conclusions.—In adults with AML, A+I therapy appears to be superior to A+D induction therapy. The 2 regimens have similar toxicity. A direct, prospective comparison of A+D, A+I, and A+mitoxantrone.

► In contrast to randomized studies of 2 different doses of cytarabine, which did not show significant differences in CR rate or remission duration (1), idarubicin is more active in combination with cytarabine than daunorubicin. Idarubicin plus cytarabine (A+I) should now be considered the treatment of choice for patients seen with AML. The effects of idarubicin are particularly notable in patients with initially high levels of white blood cells, a group that generally has a poorer prognosis after therapy. Although cell surface phenotype was not examined in these studies, it may influence treatment outcome. Myeloid leukemias that express lymphoid markers (e.g., CD2 or CD19) appear to have a more favorable prognosis (2), and those that express the hematopoietic stem-cell marker CD34 have a poorer prognosis (3). Expression of multidrug resistance gene-1 has an adverse impact on treatment outcome.—D.L. Longo, M.D., F.A.C.P.

References

1. Dillman RO, et al: *Blood* 78:2520, 1991.
2. Ball ED, et al: *Blood* 77:2242, 1991.
3. Geller RB, et al: *Br J Haematol* 76:340, 1990.

MDR1 Gene Expression and Treatment Outcome in Acute Myeloid Leukemia

Pirker R, Wallner J, Geissler K, Linkesch W, Haas OA, Bettelheim P, Hopfner M, Scherrer R, Valent P, Havelec L, Ludwig H, Lechner K (Univ of Vienna; St Anna Kinderspital, Vienna)
J Natl Cancer Inst 83:708–712, 1991 4–19

Background.—Multidrug resistance—an important type of resistance in cell lines—results from expression of the multidrug resistance-1 (MDR1) gene and its 170-kd protein product, P-glycoprotein. The protein acts as an energy-dependent drug efflux pump for anthracyclines, vinca alkaloids, and other hydrophobic compounds.

Study Design.—The role of MDR1 gene expression in the outcome of treatment was examined prospectively in 68 consecutive patients with de novo acute myeloid leukemia (AML). The levels of MDR1 RNA were determined in blast cells at the time of diagnosis and were correlated with the outcome in 63 patients. Remission was induced with an anthracycline combined with cytarabine. Daunorubicin was used in most patients.

Observations.—The MDR1 RNA was identified in 71% of the patients. Complete remission was achieved by 53% of these patients and by 89% of those who were negative for MDR1 RNA. The MDR1 gene was expressed by most of the patients who had resistant disease or died early. Both the overall survival and the disease-free survival were lower in patients who expressed MDR1 than in MDR1 RNA-negative patients.

Conclusions.—Expression of the MDR1 gene in patients with de novo AML has a negative prognostic influence. Multidrug resistance appears to be a significant factor in AML.

▶ The adverse impact of MDR1 expression on treatment outcome in acute leukemia has also been documented by other groups (1,2). In one study of cell lines, the correlation was less clear (3); however, expression of MDR1 appears to be increased in patients who relapse. It will be important to look for the possible effects of MDR1 on idarubicin response, because its more lipophilic properties may make MDR1 less effective at pumping it out of cells.

Investigators at Stanford are planning to use the expression of MDR1 purge bone marrow of drug resistant leukemic cells (4). Three rounds of treatment with antibody to MDR1 plus complement together with etoposide treatment in vitro appears capable of removing 4+ logs of tumor cells without inhibiting marrow-committed precursors. Whether this amount of activity will allow autologous transplantation in acute leukemia is not yet clear.—D.L. Longo, M.D., F.A.C.P.

References

1. Marie J-P, et al: *Blood* 78:586, 1991.
2. Musto P, et al: *Br J Haematol* 77:50, 1991.
3. Kato S, et al: *Eur J Haematol* 47:146, 1991.
4. Aihara M, et al: *Blood* 77:2079, 1991.

Recombinant Human Granulocyte-Macrophage Colony-Stimulating Factor in Combination With Standard Induction Chemotherapy in De Novo Acute Myeloid Leukemia

Bettelheim P, Valent P, Andreeff M, Tafuri A, Haimi J, Gorischek C, Muhm M, Sillaber C, Haas O, Vieder L, Maurer D, Schulz G, Speiser W, Geissler K, Kier P, Hinterberger W, Lechner K (Univ of Vienna; St Anna Children's Hosp, Vienna; Sloan Kettering Cancer Ctr, New York; Behring Corp, Marburg, Germany)

Blood 77:700–711, 1991 4–20

Introduction.—Several studies have shown that recombinant human granulocyte-macrophage colony-stimulating factor (rhGM-CSF) is capable of stimulating quiescent acute myeloid leukemia (AML) blast cells in vitro to become more sensitive to cell-cycle-specific drugs and promote drug-induced cell kill. A phase I-II study of rhGM-CSF was conducted in 18 patients with newly diagnosed AML.

Patients.—The 10 men and 8 women (age range, 25–77 years) were treated with continuous intravenous infusion of rhGM-CSF in combination with standard induction chemotherapy. The infusion of rhGM-CSF was started 48 or 24 hours before chemotherapy in 14 patients and after chemotherapy-induced cell reduction in 4 patients with initially high white blood cell counts. It was administered until recovery from chemotherapy-induced myelosuppression.

Results.—Fifteen patients (83.3%) had complete remission, 12 after 1 cycle and 3 after a second cycle. The duration of neutropenia was shorter in these patients than in historical controls. One patient had no remission after 2 cycles of rhGM-CSF therapy. Two patients died of invasive pulmonary aspergillosis during bone marrow aplasia. Side effects were mild and tolerable.

Conclusion.—When combined with standard induction chemotherapy in the treatment of AML, rhGM-CSF is a potentially useful agent.

▶ These results do not prove the hypothesis that rhGM-CSF sensitizes leukemic cells to subsequently administered antimetabolites, but they do suggest that the question may be worth addressing in a prospective randomized trial. A major concern is whether the dose and schedule of administration of rhGM-CSF in this study are optimal. Unfortunately, no effort was made to measure the fraction of leukemic cells entering the cell cycle during rhGM-CSF therapy. Such a study would seem prudent before committing resources to a randomized study.—D.L. Longo, M.D., F.A.C.P.

Recombinant Human Granulocyte-Macrophage Colony-Stimulating Factor After Chemotherapy in Patients With Acute Myeloid Leukemia at Higher Age or After Relapse

Büchner T, Hiddemann W, Koenigsmann M, Zühlsdorf M, Wörmann B, Boeckmann A, Freire EA, Innig G, Maschmeyer G, Ludwig W-D, Sauerland M-C, Heinecke A, Schulz G (Univ of Münster; Free Univ Hosp Steglitz West Berlin, Germany)

Blood 78:1190–1197, 1991 4–21

Background.—Chemotherapy for patients with leukemia might be improved by reducing the phase of critical neutropenia. Granulocyte-macrophage colony-stimulating factor (GM-CSF) has effectively stimulated granulopoiesis in other conditions but has not been applied in acute myeloid leukemia (AML). A trial of recombinant human GM-CSF was carried out in patients with primary or late relapsed AML.

Methods.—The subjects included 36 patients (median age, 68 years) with newly diagnosed or relapsed AML. Twenty-five patients had newly diagnosed AML and were 65 years of age or older. Those patients with newly diagnosed disease received 9 days of treatment with 6-thioguanine, ara-C, and daunorubicin (TAD9). The patients with relapse received sequential high-dose ara-C and mitoxantrone (S-HAM). When the bone marrow became free from blasts, GM-CSF was given in a continuous infusion of 250 $\mu g/m^2$/day, beginning 4 days after chemotherapy. The results were compared with those of 56 historical controls.

Results.—Thirty patients received GM-CSF, and the other 6 had persistent bone marrow blasts. Complete remission was achieved in 50% of the patients compared with 32% of the controls, and early death occurred in 14% of the patients compared with 39% of the controls. There were no major adverse effects of GM-CSF. There were 2 cases of marked leukemic regrowth; 1 was completely reversible and the other appeared to be independent of GM-CSF. Treatment with GM-CSF did not seem to decrease the duration of remission. In patients who received GM-CSF, blood neutrophils recovered 6 days earlier in the TAD9 group and 9 days earlier in the S-HAM group, with rapid clearance of infection in most patients.

Conclusions.—It appears that GM-CSF can be administered after chemotherapy to patients with AML to accelerate the recovery of neutrophils and thus improve therapeutic outcome. The incidence of significant adverse effects is less than expected. The authors encourage larger controlled trials.

▶ The use of GM-CSF after therapy for acute leukemia has at least 1 theoretical drawback that became real during the course of this study. The rapid regrowth of tumor in 2 patients makes one concerned about using a potential tumor growth factor without the protection of contemporaneous chemotherapy. Nevertheless, there is a suggestion that this older group of patients had less treatment-related morbidity and mortality than the historical control group. It will be of interest to see whether the use of GM-CSF will improve survival of older patients.—D.L. Longo, M.D., F.A.C.P.

A Phase II Clinical Trial of Carboplatin Infusion in High-Risk Acute Nonlymphoblastic Leukemia

Martínez JA, Martín G, Sanz GF, Sempere A, Jarque I, de la Rubia J, Sanz MA (Hosp La Fe, Valencia, Spain)

J Clin Oncol 9:39–43, 1991 4–22

Objective.—Carboplatin (CBDCA) is a second-generation platinum drug that is effective when used as a continuous infusion in the treatment of refractory adult leukemia. The effects of a continuous infusion of CBDCA, 300 mg/m^2, given daily for 5 days, was assessed in 9 patients who had secondary acute nonlymphocytic leukemia (ANLL).

Patients.—Seven patients initially had myelodysplastic syndrome, and 2 had treatment-related ANLL. Three patients in first relapse of ANLL, 6 with refractory ANLL, and 9 in the blastic phase of chronic myelogenous leukemia also were treated.

Outcome.—Eight patients had a complete remission, and 4 had a partial remission, for an overall response rate of 44%. Treatment was generally well tolerated. Posttreatment neutropenia lasted a median of 36 days. Severe infection was rare. One patient had reversible renal toxicity, and another had reversible ototoxicity. Three patients had fatal bleeding.

Conclusions.—The use of CBDCA appears to be effective in patients with secondary ANLL, and it causes little serious extrahematologic toxicity. Severe infection and gram-negative bacteremia occur infrequently.

▶ The activity of infusional carboplatin in the salvage setting is impressive; however, the toxicity was sufficiently severe to make it difficult to ascertain how one might integrate other active agents such as etoposide, which could have synergistic antitumor effects but would be expected to increase the toxicity. Mitoxantrone-based combinations were also reported this year. Archimbaud and colleagues (1) used mitoxantrone, continuous infusion etoposide, and cytarabine in 72 patients younger than 60 years of age with relapsed acute myelogenous leukemia. The complete response rate was 61%. Amadori and colleagues (2) used mitoxantrone, etoposide, and cytarabine in 32 patients with refractory acute myelogenous leukemia. The complete response rate to this regimen was 66%. This level of activity in the salvage setting warrants comparison of these regimens to idarubicin plus cytarabine in untreated patients.—D.L. Longo, M.D., F.A.C.P.

References

1. Archimbaud E, et al: *Blood* 77:1894, 1991.
2. Amadori S, et al: *J Clin Oncol* 9:1210, 1991.

Safety of Stringent Prophylactic Platelet Transfusion Policy for Patients With Acute Leukaemia

Gmür J, Burger J, Schanz U, Fehr J, Schaffner A (Univ Hosp of Zürich, Zürich, Switzerland)

Lancet 338:1223–1226, 1991 4–23

Introduction.—In acute leukemia, the risk of hemorrhagic complications appears to become unacceptably high when the platelet counts decrease below 20×10^9/L. However, there is insufficient evidence to establish this as the threshold for prophylactic platelet transfusions. The

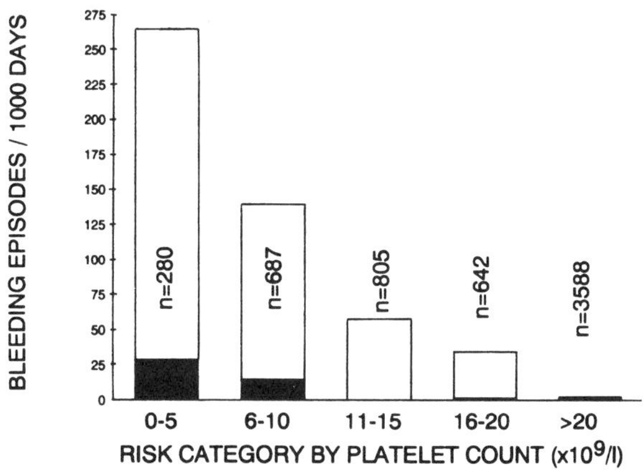

Fig 4–7.—Relation of bleeding risk to blood platelet counts: computed per 1,000 days at risk. *Open bars* = minor bleeding complications. *Filled bars* = major bleeding complications. The *numbers in the bars* are the numbers of observed days at risk in a given class. The correlation coefficient between class 1–4 and the incidence of bleeding is r = .963, $P < .01$. Risk category platelets $>20 \times 10^9$/L were not included in the correlation coefficient because the few bleeding complications in this group were related to factors other than solely the platelet count, and because of the broad range of counts in this category. (Courtesy of Gmür J, Burger J, Schanz U, et al: *Lancet* 338:1223–1226, 1991.)

practicability of a more restrictive transfusion policy was assessed in patients undergoing treatment for acute leukemia.

Methods.—A total of 102 patients took part in a prospective study of platelet transfusions in newly diagnosed acute leukemia. Evidence of hemorrhage was assessed every day as long as the platelet count was below 50×10^9/L. The protocol also considered such factors as bleeding, fever, coagulation disorders, and the intention to perform therapeutic procedures.

Findings.—There were 28 major nonlethal and 3 lethal bleeding episodes in 23 patients. Eighteen of these episodes occurred at platelet counts of 10×10^9/L or more. Bleeding episodes occurred on 1.9% of the days when platelet counts were at or below this level and .07% of the days when the platelet counts were $10-20 \times 10^9$/L (Fig 4–7).

Conclusions.—In patients with acute leukemia, the threshold for prophylactic transfusion can be safely set at 5×10^9/L in patients with no fever or manifestations of bleeding and at 10×10^9/L in patients with such signs. The threshold should be increased to at least 20×10^9/L for patients with coagulation disorders or anatomical lesions or those receiving heparin. A restrictive policy of this type applies to all types of hypoproliferative thrombocytopenia, reduces exposure to blood donors, and saves considerable resources.

▶ Our standard practices regarding the use of prophylactic platelet transfusions had their origin in the pioneering studies of Freireich and his colleagues on the National Cancer Institute Adult Leukemia Service in the 1950s and 1960s (1). In the original series, bleeding was noted on 38% of the hospital days during which the platelet count was between 10×10^9/L and 20×10^9/L. It was noted on an even higher percentage of days when the platelet count decreased below 10×10^9/L. Why were the bleeding episodes so much more rare in this study? It is possible that empiric antibiotics allow the patient to spend considerably less time febrile, and without increased temperature, platelet consumption should be lower. It also is possible that the supportive care measures in the 1960s used more agents that inhibit platelet function, including aspirin, other pain relievers, and antipyretics.

Whatever the contributions, it seems quite clear that setting the platelet transfusion threshold higher (holding platelets until the counts decreased to 5×10^9/L in patients without fever or bleeding and at 10×10^9/L in those patients with fever or bleeding) did not greatly (or at all) increase the incidence of fatal hemorrhage. It also resulted in sparing the patient the problem of allosensitization, reduced expense, and optimized the chances that the patient would respond to platelet transfusions when they were needed. Here is another old habit that may be hard for some of us old docs to break—or at least break comfortably. Nevertheless, the benefits may be worth a few more anxious moments for the physician. I wonder what the lawyers will do with this.—D.L. Longo, M.D., F.A.C.P.

Reference

1. Gaydos LA, et al: *N Engl J Med* 266:905, 1962.

Chemotherapy Compared With Bone Marrow Transplantation for Adults With Acute Lymphoblastic Leukemia in First Remission

Horowitz MM, Messerer D, Hoelzer D, Gale RP, Neiss A, Atkinson K, Barrett AJ, Büchner T, Freund M, Heil G, Hiddemann W, Kolb H-J, Löffler H, Marmont AM, Maschmeyer G, Rimm AA, Rozman C, Sobocinski KA, Speck B, Thiel E, Weisdorf DJ, Zwaan FE, Bortin MM (Med College of Wisconsin, Milwaukee; Biometric Ctr for Therapeutic Studies, Munich, Germany; Johann Wolfgang Goethe Univ, Frankfurt, Germany; Univ of California, Los Angeles; Universitat Innsbruck, Innsbruck, Austria, et al)
Ann Intern Med 115:13–18, 1991 4–24

Introduction.—Chemotherapy and allogeneic or autologous bone marrow transplants are primary treatments for patients with acute lymphoblastic leukemia (ALL). The results of these 2 approaches have not been adequately reported in the literature. Therefore, patients in remission received intensive chemotherapy or allogeneic bone marrow transplantation to prevent relapse, and the results were studied retrospectively.

Methods.—One patient group including 484 patients received intensive postremission chemotherapy for ALL, whereas the other group of 251 patients received HLA-identical sibling bone marrow transplants for ALL in first remission. The treatment took place between 1980 and 1987, with chemotherapy being done in 44 hospitals in Germany and transplants being performed in 98 hospitals worldwide. The results were reported to the International Bone Marrow Transplant Registry.

Results.—The 5-year survival for both the transplant and chemotherapy groups was similar (Fig 4–8). The leukemia-free survival probability at 5 years was 38% for patients receiving chemotherapy and 44% for those receiving transplants. For both treatments, similar prognostic factors predicted treatment failures. There was no benefit of 1 treatment group over the other for any prognostic factor.

Discussion.—There were no significant 5-year survival differences in patients with ALL in first remission receiving either chemotherapy or bone marrow transplant. The relapse rates were lower in the transplant group, but the 5-year survival for both groups was still similar.

▶ These data do not provide convincing evidence that the relapse rate in adult patients with ALL is favorably affected by allogeneic bone marrow transplantation. On the other hand, single-center studies usually report better results. For example, a report from Stanford demonstrated that patients undergoing marrow transplantation have a disease-free survival of 61% (1). Chemotherapy alone appears to result in the long-term survival of 30% to 40% of the patients (2,3). A 6-drug regimen called HEAVD is capable of achieving an 80% complete response rate, but its overall survival is 35% (2). The addition of postinduction intensification also does not improve results (3). The persistent dilemma is that those patients who are selected for transplantation fare 20% to 30% better than the patients treated with chemotherapy alone, but it is not clear whether this improvement reflects a selection bias.—D.L. Longo, M.D., F.A.C.P.

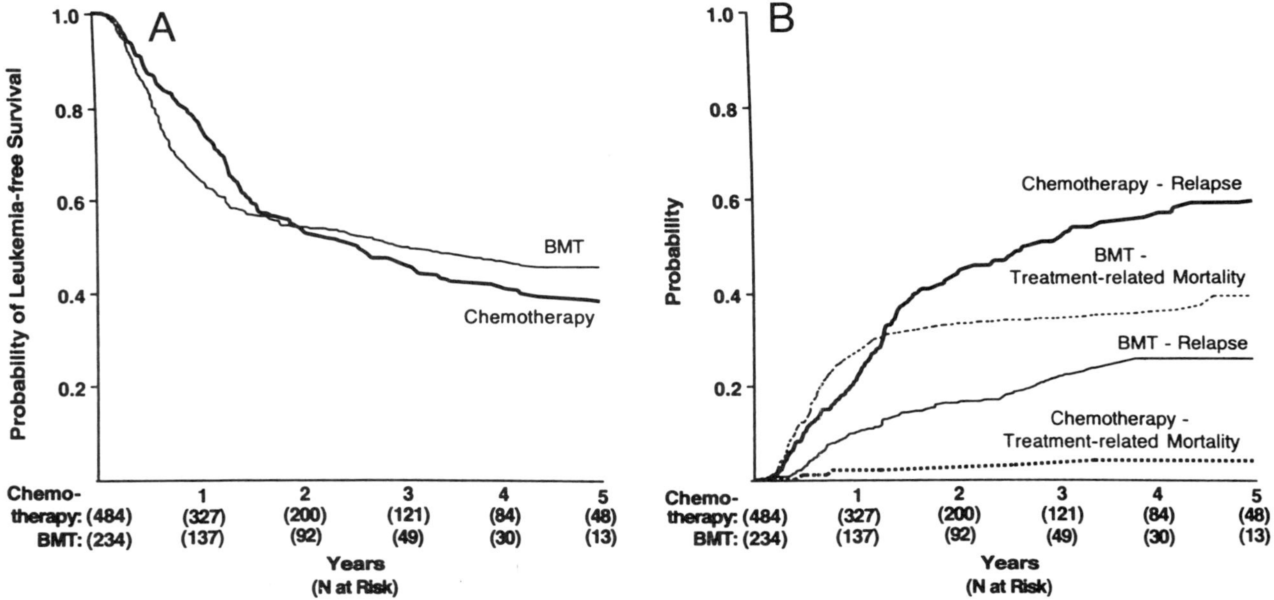

Fig 4–8.—Adjusted probabilities for adults with ALL in first remission according to type of post-remission therapy. **A,** leukemia-free survival; **B,** relapse and treatment-related mortality. The *numbers in parentheses* indicate the number *(N)* of patients remaining at risk (alive in remission). *Abbreviation: BMT,* bone marrow transplant. (Courtesy of Horowitz MM, Messerer D, Hoelzer D, et al: *Ann Intern Med* 115:13–18, 1991.)

References

1. Chao NJ, et al: *Blood* 78:1923, 1991.
2. Bassan R, et al: *Eur J Cancer* 27:441, 1991.
3. Ellison RR, et al: *J Clin Oncol* 9:2002, 1991.

Chronic Leukemia

Prognostic Significance of Philadelphia Chromosome-Positive Cells Detected by the Polymerase Chain Reaction After Allogeneic Bone Marrow Transplant for Chronic Myelogenous Leukemia

Roth MS, Antin JH, Ash R, Terry VH, Gotlieb M, Silver SM, Ginsburg D (Univ of Michigan, Ann Arbor; Howard Hughes Med Inst, Ann Arbor; Brigham and Women's Hosp, Boston; Med College of Wisconsin, Milwaukee)
Blood 79:276–282, 1992 4–25

Background.—Rare cells expressing the *bcr/abl* fusion transcript can be detected by the polymerase chain reaction (PCR) in blood or marrow after allogeneic bone marrow transplant (BMT) for Philadelphia chromosome-positive chronic myelogenous leukemia. However, their prognostic significance remains unclear.

Methods.—Clinical, cytogenetic, and molecular data from 64 patients with chronic myelogenous leukemia after allogeneic BMT were analyzed. Nested primer PCR was done on the blood and bone marrow samples from patients considered to be in clinical remission.

Findings.—The *bcr/abl* transcripts were found in 37 patients for at least 1 timepoint after BMT. Thirteen of these patients subsequently relapsed. None of the 27 patients without the transcripts relapsed. The interval from first *bcr/abl* PCR signal to relapse ranged from 90 to 832 days, with a median of 150 days. Of the 54 patients studied at 2 or more timepoints after BMT, 5 of 8 who were persistently positive for *bcr/abl* had a relapse; 5 of 23 with both positive and negative assays during fol-

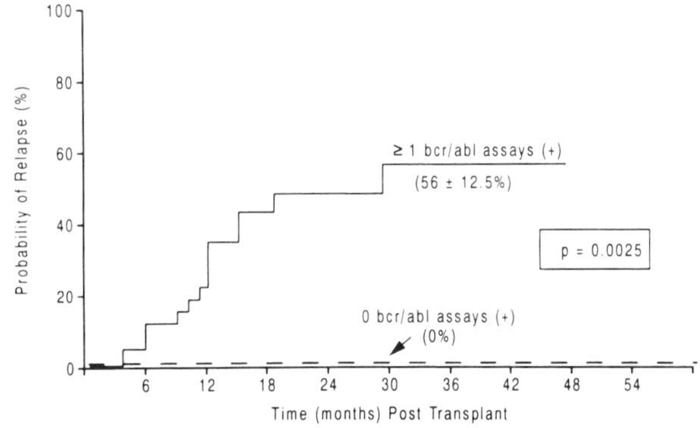

Fig 4–9.—A Kaplan-Meier plot of the actuarial probability of relapse for all 64 patients, comparing those with no (+) assays to those with 1 or more (+) assays. The difference in the probability of relapse is statistically significant (P = .0025). (Courtesy of Roth MS, Antin JH, Ash R, et al: *Blood* 79:276–282, 1992.)

low-up relapsed; and none of the 23 persistently negative patients had a relapse. The cumulative actuarial relapse rates for these 3 subgroups were 77%, 20, and 0%, respectively (Fig 4–9).

Conclusions.—Nested primer *bcr/abl* PCR can define subgroups of patients with chronic myelogenous leukemia in apparent clinical remission after BMT that have low, intermediate, and high risks of relapse. The pattern of *bcr/abl* PCR detection in such patients may help physicians create trials designed to reduce the risk of relapse and may also enable early intervention for those who do not clear the malignant clone.

Clinical Significance of *bcr-abl* Gene Rearrangement Detected by Polymerase Chain Reaction After Allogeneic Bone Marrow Transplantation in Chronic Myelogenous Leukemia

Delage R, Soiffer RJ, Dear K, Ritz J (Dana-Farber Cancer Inst, Boston; Harvard Med School, Boston)

Blood 78:2759–2767, 1991 4–26

Background.—Amplification of a segment of *bcr-abl* messenger RNA by polymerase chain reaction (PCR) can be used to demonstrate minimal residual disease after bone marrow transplantation (BMT) in patients with chronic myelogenous leukemia. This method can detect few cells, but most patients with a positive PCR remain free of disease for a long time. Patients with CML who underwent allogeneic BMT were studied to determine the clinical significance of PCR-detectable *bcr-abl* messenger RNA.

Patients.—The study sample comprised 14 men and 10 women (median age, 34 years). All had allogeneic BMT using CD6 T-cell–depleted marrow. A total of 100 serial blood or marrow samples was analyzed by PCR for *bcr-abl*–positive cells. A titration assay of the PCR-amplified product was performed to estimate the number of residual tumor cells in 8 selected patients.

Findings.—Polymerase chain reaction was positive in 83.3% of the patients during complete cytogenetic or clinical remission. Chronic myelogenous leukemia was more likely to relapse in patients who had sustained PCR positivity, as opposed to those in whom it was intermittently negative (Fig 4–10). Relapse was also more likely in patients in whom PCR detected *bcr-abl* transcript between 2 and 10 weeks after BMT. In 4 of the patients who had titration assay, the number of leukemic cells increased continually from shortly after BMT until cytogenetic or clinical relapse 1–2 years later. In the other 4 patients who stayed in clinical remission, PCR detected either no leukemic cells or relatively low and stable numbers.

Conclusions.—In chronic myelogenous leukemia, important prognostic information can be gained by detection of the *bcr-abl* transcript by PCR after allogeneic BMT. The proliferation of the residual leukemic cell population can be followed by serial estimation of the number of such

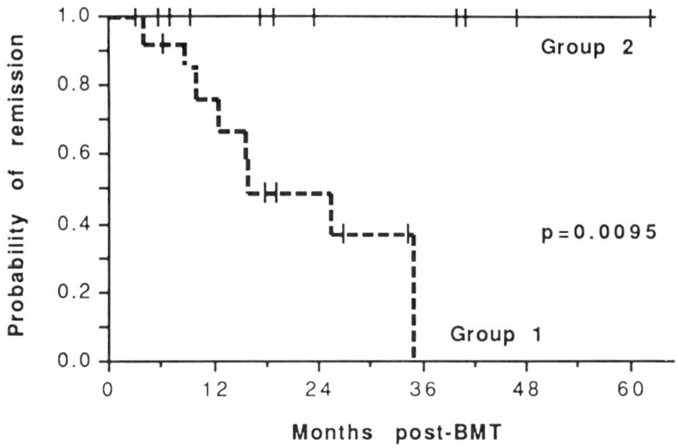

Fig 4–10.—The probability of maintaining remission after allogeneic bone marrow transplantation (BMT) in patients with sustained PCR positivity (group 1) and in patients with at least 1 negative PCR analysis (group 2). (Courtesy of Delage R, Soiffer RJ, Dear K, et al: *Blood* 78:2759–2767, 1991.)

cells. These analyses can help to assess the effectiveness of the preparative regimen and direct therapy after BMT, before overt clinical relapse occurs.

▶ Hughes and colleagues (1) studied the capacity of PCR to detect *bcr-abl* transcripts in 3 groups of patients: those transplanted with unmanipulated matched allogeneic marrow in the chronic phase 3–6 months after the transplant; those transplanted with unmanipulated matched allogeneic marrow in the chronic phase 8 months–8 years after the transplant; and patients transplanted in the chronic phase with T-cell–depleted marrow. They found that PCR may detect residual *bcr-abl* within 6 months of transplant without necessarily affecting the probability of relapse adversely. However, PCR positivity occurring later after transplant is a harbinger of relapse.

The optimal timing of allogeneic transplantation is still unclear. However, 2 groups have reported that acceleration of the disease correlates with hypermethylization of the calcitonin gene (2,3). The use of this technique to assess the optimal timing of transplantation in the chronic phase may further improve survival in chronic myelogenous leukemia.—D.L. Longo, M.D., F.A.C.P.

References

1. Hughes TP, et al: *Blood* 77:874, 1991.
2. Nelkin BD, et al: *Blood* 77:2431, 1991.
3. Malinen T, et al: *Blood* 77:2435, 1991.

Interferon-Alpha Produces Sustained Cytogenetic Responses in Chronic Myelogenous Leukemia: Philadelphia Chromosome-Positive Patients

Talpaz M, Kantarjian H, Kurzrock R, Trujillo JM, Gutterman JU (Univ of Texas MD Anderson Cancer Center, Houston)

Ann Intern Med 114:532–538, 1991 4–27

Background.—In 1981, a study was begun of 96 patients in the early benign stage of chronic myelogenous leukemia who were receiving interferon-α (IFN-α)-treatment. The follow-up of those patients who showed durable karyotypic conversion to diploid hemopoiesis was reported.

Methods.—The patients were treated with IFN-α until hematologic remission occurred; they were then returned to their homes, where they continued to report complete blood counts and platelet counts. Every 3 or 4 months, each patient underwent a physical examination, blood and bone marrow analysis, and a cytogenetic evaluation.

Results.—Of the 96 patients, 73% had a complete hematologic response and 19% had a complete cytogenetic response. The complete cytogenetic response rate was 14% among the 51 patients treated with partially pure IFN-α and 24% among the 45 treated with recombinant IFN-α-2a. The difference in the cumulative incidence of complete cytogenetic remission based on 50-month follow-up was not substantial between the 2 groups. The overall duration of hematologic remission in the 70 patients who achieved such remission was 41 months, with no difference between the 2 groups. Hematologic remission did last substantially longer in those patients who had either partial or complete cytogenetic remission. The overall survival rate of 62 months did not differ substantially between the 2 treatment groups. Side effects, which most often were mild fatigue and weight loss, occurred in both groups.

Discussion.—Unlike the responses achieved with chemotherapy or bone marrow transplant, the IFN-α–induced complete cytogenetic responses did not require profound myelosuppression. The 62-month median survival in patients treated with IFN-α is better than the 39-month median survival of the 303 patients treated with various chemotherapies at the same institution. If continued follow-up shows a subset of patients with ongoing remission at the 10-year point, then a change in the survival outlook for some patients treated with IFN-α would be in order.

▶ This long-term follow-up of patients treated with IFN-α is interesting and important. These data suggest that patients who respond to interferon have more prolonged survival; this is not necessarily a valid conclusion, because a subset of patients who are responsive to therapy is being compared to all historical controls. However, it is possible that interferon prolongs survival, and this should be tested prospectively. It would be of interest to use the PCR technique for the detection of *bcr-abl* transcripts that have been used in patients undergoing bone marrow transplantation, because examination of cytogenetics in peripheral blood or marrow metaphases may not be sufficiently sensitive.

The group at the M.D. Anderson Cancer Center has also studied the use of interferon to maintain a chemotherapy-induced response in patients with chronic myelogenous leukemia (1). In 32 patients, the group did not discern any evidence that the use of chemotherapy added anything to the response that was expected from interferon alone. Intensive chemotherapy with autologous bone marrow was also evaluated in patients who were ineligible for allogeneic transplantation or who were resistant to interferon therapy (2). They found that some patients obtained partial cytogenetic responses but, interestingly, after autologous transplantation, 3 of 7 patients who were formerly resistant to interferon recovered interferon sensitivity.—D.L. Longo, M.D., F.A.C.P.

References

1. Kantarjian HM, et al: *Cancer* 68:1201, 1991.
2. Kantarjian HM, et al: *Cancer* 67:2959, 1991.

Suppression of Chronic Myelogenous Leukemia Colony Growth by Interleukin-1 (IL-1) Receptor Antagonist and Soluble IL-1 Receptors: A Novel Application for Inhibitors of IL-1 Activity

Estrov Z, Kurzrock P, Wetzler M, Kantarjian H, Blake M, Harris D, Gutterman JU, Talpaz M (Univ of Texas MD Anderson Cancer Ctr, Houston)

Blood 78:1476–1484, 1991 4–28

Background.—The suppressive effect of interferon-α (IFN) in chronic myelogenous leukemia may result in part from its suppressive effects in interleukin-1 (IL-1) autocrine loops. The part played by IL-1β in the malignant evolution of chronic myelogenous leukemia and the functional activity of IL-1 inhibitors were assessed.

Methods.—Peripheral blood and bone marrow samples from 38 patients with chronic myelogenous leukemia were studied. All had received no treatment for at least 2 weeks. Eighteen patients were sensitive to IFN and 20 were resistant. Specimens from both patients and hematologically normal controls were studied by the colony-forming unit-granulocyte, erythrocyte, monocyte, megakaryocyte colony culture assay. In addition, lysates of 2.5×10^7 low-density cells from 6 patients who were IFN-resistant, 6 patients who were IFN-sensitive, and 3 normal volunteers were tested by enzyme-linked immunosorbent assay technique for intrinsic IL-1β content.

Results.—Distinct responses were seen in samples from IFN-sensitive and IFN-resistant patients. In the IFN-sensitive group, hematopoietic colonies formed in the presence of fetal calf serum, erythropoietin, and either granulocyte-macrophage colony-stimulating factor, IL-3, or both, or phytohemagglutinin-conditioned medium. At concentrations of 10–100 units/mL, IL-1β augmented colony growth in dose-dependent fashion. In the patients who were resistant to IFN, growth factors did not augment the growth-promoting effects of fetal calf serum and erythropoietin. The "autonomous" colony growth was even attenuated by adherent cell fractionation or T-lymphocyte depletion. Interleukin-1β content was 610 pg in IFN-resistant patients, 54.6 pg in IFN-sensitive patients, and 49.4 pg in controls. Both soluble IL-1 receptors (at 5–100 ng/mL) and IL-1 receptor antagonist (at 10–500 ng/mL) inhibited chronic myelogenous leukemia colony growth in a dose-dependent manner. Maximal inhibition was 64% and 65%, respectively, and anti–IL-β-neutralizing antibodies had a similar effect.

Conclusions.—Interleukin-1β appears to have some role in the progression of chronic myelogenous leukemia. Proliferation may be reduced by blocking of the interaction between IL-1β and its receptor. A clinical trial of IL-1 receptor antagonist is planned in patients with chronic myelogenous leukemia.

▶ It appears that IFN may represent a treatment advance for chronic myelogenous leukemia. If it works by inhibiting an autocrine growth pathway, then there may be even more specific ways of interfering with the growth of the cells. The IL-1 receptor antagonist shows some activity against tumor cell proliferation in vitro and may be effective in vivo.—D.L. Longo, M.D., F.A.C.P.

Cost Effectiveness of Prophylactic Intravenous Immune Globulin in Chronic Lymphocytic Leukemia

Weeks JC, Tierney MR, Weinstein MC (Dana-Farber Cancer Inst; Massachusetts Gen Hosp; Harvard School of Public Health, Boston)

N Engl J Med 325:81–86, 1991 4–29

Background.—A recent double-blind randomized controlled trial by the Cooperative Group for the Study of Immunoglobulin in Chronic Lymphocytic Leukemia demonstrated a statistically significant reduction in bacterial infections after intravenously administered immunoglobulin therapy in patients with chronic lymphocytic leukemia and hypogammaglobulinemia. Because this treatment strategy is very costly, the data from this study were used to evaluate whether prophylactic intravenously administered immunoglobulin is likely to result in a net clinical benefit and to examine its cost effectiveness.

Methods.—A decision-analysis model was constructed to compare 2 strategies: treatment with intravenously administered immunoglobulin, 400 mg/kg, given every 3 weeks for 1 year and no immunoglobulin therapy. The data on the efficacy of the intravenously administered immunoglobulin were derived from the results of the Cooperative Group trial, and the estimates of treatment cost, complications, and infections were derived from component costs. The health outcomes were measured in terms of the gains in quality-adjusted life expectancy.

Data Analysis.—Assuming that intravenously administered immunoglobulin entails no inconvenience, therapy results in a gain of .8 quality-adjusted day per patient per year of therapy, at a cost of $6 million per quality-adjusted life-year gained. In contrast, when the inconvenience of treatment is taken into account, intravenously administered immunoglobulin therapy results in a loss of quality-adjusted life expectancy. Therefore, treatment is not cost-effective and would not be used—even if it were free.

Summary.—Intravenously administered immunoglobulin therapy in patients with chronic lymphocytic leukemia and hypogammaglobulinemia may not result in improved quality or length of life, and this treatment is extraordinarily expensive in relation to other treatments that are generally accepted as cost-effective. Decision-analysis modeling provides a method of evaluating the potential clinical and financial effects of adopting an intervention in medical practice.

▶ When a prospective randomized trial demonstrates that a particular safe intervention exerts a significant beneficial effect on a population of patients, physicians generally make a decision to try to obtain the beneficial effect for their own patients. I really resent being told that a drug that has been shown to help some patients cannot be used in my patient because it is too expensive. Although it may make economic sense to let some fraction of patients get seriously ill and perhaps even die because of the expense of preventing infections in patients who were not ever going to get infections, it is immoral. We make an implicit contract with our patients to offer treatments that may improve the quality or length of their lives. We also run a very serious risk of permitting serious illnesses or death to occur in a minority of patients because the majority does not need a life-saving intervention. This is social Darwinism run amok. Shouldn't we be permitted to make our best recommendations to an individual patient without taking into account the effects of that treatment on both the entire population of patients and the economics of the health care system.— D.L. Longo, M.D., F.A.C.P.

Myeloma

High Serum Lactate Dehydrogenase Level as a Marker for Drug Resistance and Short Survival in Multiple Myeloma

Dimopoulos MA, Barlogie B, Smith TL, Alexanian R (Univ of Texas MD Anderson Cancer Ctr, Houston)

Ann Intern Med 115:931–935, 1991 4–30

Background.—There are many useful predictors of survival in multiple myeloma, but there are few tests that will predict the likelihood of a response to chemotherapy. Serum lactate dehydrogenase (LDH) was studied as a prognostic factor in multiple myeloma.

Methods.—The subjects were 391 consecutive, previously untreated patients with multiple myeloma; they were evaluated during a 10½-year period. All patients were treated with a chemotherapy regimen including doxorubicin, high-dose glucocorticoid combinations, or both. The response rates were consistently near 45% to 55%. A number of pretreatment characteristics, including LDH, were assessed to evaluate the likelihood of response and survival time. Levels of lactate dehydrogenase more than 300 units per L were considered significantly increased; clinical response was based on a 75% reduction in the calculated tumor load. Patients were followed for a median of 28 months, and 63% of the patients were followed until death.

Results.—A significant elevation in serum LDH was seen in 11% of all patients and 26% of the patients with high tumor mass. Those patients with a high level of LDH were more likely to have other abnormal laboratory results as well. Of the patients with a high level of LDH, 43% had plasma cell leukemia or clinical features resembling lymphoma, and 17% had plasma cell hypodiploidy. The rate of response to chemotherapy was only 20% for patients with high levels of LDH vs. 57% for those with low levels of LDH. Lactate dehydrogenase was a significant independent predictor of response, carrying an odds ratio of .25. Those patients with a high level of LDH survived a median of 9 months vs. 39 months for those with a low level of LDH; they also had the highest relative risk—2.63.

Conclusions.—In multiple myeloma, elevation of LDH indicates occult extraosseous disease and high tumor mass. A high level of LDH predicts a poor prognosis, and patients with this finding should be considered for early intensive treatment. Lactate dehydrogenase is a convenient and inexpensive marker that provides a practical alternative to more complex studies.

▶ Levels of serum LDH now join levels of serum β2-microglobulin as markers of prognosis in patients with myeloma. In other series, levels of serum neopterin (1,2) and levels of serum IL-6 (2) have been found to correlate with prognosis. The neopterin levels are particularly highly correlated with the stage of disease. Levels of serum β2-microglobulin cannot be used to assess tumor burden in patients being treated with interferon, because they augment secretion of β2-microglobulin from the tumor cells (3); in patients given interferon, the increasing levels of serum β2-microglobulin do not necessarily indicate progressive disease. Other assessments of tumor burden need to be used to monitor the response to interferon.—D.L. Longo, M.D., F.A.C.P.

References

1. Boccadoro M, et al: *Eur J Haematol* 47:305, 1991.
2. Reibnegger G, et al: *Cancer Res* 51:6250, 1991.
3. Tienhaara A, et al: *Br J Haematol* 77:335, 1991.

Monoclonal Antibody-Purged Autologous Bone Marrow Transplantation Therapy for Multiple Myeloma

Anderson KC, Barut BA, Ritz J, Freedman AS, Takvorian T, Rabinowe SN, Soiffer R, Heflin L, Coral F, Dear K, Mauch P, Nadler LM (Dana-Farber Cancer Inst, Boston)

Blood 77:712–720, 1991 4–31

Background.—Despite the sensitivity of myeloma cells to radiotherapy and chemotherapy, durable complete responses are rare. The results of treatment of 11 patients with plasma cell dyscrasias with high-dose chemoradiotherapy and anti–B-cell monoclonal antibody-purged autologous bone marrow transplantation (ABMT) were evaluated.

Patients.—Ten patients with multiple myeloma and 1 patient with recurrent extramedullary plasmacytomas were treated. Most patients had advanced Durie-Salmon stage myeloma at diagnosis; all were pretreated with chemotherapy; and 6 had received prior radiotherapy.

Findings.—At the time of transplantation, all patients had good performance status, with a Karnofsky score of 80% or greater; they also had less than 10% marrow tumor cells. Eight patients had residual monoclonal marrow plasma cells and 10 had paraprotein. After treatment with high-dose melphalan and total body irradiation, 7 patients had complete responses, 3 had partial responses, and 1 died. Engraftment post-ABMT was prompt, with granulocytes greater than 500/mm^3 at a median of 21 days posttransplant. Untransfused platelets greater than 200,000/mm^3 were seen at a median of 23 days posttransplant in 10 of 11 patients. There was an early predominance of natural killer cells and cytotoxic/suppressor T cells, with a return of B cells at 3 months and normalization of the T4:T8 ratio at 1 year posttransplant. Less than 5% of the polyclonal marrow plasma cells were seen in all responders after treatment. Three of 7 patients with complete response had return of paraprotein (2 with myeloma), but all responded to α2-interferon therapy. At the latest follow-up, 8 patients were alive at 18.9 months posttransplant. Four patients were free of disease at 12.3, 17.5, 18.9, and 29 months posttransplant.

Conclusion.—High-dose melphalan and total body irradiation can achieve high response rates without unexpected toxicity in patients with sensitive disease. Engraftment is not inhibited by monoclonal antibody-purging techniques. Relapses still occur; however, because of the significant response rates in these patients with sensitive disease, the possibility that ABMT or other alternative strategies may be used earlier in the disease course (at a time when there is less tumor burden and fewer sensitive cells) should be evaluated. The result may be higher complete responses.

▶ The trend toward more aggressive therapy for multiple myeloma continues. Four of the 11 patients studied remained in initial remission for relatively short periods of follow-up. In another study of aggressive therapy, Attal and colleagues (1) treated 35 patients with either VAD (vincristine, doxorubicin, dexamethasone) or VMCP (vincristine, melphalan, cyclophosphamide, prednisone) induction therapy. Thirty-two patients went on to receive high-dose therapy with autologous bone marrow support and then received maintenance interferon after count recovery. Fifteen patients (43%) had a complete response, and 85% of the complete responders remained in complete remission at approximately 3 years after the transplant. In light of the advanced age of many patients with myeloma, it is clear that this approach is applicable only to a subset of patients. However, the prospect that some fraction of patients may be curable is worth further investigation.—D.L. Longo, M.D., F.A.C.P.

Reference

1. Attal M, et al: *Blood* 79:1130, 1992.

Second and Third Responses to the Same Induction Regimen in Relapsing Patients With Multiple Myeloma

Paccagnella A, Chiarion-Sileni V, Soesan M, Baggio G, Bolzonella S, De Besi P, Casara D, Frizzarin M, Salvagno L, Favaretto A, Fiorentino MV (Padova Gen Hosp, Padova, Italy; Slotervaart Hosp, Amsterdam; Padova Univ, Padova, Italy)
Cancer 68:975–980, 1991 4–32

Background.—The use of melphalan improved the median survival time (MST) of patients with multiple myeloma. In 1975, physicians began treating multiple myeloma with a combination chemotherapy regimen consisting of melphalan, cyclophosphamide, vincristine, carmustine, and prednisone (M-2), with no maintenance therapy. When relapse occurred, the patients received the same regimen. The response rate and the MST with the M-2 regimen were studied, including whether this regimen could achieve a second or third response in patients who relapsed.

Patients.—A group of 115 consecutive, previously untreated patients received the M-2 regimen during an 11-year period. Of the 115, 75 were men and 40 were women; the mean patient age was 64 years. According to the system of Durie and Salmon, 3.5% were in stage I, 39% were in stage II, and 57.5% were in stage III. A total of 67% of the patients were in renal function stage A. Chemotherapy was discontinued 1 year from the start when the patient responded. When relapse occurred, the same regimen was begun and then stopped at 5–10 months when stable remission was achieved. The follow-up was complete.

Findings.—Of the patients, 82% achieved an objective response to induction therapy; a median of 5 courses was needed to obtain maximum response. The median duration of first response was 22 months. Thirty-eight patients were retreated after a first relapse, and 69% responded to the same regimen. The median duration of response in this group was 11 months; both the response rate and the median duration of response were significantly lower than with induction chemotherapy. Sixteen patients had a second relapse; 44% responded again, for a median duration of response of 3.5 months. For all patients, the mST was 50.5 months, with a range of 31 months in stage IIIB to 62 months in stage IIA. Leukopenia was the only relevant side effect of induction therapy.

Conclusions.—Patients with multiple myeloma can achieve a high response rate in first and second relapses using M-2 chemotherapy without maintenance therapy. Survival is not lessened by a planned treatment pause at remission that improves quality of life. Secondary leukemia is uncommon.

▶ This report stands in contrast to the previous abstracts describing the results with high-dose therapy in a selected subset of patients. Conventional-dose combination chemotherapy can be effective in controlling the disease for long periods of time, even when complete eradication of disease is not the goal. However, there is evidence that the emergence of resistant disease over time may be caused, at least in part, by the expression of the median duration of response (1). Administration of chemotherapeutic agents by continuous infusion or with agents to reverse drug resistance may further improve the efficacy of conventional-dose treatment approaches.

It is important to keep in mind the 69% response rate to retreatment with the M-2 regimen reported in this paper when evaluating the results of other conventional-dose salvage chemotherapy programs. For example, Leoni and colleagues (2) report that 8 of 15 "relapsed and resistant" patients responded to teniposide, dexamethasone, and continuous-infusion cyclophosphamide. It is difficult to know whether this is better or worse than would be expected with retreatment using primary chemotherapy regimens; however, it may be of use to more carefully evaluate infusional regimens in previously treated patients with myeloma.—D.L. Longo, M.D., F.A.C.P.

References

1. Salmon SE, et al: *Blood* 78:44, 1991.
2. Leoni F, et al: *Br J Haematol* 77:180, 1991.

Nephrotoxic Potential of Bence Jones Proteins

Solomon A, Weiss DT, Kattine AA (Univ of Tennessee Med Ctr/Graduate School of Medicine, Knoxville)

N Engl J Med 324:1845–1851, 1991 4–33

Introduction.—The renal manifestations of myeloma nephropathy, light-chain deposition disease, and amyloidosis AL result from the deposition of Bence Jones proteins as tubular casts, basement-membrane precipitates, or fibrils, respectively. The severity of renal manifestations vary greatly among patients for unknown reasons.

Methods.—The pathologic importance of various Bence Jones proteins was studied in mice injected with Bence Jones proteins obtained from 40 patients with multiple myeloma or amyloidosis AL. The mice were killed 48 hours later, and their kidneys were examined.

Results.—Of the 40 different human Bence Jones proteins, 26 were deposited in the mouse kidneys—mainly as tubular casts, basement-membrane precipitates, or crystals; there were no light-chain deposits. Of the 18 patients for whom renal tissue was available for study, 14 had findings comparable to those in the mice. The protein obtained from 22 of the 27 patients whose serum creatinine levels equaled or exceeded 168 μmol/L were deposited in mouse kidneys, whereas protein deposition occurred after the injection of proteins from only 4 of the 13 patients with serum creatinine levels less than 168 μmol/L. Repeated protein injection using protein from the 2 patients with amyloidosis AL resulted in the deposition of the protein in mouse kidneys as amyloid.

Conclusion.—Certain Bence Jones proteins are primarily responsible for producing the distinctive types of protein deposition in renal tissue in patients with diseases associated with the production of monoclonal light chains. This experimental model may be valuable for identifying nephrotoxic or amyloidogenic light chains.

▶ The deposition of monoclonal light chains (i.e., Bence Jones proteins) in the kidney results in impairment of renal function and is primarily responsible for the morbidity and mortality of light-chain disease. However, not all patients with Bence Jones proteinurea have renal damage. It appears that the physical and chemical properties of the proteins themselves may account for the "benign" nature of some Bence Jones proteins as compared with the "malignant" propensity of others to form deposits or precipitates that impair renal function. The specific molecular features responsible for the renal deposition of certain Bence Jones proteins need to be determined. This model provides investigators the opportunity to identify the nephrotoxic and amyloidogenic light chains that may provide insights toward more effective treatment.—R.F. Ozols, M.D., Ph.D.

Murine Anti-Interleukin-6 Monoclonal Antibody Therapy for a Patient With Plasma Cell Leukemia

Klein B, Wijdenes J, Zhang X-G, Jourdan M, Boiron J-M, Brochier J, Liautard J, Merlin M, Clement C, Morel-Fournier B, Lu Z-Y, Mannoni P, Sany J, Bataille R (INSERM U291, Montpellier, France; CRTS, Besançon; Institut Paoli Calmettes, Marseilles, France; Hôpital Saint Eloi, Montpellier, France)

Blood 78:1198–1204, 1991 4–34

Background.—In vitro, interleukin-6 (IL-6) shows potent growth activity for fresh tumor cells in human multiple myeloma. The therapeutic effect of injecting anti–IL-6 monoclonal antibodies (MoAbs) was evaluated in a patient with primary plasma cell leukemia that was resistant to chemotherapy.

Case Report.—Man, 61, had primary plasma cell leukemia, extensive bone lesions, massive bone marrow invasion by malignant plasma cells, and 25% myeloma cells in peripheral blood. Symptomatic treatment and 2 VAD (vincristine, doxorubicin, and dexamethasone) regimens improved his condition slightly; however, thereafter, he had a fulminant progression with symptoms identical to those seen at diagnosis. He was then started on daily injection of murine anti–IL-6 MoAbs, administered in an 1-hour infusion in 100 mL physiologic serum and .5% human serum albumin. The doses were calculated to achieve serum MoAb concentrations known to inhibit myeloma cell proliferation in vivo and were adjusted thereafter. The patient was treated for 2 months; his clinical status improved and there were no major side effects. Myeloma cell proliferation in the bone marrow was blocked, from 4.5% to 0% myeloma cells in S-phase in vivo. There was approximately a 30% correction in serum calcium and monoclonal IgG, and a correction to undetectable levels in C-reactive protein. The platelet and circulating neutrophil counts decreased, and a transient immunization was detected 15 days after the start of treatment. This finding was thought to explain the recovery of myeloma cell proliferation after 2 months of treatment. After treatment, 2 more VAD regimens were given. The patient died of infection 1½ months after the end of MoAb treatment.

Conclusions.—The first clinical trial of anti–IL-6 MoAbs was studied. The MoAbs appear to be feasible for injection, cause transient tumor cytostasis, and reduce IL-6–related toxicities. These findings may serve as a basis for further development of anti–IL-6 therapy.

▶ The data suggesting that IL-6 is an autocrine growth factor for myeloma is actually considerably stronger for murine than for human myeloma. Indeed, only 1 authentic human myeloma cell line has been reported to secrete and respond to IL-6, and it required considerable effort to demonstrate the presence of small amounts of IL-6 production in this line (1). It appears that the phase of human myeloma growth that is IL-6–dependent is a transient phase occurring early in the natural history. The anecdotal response to an IL-6 antibody is somewhat surprising, because it is not clear whether there is a physiological basis for an antibody to be retained in the vicinity of IL-6 production and to act as a sponge to prevent it from binding its cellular receptor. It is possible that an antibody to the high-affinity IL-6 receptor might produce some antitumor effects, at least transiently; however, the greater likelihood would seem to be that alternative pathways for growth stimulation will be selected as the IL-6 pathway is blocked.—D.L. Longo, M.D., F.A.C.P.

Reference

1. Schwab G, et al: *Blood* 77:587, 1991.

Additional Reading

Shimamoto Y, Anami Y, Yamaguchi M: A new risk grouping for IgD myeloma based on analysis of 165 Japanese patients. *Eur J Haematol* 47:262–267, 1991.

▶ Everything you ever wanted to know about a rare myeloma; light-chain isotype (λ is worse than κ) and white blood cell count (a higher count is worse) are the 2 main prognostic factors.

Vallespi T, Montserrat E, Sanz MA: Chronic lymphocytic leukaemia: Prognostic value of lymphocyte morphological subtypes. A multivariate survival analysis in 146 patients. *Br J Haematol* 77:478–485, 1991.

▶ The number of prolymphocytes in the peripheral blood greater than 5×10^9/L separates the patients into prognostic groups.

Kantjarian HM, Childs C, O'Brien S, et al: Efficacy of fludarabine, a new adenine nucleoside analogue, in patients with prolymphocytic leukemia and the prolymphocytoid variant of chronic lymphocytic leukemia. *Am J Med* 90:223–228, 1991.

▶ Fludarabine is considerably less effective in prolymphocytic leukemia than in chronic lymphocytic leukemia; complete responses occurred in only 3 of 17 (18%) patients.

Losada AP, Wessman M, Tiainen M, et al: Trisomy 12 in chronic lymphocytic leukemia: An interphase cytogenetic study. *Blood* 78:775–779, 1991.

▶ Using in situ hybridization techniques, the authors found that trisomy 12 is more common than would be detected by karyotype analysis.

Puccio CA, Mittelman A, Lichtman SM, et al: A loading dose/continuous infusion schedule of fludarabine phosphate in chronic lymphocytic leukemia. *J Clin Oncol* 9:1562–1569, 1991.

▶ Fludarabine induces responses in the majority of patients with chronic lymphocytic leukemia.

Motomura S, Kanamori H, Maruta A, et al: The effect of 1-hydroxyvitamin D_3 for prolongation of leukemic transformation-free survival in myelodysplastic syndromes. *Am J Hematol* 38:67–68, 1991.

▶ Administration of 4–6 μg/day of 1-hydroxyvitamin D_3 significantly prolonged the period without leukemia in patients with myelodysplasia; there was also a significant survival advantage.

Kastner P, Perez A, Lutz Y, et al: Structure, localization and transcriptional properties of two classes of retinoic acid receptor alpha fusion proteins in acute promyelocytic leukemia (APL): Structural similarities with new family of oncoproteins. *EMBO J* 11:629–642, 1992.

▶ There is emerging evidence that the chimeric receptor generated by the fusion of the *myl* gene with the retinoic acid receptor α-gene interferes with normal retinoic acid receptor gene function; the addition of retinoic acid causes the chimeric protein to move to the nucleus.

Frickhofen N, Kaltwasser JP, Schrezenmeier H, et al: Treatment of aplastic anemia with antilymphocyte globulin and methylprednisolone with or without cyclosporine. *N Engl J Med* 324:1297–1304, 1991.

▶ Approximately two thirds of patients with aplastic anemia will respond to triple therapy with antilymphocyte globulin, steroids and cyclosporine.

Pallesen G, Sandvej K, Hamilton-Dutoit SJ, et al: Activation of Epstein-Barr virus replication in Hodgkin and Reed-Sternberg cells. *Blood* 78:1162–1165, 1991.

▶ More handwaving about the possible role of Epstein-Barr virus in the pathogenesis of Hodgkin's disease.

McMaster ML, Johnson DH, Greer JP, et al: A combination chemotherapy of brief duration for elderly patients with poor-prognosis non-Hodgkin's lymphoma. *Cancer* 67:1487–1492, 1991.

▶ Bleomycin, etoposide, cyclophosphamide, doxorubicin, methotrexate with leucovorin, and prednisone (BECALM) were used in patients with a median age of 75 years; 7 of 26 patients are long term survivors.

Williams ME, Meeker TC, Swerdlow SH: Rearrangement of the chromosome 11 *bcl*-1 locus in centrocytic lymphoma: Analysis with multiple breakpoint probes. *Blood* 78:493–498, 1991.

▶ The diffuse, intermediately differentiated lymphocytic lymphoma (or centrocytic lymphoma in the Kiel terminology) is associated with a characteristic translocation involving t(11;14); where the *bcl*-1 gene from chromosome 11 translocations to the immunoglobulin heavy chain, joining region genes on chromosome 14.

5 Bone Marrow Transplantation

Introduction

The transplantation of bone marrow from 1 individual to another has taught us an enormous amount about normal immune function, normal hematopoiesis, and the intricate interrelationships among the various cellular components of the host defense system. In addition, allogeneic bone marrow transplantation has led to the cure of formerly incurable malignancies and has provided perhaps the most convincing encouragement that it is possible for the immune system to mediate clinically significant antitumor responses. Indeed, graft-vs.-leukemia and graft-vs.-lymphoma effects appear to be essential components of the efficacy of allogeneic transplant regimens, and they provide much, if not all, of the incremental improvements in survival seen with this approach as compared with conventional chemotherapy or high-dose therapy with autologous marrow support. The problems associated with bone marrow transplantation include the expense of delivering the complicated, hospital-care–intensive support that is required, failure of the donor immune system to adequately reconstitute the immune functions of the host (leading to infections), and the relative inseparability of graft-vs.-tumor and graft-vs.-host reactions (leading to immune-mediated organ damage).

Because this chapter focuses on the advances in the management of the various problems associated with allogeneic bone marrow transplantation—rather than on the improvements in disease-free survival that are associated with its use in various tumors (which tend to be referred to in this YEAR BOOK in the chapters dealing with the particular tumor types)— it might be possible for the reader who is not involved with delivering this type of therapy to conclude that it is too toxic and more trouble than it is worth. Wrong!

In the 1991 YEAR BOOK OF ONCOLOGY, we cited the study of Wingard and colleagues (1), which documented that most of the 135 patients studied 6 months–12 years after transplantation had excellent performance status; 93% reported that they could do normal activities with no (or only minor) physical problems. Two thirds of the patients considered themselves to be in good-to-excellent health. A total of 65% had returned to work, and another 12% were attending school. Unfortunately, 23% had experienced job discrimination and 39% had trouble obtaining insurance. Thus, the conventional image of patients who have survived bone marrow transplantation is that they are fragile victims who deserve pity—but not an opportunity to be normal. Of course, one third of patients do have medical problems related to chronic graft-vs.-host disease.

However, discrimination on the basis of health history is a consequence of being poorly informed. Physicians should strive to correct the mistaken impression that patients who have undergone transplantation are uniformly less able to function than individuals without such a health history.

Dan L. Longo, M.D., F.A.C.P.

Reference

1. Wingard JR, et al: *Ann Intern Med* 114:113, 1991.

Hematologic Malignancies

Increased Incidence of Solid Malignant Tumors After Bone Marrow Transplantation for Severe Aplastic Anemia

Socié G, Henry-Amar M, Cosset JM, Devergie A, Girinsky T, Gluckman E (Hôpital Saint-Louis, Paris; Institut Gustave Roussy, Villejuif, France)
Blood 78:277–279, 1991. 5–1

Background.—Allogeneic marrow transplantation is practiced increasingly in cases of hematologic malignancy and nonmalignant hemtologic disease. Because secondary neoplasia has been described after chemoradiotherapy, and because tumors can develop after solid organ transplantation, human marrow recipients who receive high-dose chemotherapy and/or radiotherapy as well as postgraft immunosuppression may be at high risk of having a secondary malignancy develop.

Findings.—Marrow transplantation was performed after conditioning with cyclophosphamide and thoracoabdominal irradiation in 107 patients with nonconstitutional severe aplastic anemia and in 40 with Fanconi anemia. During a mean follow-up of approximately 5 years, a solid malignancy developed within the field of radiation in 4 patients. The median interval from marrow transplantation to tumor development was 7 years. No clinical correlates of tumor development were identified. The cumulative 8-year incidence rate was 22%.

Conclusion.—The possibility of a solid malignancy should be considered when following patients for severe anemia after marrow transplantation.

▶ The inclusion of this paper is testimony to the incredible therapeutic benefit of allogeneic bone marrow transplantation. Severe aplastic anemia is a fatal disease; with supportive care alone, nearly half the patients die within 6 months of bleeding or infection. However, a large fraction of patients are now living so long that we must now worry about the late effects of the bone marrow transplant preparative regimen. It appears that the use of radiation therapy in these patients leads to a higher-than-expected rate of developing solid tumors, as has been seen in patients with Hodgkin's disease who receive radiation therapy (1, 2). In this cohort from France, the secondary tumors were not related to the presence of graft-vs.-host disease or other patient-related prognostic factors. In contrast, the incidence of secondary solid tumors developing in the Seattle patients with aplastic anemia was 6% at 15 years (3). All 4 patients in the Seattle series had chronic graft-vs.-host disease. However, perhaps a key difference was the absence of radiation from the Seattle conditioning regimen. It is possible to speculate that elimination of radiation therapy from the conditioning regimen and control of graft-vs.-host disease might significantly reduce the incidence of secondary solid tumors in patients with aplastic anemia who undergo allogeneic bone marrow transplantation.

It is a bit surprising that the risk of secondary malignancies did not appear to be different in patients with aplastic anemia compared with those with Fanconi's anemia. Fanconi's anemia is associated with chromosomal fragility that might have predisposed the patients to radiation-induced malignant transformation. However, based on the small number of patients in this paper by Socié and colleagues, no increased risk was noted.—D.L. Longo, M.D., F.A.C.P.

References

1. Tucker MA, et al: *N Engl J Med* 318:76, 1988.
2. Meadows AT, et al: *Med Pediatr Oncol* 17:477, 1989.
3. Storb R, et al: in Gale RP, Champlin RE (eds): *New Strategies in Bone Marrow Transplantation*. New York, Wiley-Liss, 1991.

Engraftment After Infusion of CD34$^+$ Marrow Cells in Patients With Breast Cancer or Neuroblastoma

Berenson RJ, Bensinger WI, Hill RS, Andrews RG, Garcia-Lopez J, Kalamasz DF, Still BJ, Spitzer G, Buckner CD, Bernstein ID, Thomas ED (Univ of Washington, Seattle; MD Anderson Cancer Ctr, Houston; Hospital de Sant Pau, Barcelona, Spain)

Blood 77:1717–1722, 1991 5–2

Background.—The CD34 antigen is expressed by 1% to 4% of human marrow cells, but it is not expressed on mature peripheral blood cells. It also is found on nearly all colony-forming cells and blast colony-forming cells. Those marrow cells that express CD34 can engraft lethally irradiated baboons. The antigen is not found on tumor cells from most patients with solid tumors. Positive selection of CD34$^+$ cells, therefore, may provide marrow cells that are capable of engraftment but are not associated with tumor.

Procedures.—Seven patients with stage IV breast cancer and 2 with stage IV neuroblastoma had their marrow cells separated by immunoadsorption with the anti-CD34 antibody 12-8. Of the positively selected cells, 64% were CD34$^+$. After marrow ablation, the patients received 1×10^6 5×10^6 of CD34-enriched cells per kg.

Results.—Evidence of engraftment was found in 6 of the 9 patients. The granulocyte counts exceeded 500/mm^3 in these cases, and the platelets exceeded 20,000/mm^3 at 30–45 days after transplantation. Five of the patients had durable engraftment. Three patients, 2 of whom had early engraftment, died within 3 weeks of marrow transplantation.

Discussion.—Marrow preparations enriched in $CD34^+$ cells can reconstitute hematopoiesis after myeloablation in patients with metastatic breast cancer or neuroblastoma. More effective conditioning regimens may be needed to eradicate residual tumor and prevent relapse after autologous marrow transplantation.

▶ An alternative to allogeneic transplantation in patients with tumors other than acute leukemia is to purify the autologous hematopoietic stem cells for use in reconstituting marrow function after ablative therapy. Although this precludes the participation of graft-vs.-tumor effects, it also prevents graft-vs.-host effects. Berenson and colleagues used antiimmunoglobulin columns to positively select $CD34^+$ cells. Even greater purity of 85% to 99% $CD34^+$ cells has been reported using paramagnetic microspheres to partition the antibody-coated stem cells (1).—D.L. Longo, M.D., F.A.C.P.

Reference

1. Strauss LC, et al: *Am J Pediatr Hematol Oncol* 13:217, 1991.

The Optimal Timing of Autologous Bone Marrow Transplantation in Hodgkin's Disease Patients After a Chemotherapy Relapse

Desch CE, Lasala MR, Smith TJ, Hillner BE (Med College of Virginia, Richmond)

J Clin Oncol 10:200–209, 1992 5–3

Introduction.— A decision analysis model was created with which to determine the optimal sequence of salvage chemotherapy and autologous marrow transplantation for patients with Hodgkin's disease who relapse after primary chemotherapy.

Methods.—The model simulated a patient (age, 25 years) who relapsed within a year after receiving MOPP (mechlorethamine, vincristine, procarbazine, and prednisone) chemotherapy for Hodgkin's disease. Four of the possible strategies used marrow transplantation and salvage chemotherapy in various sequences, whereas a fifth strategy used salvage chemotherapy only. Clinical data were derived from 17 published reports.

Findings.—The best strategy appeared to be delaying marrow transplantation until the second relapse. The least effective approach was to perform marrow transplantation in second complete remission. When the terms of the model were altered to simulate advanced disease after the newest combined chemotherapy regimens failed, immediate marrow transplantation was the best approach. When patients were stratified by level of risk, marrow transplantation in second relapse proved best for those patients relapsing in a good prognostic group. When the prognosis was poor, marrow transplantation done only in complete resmission was best.

Conclusions.—Marrow transplantation should always be considered for patients with Hodgkin's disease who relapse. Most often, marrow transplantation at the time of second relapse will be the best strategy. It would be useful to compare the results of phase II trials on the basis of long-term overall survival on an ongoing basis.

▶ This is an ambitious and clever paper. I do not agree with the results, but that is not the fault of the authors. I believe that they were misled by the reported results of conventional-dose salvage chemotherapy programs. In general, such reports include a mixture of patients with different prognoses (according to the previously described Vancouver and National Cancer Institute analyses), and they are reported with too little follow-up to determine the fraction of patients who really benefitted from the treatment. It does not seem likely that patients with short initial remissions, stage IV initial stage, or B symptoms at relapse would benefit by delaying high-dose salvage therapy until they relapse a second time! They may not benefit from earlier high-dose therapy either, but the chances clearly do not improve with subsequent relapses. On the basis of the available data, I would follow the recommendations of Desch et al. for relapsed patients with "good prognosis," but I would administer high-dose therapy with transplantation at the time a second remission is achieved in the poor prognosis group.—D.L. Longo, M.D., F.A.C.P.

Allogeneic Bone Marrow Transplantation in Multiple Myeloma

Gahrton G, for the European Group for Bone Marrow Transplantation (Huddinge Hosp, Huddinge, Sweden)

N Engl J Med 325:1267–1273, 1991 5–4

Background.—Unlike autologous bone marrow transplants, allogeneic transplants contain no tumor cells that might cause a relapse. Allogeneic grafts might also induce a graft-vs.-tumor effect. A series of HLA-identical siblings in whom allogeneic bone marrow transplantation was performed was studied.

Patients.—Ninety patients with multiple myeloma were treated by allogeneic bone marrow grafting during a 7-year period at 76 European centers. Fifty patients were men and 40 were women (median age, 42 years). Most tumors were IgG producing, and the most common stage at diagnosis was IIIA. Conditioning and second-line treatment varied by center. The most recent follow-up was done 79 months after the start of the study.

Results.—Forty-seven patients survived to follow-up and 43 died. A total of 43% of all patients achieved complete remission, as did 58% of those who had engraftment. The actuarial 76-month survival was 40%, and the median relapse-free survival among patients who achieved complete remission was 48 months. The likelihood of complete remission was predicted by the stage of disease at diagnosis and the number of treatments tried before bone marrow transplantation. Those patients who re-

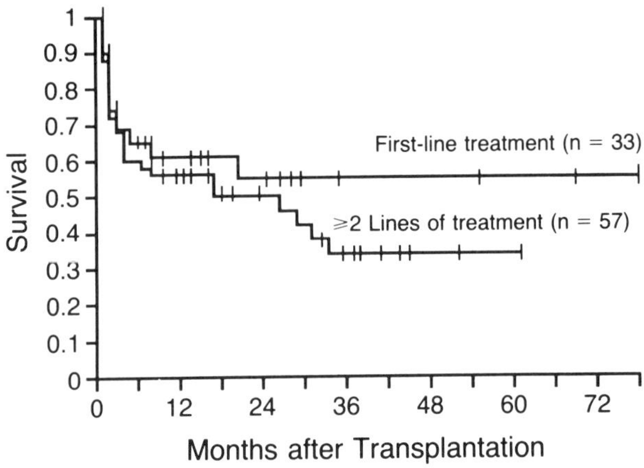

Fig 5–1.—Actuarial survival after bone marrow transplantation, according to the number of lines of treatment regimens used before transplantation. The Kaplan-Meier curves show a slight but not significant trend toward improved survival among patients who received only first-line treatment, as compared with those who received 2 or more lines of treatment. (Courtesy of Gahrton G, for the European Group for Bone Marrow Transplantation: *N Engl J Med* 325:1267–1273, 1991.)

sponded to pretransplant treatment, those with stage I disease, and those who had only first-line treatment before transplantation tended to survive longer; however, these differences were not significant (Fig 5–1). The long-term survival was significantly better in those patients who had complete remission after engraftment and grade I graft-vs.-host disease.

Conclusions.—Allogeneic bone marrow transplantation may be promising treatment for multiple myeloma. The optimal indications for treatment cannot be identified, but patients as old as 55 years of age have a success rate comparable to that of younger patients. Transplantation may be successful in those who have failed first-line treatment, and the treatment may be an option in patients with factors predicting a poor prognosis with conventional therapy.

▶ This multicenter study achieved complete responses in approximately half the patients, and the average remission lasted 4 years.—D.L. Longo, M.D., F.A.C.P.

Solid Tumors

High-Dose Alkylating Agent Chemotherapy With Autologous Bone Marrow Support in Patients With Stage III/IV Epithelial Ovarian Cancer

Shpall EJ, Clarke-Pearson D, Soper JT, Berchuck A, Jones RB, Bast RC Jr, Ross M, Lidor Y, Vanacek K, Tyler T, Peters WP (Duke Univ Med Ctr, Durham, NC)

Gynecol Oncol 38:386–391, 1990 5–5

Introduction.—Most patients with stages III and IV ovarian cancer are incurable with standard therapy, yet ovarian cancer is quite responsive to chemotherapy in patients who begin treatment with limited residual disease. A dose-intensive multiagent chemotherapy regimen might improve the prognosis in patients with advanced ovarian cancer.

Methods.—The efficacy of high-dose cyclophosphamide, thiotepa, and cisplatin followed by autologous bone marrow support was evaluated in 6 patients with stage III and 6 patients with stage IV epithelial ovarian cancer. All patients had progressive disease and had undergone a median of 3 previous chemotherapy regimens. After their initial surgery, 7 patients had residual disease greater than 1 cm.

Results.—Chemotherapy was administered to 1 patient without complications, but she died of septic shock subsequent to a platelet transfusion contaminated with *Klebsiella* bascteria; 2 other patients died of renal failure and concomitant *Candida* sepsis. In 1 patient, asymptomatic veno-occlusive disease of the liver developed, with a peak bilirubin level of 19 that normalized within 3 months. There were no other significant infectious complications or major organ damage. Of the 8 evaluable patients, 6 had a partial response lasting 3–9 months. At a median of more than 3.5 months after transplantation, 2 patients were alive. The other 6 patients died of progressive disease at a median 9 months after transplantation. The 1 patient who refused posttransplant surgical evaluation was alive and clinically and radiographically free of tumor at more than 11 months after transplant.

Conclusion.—The 75% response rate in this group suggests that the regimen is highly potent. Application of the same treatment earlier in the disease would probably produce superior antitumor effects. In this study, the initial bolus intraperitoneal infusion of cisplatin was switched to continuous administration that delivered the same total dose to reduce toxicity, which was fatal in some patients who were treated early in the study.

▶ Bone marrow transplantation in solid tumors has become an extraordinary popular research focus. It is particularly intriguing in ovarian cancer, because this tumor rarely metastasizes to the bone marrow. Despite the theoretical benefits, there have been few studies of transplantation in ovarian cancer. These authors report their initial experience with 12 patients with advanced disease who had failed cisplatin-based combination chemotherapy before transplantation. High-dose intraperitoneal cisplatin, high-dose systemic-cyclophosphamide, and thiotepa with autologous bone marrow support were used. Although 75% of the patients responded, these were all partial responses with a median duration of 6 months. Three (25%) of the patients had toxic deaths related to the transplantation itself. Although the number of patients in their study is small, this is a highly skilled transplant group, and its experience suggests that patients with advanced, progressive cisplatin-resistant disease are unlikely to benefit greatly from transplantation. Future studies will likely address more responsive populations, including untreated patients with advanced disease with poor prognostic features and those patients who are in complete remission but are at high risk for relapse. At the present time, there is no role for bone marrow transplantation in ovarian cancer outside the context of a clinical trial.—R.C. Young, M.D., F.A.C.P.

Complications

Low-Dose Amphotericin B Prophylaxis Against Invasive *Aspergillus* Infections in Allogeneic Marrow Transplantation

Rousey SR, Russler S, Gottlieb M, Ash RC (Med College of Wisconsin, Milwaukee)

Am J Med 91:484–492, 1991 5–6

Background.—Patients who undergo bone marrow transplantation (BMT) have many opportunistic infections, (e.g., recurrent *Aspergillus* blood infections). Because invasive aspergillosis has remained intractable to treatment, prophylactic antifungal therapy is being investigated. The use of low-dose intravenously administered amphotericin B prophylactically in patients undergoing BMT was studied.

Methods.—The subjects selected to receive prophylactic amphotericin B included 186 consecutive patients who were scheduled for allogeneic BMT. They were divided into 3 treatment cohorts: cohort 1, most patients were managed without specialized air filtration in single-bed hospital rooms; cohort 2, patients in a new BMT unit laminar airflow rooms; and cohort 3, patients in laminar airflow rooms who also received prophylactic, intravenously administered amphotericin B, 20 mg/day, on the initial day of pretransplant preparation and until the surgery. The amphotericin dose was then administered every other day—but not on the day cyclosporine was given. Administration of amphotericin B decreased if the patients showed signs of renal or hepatic side effects.

Results.—Those patients receiving amphotericin B had a cumulative incidence of invasive aspergillosis of 8.9% after 120 days; this was signif-

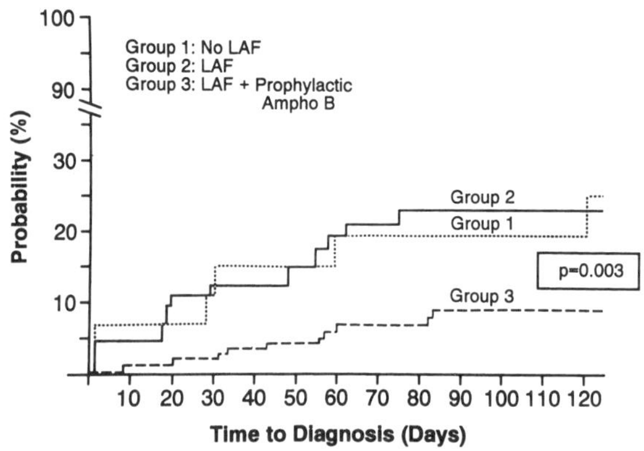

Fig 5–2.—The incidence of invasive aspergillosis according to prophylaxis group. The curves show the cumulative probability and time of diagnosis of treatment-associated aspergillosis. The patients were censored from analysis at the time of relapse or of death from transplant-related causes other than aspergillosis. There was no difference in the incidence of aspergillosis between groups 1 and 2 (P = .95). The incidence of aspergillosis in group 3 (amphotericin B chemoprophylaxis) was statistically different from that in groups 1 and 2 (no chemoprophylaxis) by global test of significance (P for trend = .01) and by pairwise comparison (P = .003). (Courtesy of Rousey SR, Russler S, Gottlieb M, et al: *Am J Med* 91:484–492, 1991.)

icantly less than the incidence of infection in groups 1 and 2, where was 24.7% and 23.2% respectively (Fig 5–2). Group 3 showed a significantly lower hepatic dysfunction and a significantly higher exposure to vancomycin than the other 2 patient groups. All patient groups demonstrated a significant overall decrease in transplant-associated deaths over time, with the lowest rate occurring in group 3. Patients given amphotericin B also had a significantly lower mortality rate associated with cytomegalovirus.

Conclusions.—The incidence of the invasive *Aspergillus* infections can respond to amphotericin B prophylaxis if the drug is administered before and during the immediate transplant surgical period.

▶ This study from the bone marrow transplant program at the Medical College of Wisconsin sought to reduce the incidence of invasive fungal infections (particularly *Aspergillus)* with the use of low-dose amphotericin B prophylaxis. Using a dose of amphotericin B, 20 mg, given intravenously from the first day of transplant-conditioning chemotherapy and continued at 20 mg every other day throughout the posttransplant period. these authors were able to demonstrate a decrease in *Aspergillus*-associated mortality compared with 2 previously managed groups. Although these trials were sequential, nonrandomized, and included different numbers of patients in each group, the authors' study does suggest that laminar airflow filtration and high-efficiency particulate air-filtered transplant facilities do not reduce the incidence of this serious complication (Fig 5–2). Because of the sequential nature of the trial, one cannot conclude that this prophylaxis is responsible for the significant reduction in overall mortality experienced by the patients who received prophylaxis in the transplant facility. It is noteworthy that the prophylactic amphotericin schedule used in their study was not associated with increased renal or hepatic dysfunction compared with other bone marrow transplant populations.—R.C. Young, M.D., F.A.C.P.

Recombinant Granulocyte-Macrophage Colony-Stimulating Factor After Autologous Bone Marrow Transplantation for Lymphoid Cancer

Nemunaitis J, Rabinow SN, Singer JW, Bierman PJ, Vose JM, Freedman AS, Onetto N, Gillis S, Oette D, Gold M, Buckner CD, Hansen JA, Ritz J, Appelbaum FR, Armitage JO, Nadler LM (Univ of Washington, Seattle; Immunex Corp, Seattle; Dana-Farber Cancer Inst, Boston; Univ of Nebraska, Omaha; Hoescht-Roussel Pharmaceuticals, Somerville, NJ)

N Engl J Med 324:1773, 1991. 5–7

Background.—Previous phase I–II clinical trials demonstrated that recombinant human granulocyte-macrophage colony-stimulating factor (rhGM-CSF) could accelerate neutrophil recovery after autologous bone marrow transplantation. Whether the effects of rhGM-CSF were clinically significant was evaluated in a randomized, double-blind study at 3 institutions.

Methods.—A group of 128 patients was randomized to receive rhGM-CSF, 250 μg/m^2 given in a 2-hour infusino daily for 21 days, starting within 4 hours after marrow infusion or placebo. Sixty-five patients received rhGM-CSF, and 63 were treated with placebo. The time to recover a neutrophil count of 500×10^6/L, infections, number of days antibiotics were administered, toxicity, and days of hospitalization were measured. All the patients had lymphoma and were treated with high-dose chemotherapy previously demonstrated to require autologous marrow support.

Results.—Toxicity from rhGM-CSF was minimal. However, patients receiving rhGM-CSF had recovery of neutrophils 7 days earlier, had fewer infections, were given antibiotics an average of 3 days less, and were hospitalized 6 days less than patients receiving placebo. Survival was comparable on the 2 arms.

Conclusion.—It appears that rhGM-CSF significantly reduces the morbidity of high-dose therapy with autologous bone marrow transplantation in patient with lymphoma.

▶ Both rhGM-CSF and granulocyte colony-stimulating factor (G-CSF) can speed the recovery of neutrophils after myelotoxic therapy. Most studies have suggested that G-CSF may be somewhat less toxic than rhGM-CSF because it produces less fever and myalgia. Both have been used in patients with aplastic anemia and myelodysplastic syndromes. The response to therapy has been heterogeneous. In many patients, the neutrophil counts increase while the patient is receiving therapy, but there are no lasting effects after therapy is stopped (1, 2). In some patients, the blast counts have been said to increase with the use of rhGM-CSF (3); in others, the blast counts have been said to decrease (2). However, most data on G-CSF suggest that brief exposures to therapy result in blast cell counts either decreasing or remaining stable (1, 4). However, blast cell counts can increase when chronic therapy with G-CSF is given (5).

There is also some indication that rhGM-CSF alone may permit certain patients to be treated with high-dose chemotherapy without autologous marrow reinfusion (6). However, there is no convincing evidence that rhGM-CSF or G-CSF can exert stimulatory effects on the platelets. There are a variety of factors in various stages of clinical development that may stimulate platelets: IL-1α, IL-1β, IL-6, and stem cell factor (or kit ligand) are all candidates.

Once it is possible to ameliorate both neutrophil and platelet toxicity, it is very important to evaluate whether the use of colony-stimulating factors will permit the dose escalation of chemotherapy regimens, i.e., to augment the maximum-tolerated doses. It will then be critical to determine whether higher doses are more effective cancer treatments.—D.L. Longo, M.D., F.A.C.P

References

1. Yoshida Y, et al: *Br J Haematol* 78:378, 1991.
2. Antin JH, et al: *Blood* 72:705, 1988.
3. Ganser A, et al: *Blood* 73:31, 1989.
4. Negrin RS, et al: *Ann Intern Med* 110:976, 1989.
5. Negrin RS, et al: *Blood* 76:36, 1990.
6. Laporte JP, et al: *Lancet* 338:601, 1991.

Clinical Features and Analysis of Risk Factors for Invasive Candidal Infection After Marrow Transplantation

Goodrich JM, Reed EC, Mori M, Fisher L, Skerrett S, Dandliker PS, Klis B, Counts GW, Meyers JD (Univ of Washington)

J Infect Dis 164:731–740, 1991 5–8

Background.—Invasive candidal infections remain a major cause of morbidity in the immunocompromised patient; however, the incidence of these infections has not been clearly determined because of the difficulty in defining the disease. The clinical features and risk factors for severe candidal disease were evaluated in patients with bone marrow transplants. Also, which subpopulation would best benefit from prophylactic antifungal drug treatment was determined.

Methods.—Patients undergoing an initial bone marrow transplant comprised the study population. The time of observation included 2 weeks before the transplant until 100 days after the procedure. Candidal infection was indicated by a positive culture result from a previously sterile location. Survival or death, including death from fungemia, was recorded and analyzed.

Results.—A total of 171 of the 1,506 patients who underwent transplantation had invasive candidal infections after the procedure, and 102 patients had 104 episodes of fungemia, representing 6.8% of the study population. Of these 102 patients, 46 showed positive blood cultures without tissue invasion, whereas 59 had infections at both sites. Of the 125 patients with tissue-invasive infections, 69 did not have fungemia. The median time between surgery and detection of the candidal or fungemia infection was 15 days. Those patients who had fungemia without tissue infection had a death rate of 39%, but those who had fungemia with tissue disease had a death rate of 88%. Patients with an autograft had less of a chance of contracting invasive candidal infections. The risk factors for these infections included a mismatched allograft donor, older age, acute myelogenous leukemia, and acute graft-vs.-host disease. Death from fungemia was associated with being female, increased irradiation conditioning, and transplant for acute lymphocytic leukemia.

Conclusions.—Patients with bone marrow transplants who have a greater risk for fungal infections include older patients, females, and those undergoing bone marrow transplantation for acute lymphocytic leukemia. These individuals may have a major benefit from prophylactic antifungal or empiric drug therapy.

▶ This analysis of the extensive transplantation experience of the Seattle group documents an 11% incidence of invasive candial infection and a high mortality (39%) resulting from this infection. The incidence of *Candida* infections increased over time and was related in part to more intensive conditioning regimens. Increased infections were seen in patients with acute graft-vs.-host disease, donor mismatches, and increasing age. Invasive candidal infections also were more frequently seen in patients who had transplantation for malignancy rather than for aplastic anemia.—R.C. Young, M.D., F.A.C.P.

Mesna Versus Hyperhydration for the Prevention of Cyclophosphamide-Induced Hemorrhagic Cystitis in Bone Marrow Transplantation

Shepherd JD, Pringle LE, Barnett MJ, Klingemann H-G, Reece DE, Phillips GL (Vancouver Gen Hosp; Univ of British Columbia, Vancouver, Canada)

J Clin Oncol 9:2016–2020, 1991 5–9

Background.—Patients who receive high-dose cyclophosphamide therapy as preparation for allogeneic or autologous bone marrow transplantation have a high incidence of hemorrhagic cystitis. This has most often been addressed by forced diuresis, but some studies have suggested that the sulfhydryl-containing compound mesna might be superior. However, in prior studies, questions about the effects of mesna on marrow engraftment were raised. The efficacy of these 2 techniques in preventing hemorrhagic cystitis was compared, and the effects of mesna on engraftment kinetics were studied.

Methods.—The subjects were 100 consecutive patients undergoing bone marrow transplantation using cyclophosphamide, 120 mg/kg or more. Each patient also was receiving at least 1 other marrow ablative and an immunosuppressive regimen to minimize the likelihood of graft rejection. The patients were randomized to receive either mesna, at 160% of the daily cyclophosphamide dose (divided into 4 doses), or hyperhydration, at least 3 L of fluid/m^2/day. Microscopic and dipstick urinalyses were monitored, and the effects of therapy on engraftment were assessed.

Results.—A total of 33% of the mesna group had consistent or severe hematuria, compared with 20% in the hyperhydration group; the difference was not significant. Severe hemorrhagic cystitis developed in 12.5% and 7.5%, respectively; this was also an insignificant difference. The median times to achieving a neutrophil count of more than $.5 \times 10^9$/L were 20 days in the mesna group and 21 days in the hyperhydration group; no patient had primary graft rejection. Also, there were no unexpected toxic effects.

Conclusions.—Mesna and hyperhydration appears to be equally effective in preventing hemorrhagic cystitis in those patients undergoing bone marrow transplantation and receiving preparative high-dose cyclophosphamide. Mesna does not appear to increase the rate of graft failure in patients undergoing allogeneic transplantation. Which preventive therapy to use will depend on cost, nursing time, and concerns about fluid overload.

▶ High-dose cyclophosphamide plus total body radiation is a tried and true preparative regimen; however, the cyclophosphamide can lead to acute hemorrhagic cystitis that may require cystectomy to control, and even if the acute inflammation heals, the patient remains at risk of bladder cancer developing. The toxic moiety is acrolein, 1 of the products of cyclophosphamide metabolism. Mesna is an investigational agent that contains a sulfhydryl group that is capable of detoxifying acrolein. It is effective in preventing or ameliorating much of the hemorrhagic cystitis; however, there has been concern that it might be capable of inhibiting engraftment. This study found that there are no obvious differences between means and vigorous hydration in the prevention of hemorrhagic cystitis, and that there is no evidence that mesna inhibits marrow engraftment.—D.L. Longo, M.D., F.A.C.P.

Anti-B-Cell Monoclonal Antibodies in the Treatment of Severe B-Cell Lymphoproliferative Syndrome Following Bone Marrow and Organ Transplantation

Fischer A, Blanche S, Le Bidois J, Bordigoni P, Garnier JL, Niaudet P, Morinet F, Le Deist F, Fischer A-M, Griscelli C, Hirn M (Hôpital des Enfants-Malades, Paris; Centre Hospitalier Régional, Nancy, France; Hôpital E Herriat, Lyons, France; Hôpital Saint-Louis, Paris; Immunotech, Marseilles, France)

N Eng J Med 324:1451–1456, 1991 5–10

Introduction.—The B-cell lymphoproliferative syndrome can cause life-threatening complications that are the consequence of profound immunosuppression in patients undergoing marrow or organ transplantation. The results of an open, multicenter, prospective trial of CD21 and CD24 monoclonal antibodies in the treatment of 26 patients with this syndrome after organ or marrow transplantation were evaluated.

Methods.—The B-cell–specific antibodies included ALB9, a mouse IgG1 specific for CD24, and BL13, a mouse IgG1 specific for CD21. Both were infused for 4–6 hours every day for 10 days at a dose of .2 mg of antibody per kg of body weight.

Findings.–Three patients had a grade 2 fever, 2 had pain, and 1 had vomiting, diarrhea, and thrombocytopenia from the monoclonal antibody infusion. No patient produced antibodies against the mouse immunoglobulins during the study period. The B cells were not detectable in the serum of the 18 patients analyzed. Some patients had received antiviral drugs during the study. The anti–B-cell antibodies produced a complete remission in 16 of the 26 patients receiving treatment in 15–45 days (median, 21 days). The complete remission occurred only in those individuals with oligoclonial B-cell lymphoproliferative syndrome, and all patients with the monoclonal B-cell lymphoproliferative syndrome died within 38 days of beginning therapy. Of the 15 patients in complete remission who were evaluated, CD21 and CD24 expression occurred on the proliferative B cells in 10 and CD21 or CD24 expression occurred in 5 patients. Of the 16 patients in complete remission, 2 marrow-transplant recipients had a relapse.

Conclusions.—The intravenous administration of the anti–B-cell antibodies can somewhat control the oligoclonal B-cell proliferation of cells, as long as the CNS is not involved. A randomized, controlled trial is recommended to further test anti–B-cell antibodies as a treatment for the B-cell lymphoproliferative syndrome.

▶ The B-cell lymphoproliferative disorders that occur after marrow or organ transplantation or iatrogenic immunosuppression are rare (risk ranges from .5% to 5%), and they generally are 1 of 2 types: oligoclonal proliferations or monoclonal lymphomas. Epstein-Barr virus is thought to be the etiologic agent. The durable complete responses with anti–B-cell monoclonal antibodies are surprising in view of the aggressive clinical course that these lymphoproliferative disorders may take. The oligoclonal proliferations appear to respond to therapy; whereas the monoclonal proliferations are refractory to therapy. If this small experience is confirmed, then oligoclonal B-cell lymphoproliferative disorders induced by Epstein-Barr virus would become rare diseases on the list of afflictions for which a biological agent is the treatment of choice.

A potential difficulty in applying the results of this study in the United States may be the regulatory issues related to the combined use of 2 monoclonal antibodies in these patients. It is not clear whether the United States Food and Drug Administration would require the use of each agent alone before permitting the use of the combination. In light of the paucity of cases seen in any 1 center, it may be unlikely that investigators in the United States would be willing to take on the task of verifying the results.—D.L. Longo, M.D., F.A.C.P.

Graft-vs.-Host Disease

T-Cell Depletion of HLA-Identical Transplants in Leukemia

Marmont AM, Horowitz MM, Gale RP, Sobocinski K, Ash RC, van Bekkum DW, Champlin RE, Dicke KA, Goldman JM, Good RA, Herzig RH, Hong R, Masaoka T, Rimm AA, Ringdén O, Speck B, Weiner RS, Bortin MM (Med College of Wisconsin, Milwaukee; Ospedale San Martino, Genoa, Italy; Univ of California at Los Angeles; Radiobiological Inst TNO, The Netherlands; MD Anderson Cancer Ctr, Houston, et la)

Blood 78:2120–2130, 1991 5–11

Background.—Acute and chronic graft-vs.-host disease (GVHD) decreases leukemia relapse and contributes to the antileukemia efficacy of allogeneic transplants. Despite this beneficial effect, GVHD is a major cause of morbidity and mortality after allogeneic bone marrow transplants. Removing T cells from donor bone marrow has been proposed as a means of preventing GVHD in humans. The effects of T-cell depletion on the outcome of HLA-identical sibling bone marrow transplants for leukemia were analyzed. The controllable variables influencing the outcome of T-cell–depleted transplants were also studied.

Patients.—The outcome of 731 T-cell–depleted HLA-identical sibling bone marrow transplants for leukemia was compared with that of 2,480 non-T-cell–depleted transplants. The patients receiving T-cell–depleted transplants were treated for acute lymphoblastic leukemia, acute myelogenous leukemia, and chronic myelogenous leukemia. The controls

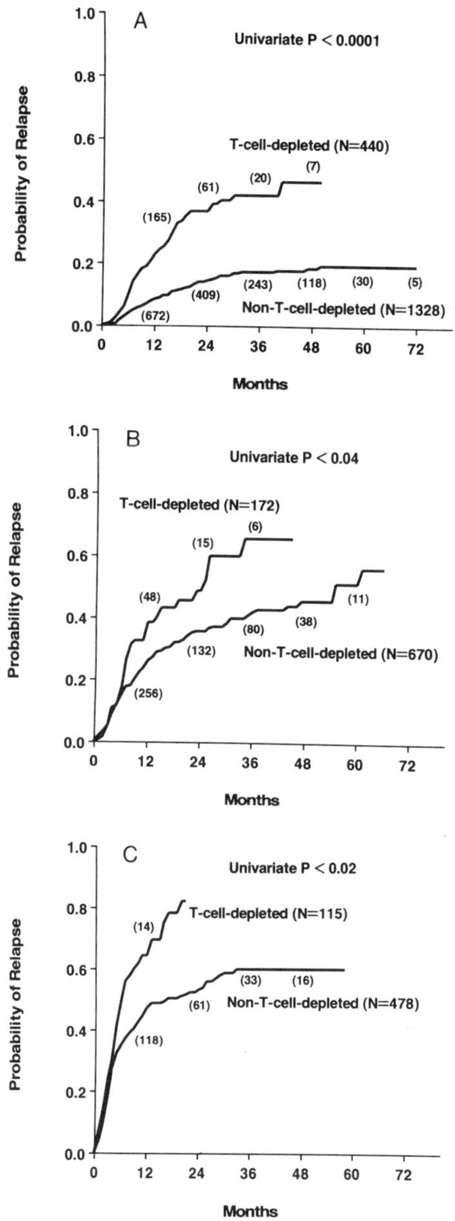

Fig 5–3.—Unadjusted probability of relapse after non–T-cell–depleted and T-cell–depleted HLA-identical sibling transplants for early (**A**), intermediate (**B**), and advanced (**C**) leukemia. The *numbers in parentheses* indicate the numbers of patients remaining at risk (alive in remission) at yearly intervals. (Courtesy of Marmont AM, Horowitz MM, Gale RP, et al: *Blood* 78:2120–2130, 1991.)

received non-T-cell–depleted transplants posttransplant immune suppression with cyclosporine and/or methotrexate to prevent GVHD.

Findings.—The T-cell depletion decreased GVHD, but it increased graft failure and leukemia relapse (Fig 5–3). Leukemia-free survival was not improved by T-cell depletion and was decreased in some settings. Among recipients of T-cell–depleted transplants for early leukemia, higher doses and dose rates of radiation, avoidance of fractionation, physical techniques of T-cell depletion, and posttransplant immune suppression with cyclosporine were associated with fewer treatment failures.

Conclusions.—The T-cell depletion in HLA-identical sibling bone marrow transplants for leukemia decreases GVHD but increases graft failure and leukemia relapse. By selecting subjects who are at greatest risk for GVHD and optimizing the controllable variables, outcome of T-cell–depleted transplants may be improved.

▶ Graft-vs.-lyphoma effects are probably similar in magnitude to graft-vs.-leukemia effects. In 1 series of lymphoma patients, relapse of Hodgkin's disease or lymphoma was half as likely in patients receiving allogeneic transplants than in those receiving autologous transplants with similar pretransplant therapy (1). The major question is whether the graft-vs.-tumor effects are separable from the effects of GVHD. In general, the advantage in disease-free survival associated with allogeneic tranpslants is counteracted by morbidity and mortality related to chronic GVHD.—D.L. Longo, M.D., F.A.C.P.

Reference

1. Jones RJ, et al: *Blood* 77:649, 1991.

Increased Risk of Leukemia Relapse With High-Dose Cyclosporine A After Allogeneic Marrow Transplantation for Acute Leukemia

Bacigalupo A, Van Lint MT, Occhini D, Gualandi F, Lamparelli T, Sogno G, Tedone E, Frassoni F, Tong J, Marmont AM (Ospedale San Martino, Genoa, Italy)

Blood 77:1423–1428, 1991 5–12

Background.—Currently, the most widely used agent for prophylaxis of graft-vs.-host disease (GVHD) after allogeneic bone marrow transplantation (BMT) is cyclosporine A (CyA). Two different doses of intravenous CyA were compared in patients with acute leukemia receiving matched allogeneic marrow transplants.

Study Design.—Forty-four patients (aged 10–50 years) with acute myeloid leukemia and 37 with acute lymphoblastic leukemia were randomly assigned to receive CyA, 1 mg/kg/day or 5 mg/kg/day, from day −1 to +20 after BMT. Thereafter, all patients took CyA orally. The patients were prepared with cyclophosphamide, 120 mg/kg, and fractionated total body irradiation (TBI), and all received unfractionated bone marrow from an HLA-identical sibling.

Results.—The media follow-up for survivors in the first group was 983

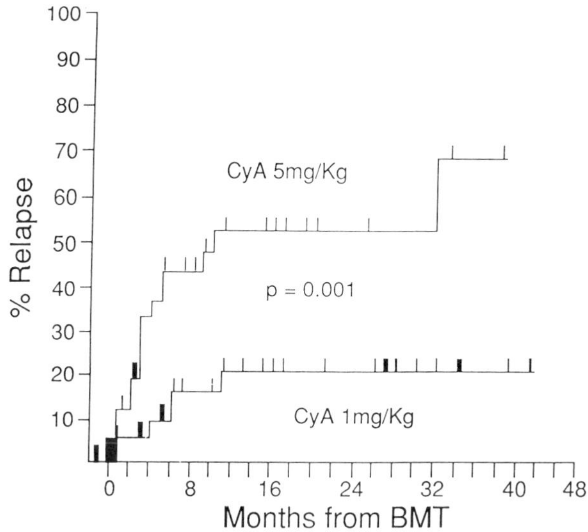

Fig 5–4.—The actuarial risk of leukemia relapse for all patients randomized: patients receiving CyA, 5 mg/kg/day, had a significantly higher risk of relapse (P = .001). (Courtesy of Bacigalupo A, Van Lint MT, Occhini D, et al: *Blood* 77:1423–1428, 1991.)

days; for survivors on the second group, it was 632 days. The patients in the first group had lower serum levels of CyA, lower bilirubin levels, lower creatinine levels, and a lower proportion of CD8+ cells in peripheral blood within 21 days. First day to .5 × 10^9/L neutrophils in the 2 groups were comparable. According to a Cox model, the actuarial risk of GVHD grade II+, after stratification for age, was significantly lower in patients in the second group. Patients in both groups had a comparable actuarial risk of chronic GVHD developing. Actuarial transplant-related mortality at 1,240 days was 28% in the first group and 26% in the second group. The major cause of death was GVHD in group 1 and multiorgan toxicity in group 2. Overall, the actuarial risk of relapse at 2 years was 20% and 52% in groups 1 and 2, respectively. This risk was 9% and 43% in the 2 groups, respectively, for patients in their first remission; it was 48% and 63%, respectively, for those in a latter complete remission. The actuarial 2-year disease-free survival overall in groups 1 and 2 was 58% and 32%, respectively: 71% and 35% in first remissions, and 30% and 23% in advanced disease (Fig 5–4).

Conclusions.—Protection from GVHD-related death with high-dose CyA is offset by significant organ toxicity and leukemia relapse. Long-term disease-free survival is clearly better in patients given low doses of CyA after CY and fractionated TBI.

▶ This study does not offer much encouragement that graft-vs.-tumor effects are separable from the effects of GVHD. When therapy for GVHD is improved, the tumor relapse rate increases. The precise natures of the GVHD and the graft-vs.-tumor reaction are not known. Because the donor and the host are matched at the major histocompatibility complex loci, the differences in minor histocompatibility antigens are thought to be important. The group in Seattle observed that HLA-matched, mixed-lymphocyte, culture-compatible, unrelated donor transplants were complicated by grade II–IV acute GVHD twice as frequently as HLA-identical sibling donor transplants (1). The increased incidence and severity of GVHD were not associated with an improved antitumor effect in the Seattle series. Only approximately 40% of the patients who might benefit from a transplant have a sibling matched donor; therefore, the study of unrelated donors and the determinants of success or failure in this setting are very important.

Weisdorf and colleages (2) examined the risk factors for acute GVHD in 469 patients who were given histocompatible sibling marrow. The overall incidence was 46%; patients older than 18 years of age were twice as likely to develop GVHD (63% vs. 27%). Graft-vs.-host disease was less frequent in female-to-female transplants and was more frequent in patients seropositive for cytomegalovirus and in those who had received alloimmunization in the form of prior pregnancy or transfusion. The patients who expressed HLA-A26 had a higher incidence of GVHD, and those whose expressed HLA-DR3 had a lower incidence.

Like other problems occurring in transplant patients, prophylaxis is more effective than treatment. At Seattle, Martin and colleagues have reviewed their considerable experience in both the primary (3) and secondary (4) treatment of acute GVHD. Primary therapy was more effective in those patients who had undergone prophylaxis with cyclosporine and methotrexate. Steroids and cyclosporine were the most effective primary therapy and were superior to antithymocyte globulin. The severity of GVHD and the presence of a liver complication other than GVHD were poor prognostic factors for both primary and secondary treatment. In the setting of an exacerbation of GVHD in the face of tapering steroids, dose escalation of the steroids was the most effective therapy. Other patients who failed primary therapy responded poorly to secondary therapy.

An approach to prophylaxis that appears to lessen the degree of hepatic dysfunction is the use of half the usual dose of cyclosporine. Stockschlaeder et al. (5) showed that the lower dose of cyclosporine (1.5 mg/kg/day rather than the usual 3 mg/kg/day) in the first 2 weeks after transplantation did not increase the risk of acute GVHD, but it was associated with reduced bilirubin values during the first month after transplantation. Survival was not adversely affected by the lower dose when the study patients were compared with a matched cohort of historical controls.

One strategy for preventing GVHD has been to deplete the T cells from the donor bone marrow. This has been accomplished in a variety of ways, including with antibodies and complement (6) or immunotoxins (7), or by using physical separation methods such as elutriation (8). Such techniques do appear to reduce the severity of GVHD, but there are also increased problems with failure to engraft, higher rates of tumor relapse, and increased incidence of secondary lymphoma induced by Epstein-Barr virus.—D.L. Longo, M.D., F.A.C.P.

References

1. Beatty PG, et al: *Transplantation* 51:443, 1991.
2. Weisdorf D, et al: *Transplantation* 51:1197, 1991.

3. Martin PJ, et al: *Blood* 76:1464, 1990.
4. Martin PJ, et al: *Blood* 77:1821, 1991.
5. Stockschlaeder M, et al: *Br J Haematol* 80:49, 1992.
6. Antin JH, et al: *Blood* 78:2139, 1991.
7. Filipovich AH, et al: *Transplantation* 50:410, 1990.
8. Wagner JE, et al: *Blood* 75:1370, 1990.

Phase I–II Trial of Pentoxifylline for the Prevention of Transplant-Related Toxicities Following Bone Marrow Transplantation

Bianco JA, Appelbaum FR, Nemunaitis J, Almgren J, Andrews F, Kettner P, Shields A, Singer JW (Univ of Washington, Seattle)

Blood 78:1205–1211, 1991 5–13

Background.—The usefulness of bone marrow transplantation (BMT) in the treatment of hematologic malignancies has been limited by disease relapse and transplant-related toxicity. Previous reports have shown a correlation between elevated levels of tumor necrosis factor-α (TNF-α) and the development of transplant-related complications. The xanthine derivative pentoxyfylline (PTX), which inhibits TNF-α production, was evaluated in patients undergoing BMT for hematologic malignancies.

Methods.—The subjects were 30 consecutive patients with hematologic malignancy (median age, 34 years). Twenty-six patients received an allogeneic graft, and 4 received an autologous graft. Pentoxifylline, which can down-regulate production of TNF-α, was given at doses of 1,200, 1,600, and 2,000 mg/day orally in 3, 4, and 5 divided daily doses. The patients were enrolled in groups of 10 at increasing dose levels, from 10 days before to 100 days after BMT. They were evaluated along with a control group of "good-risk" patients.

Results.—There were no significant adverse effects of PTX at any dose level. Overall, the 100-day actuarial survival was 90%. Mucositis lasted a mean of 3.7 days in the PTX-treated patients compared with 18.7 days in the controls. Ten percent of the PTX group had hepatic veno-occlusive disease compared with 65% of the controls; only 3% of the PTX group had renal insufficiency, compared with 65% of the controls. Pentoxifylline-treated patients also required fewer days of total parenteral nutrition and were discharged from the hospital earlier than the controls. Of the PTX group, 35% had graft-vs.-host disease of grade II or worse compared with 68% of controls. At the 2 higher dose levels, there were further reductions in severity of mucositis and nutrition requirements and therefore, a further reduction in the need for hospitalization.

Conclusions.—In patients receiving BMT for hematologic malignancies, orally administered PTX, as much as 2,000 mg/day, is well tolerated and reduces morbidity and mortality. When used alone or in combination with cytokines, PTX may allow delivery of higher doses of chemoradiotherapy. Prospective, randomized trials are underway.

▶ It is increasingly clear that many of the manifestations of graft-vs.-host disease (GVHD) are mediated by TNF. This trial with PTX showed impressive effects in lowering the incidence of mucositis, veno-occlusive disease of the liver, renal failure, and GVHD. In Seattle, another subgroup of patients receiving the nephrotoxic drugs amphotericin B and cyclosporine also had improved renal dysfunction after receiving PTX, probably because of its effects on the blood vessels (1). The use of PTX promises to further improve the outcome of allogeneic transplantation.

A variety of immunosuppressive agents are being developed for the prevention and treatment of GVHD, and most are more specific in their mechanism of action than the nonspecific immunosuppressive agents that are currently being used (steroids, methotrexate, and cyclosporine). Animal studies have suggested that interleukin-1 receptor antagonists may be therapeutic (2). Antibodies to TNF have been piloted in patients with good success. Thalidomide, an old agent now being put to new uses, also antagonizes TNF action and has a number of other effects. It has been used in patients with acute GVHD (3) and in patients with chronic GVHD (4, 5) with some positive results. However, the effects of PTX appear to be impressive, and its side effects are minimal. Randomized clinical trials testing the effects of PTX are in progress.—D.L. Longo, M.D., F.A.C.P.

References

1. Bianco JA, et al: *Transplantation* 51:925, 1991.
2. McCarthy PL Jr, et al: *Blood* 78:1915, 1991.
3. Vogelsang GB, et al: *Transplantation* 41:644, 1986.
4. Heney D, et al: *Br J Haematol* 78:23, 1991.
5. Vogelsang GB, et al: *N Engl J Med* 326:1055, 1992.

Additional Reading

Martin PJ, Schoch F, Fisher L, et al: A retrospective analysis of therapy for acute graft-vs-host disease: Secondary treatment. *Blood* 77:1821–1828, 1991.

▶ A careful review of the extensive experience at the University of Washington, in which the factors contributing to the success or failure of salvage therapy of acute graft-vs.-host disease are outlined.

Weisdorf D, Hakke R, Blazar B, et al: Risk factors for acute graft-vs-host disease in histocompatible donor bone marrow transplantation. *Transplantation* 51:1197–1203, 1991.

▶ This is both an analysis of factors contributing to acute graft-vs.-host disease in 469 patients and an identification of HLA-A26 as a high-risk factor and HLA-DR3 as a low-risk factor for the disease. Age older than 18 years is also a serious contributor to the appearance of acute graft-vs.-host disease.

Beatty PG, Hansen JA, Longton GM, et al: Marrow transplantation from HLA-matched unrelated donors for treatment of hematologic malignancies. *Transplantation* 51:443–447, 1991.

▶ Graft-vs.-host disease is more frequent and more severe in unrelated donors, but it is not so common or fatal that patients without sibling donors should be denied the potential therapeutic benefit of high-dose therapy and allogeneic transplantation.

Rabinowe SN, Soiffer RJ, Tarbell NJ, et al: Hemolytic-uremic syndrome following bone marrow transplantation in adults for hematologic malignancies. *Blood* 77:1837–1844, 1991.

▶ Sixteen of 168 patients had a sudden decrease in hematocrit and an increase in serum creatinine between 3 and 11 months after bone marrow transplantation. In twelve patients, heart failure, peripheral edema or hypertension developed, but none of the patients have died.

Clay TM, Bidwell JL, Howard MR, Bradley BA: PCR-fingerprinting for selection of HLA matched unrelated marrow donors. *Lancet* 337:1049–1052, 1991.

▶ Despite serologic typing suggesting identity, clinical experience identifies a substantial incidence of graft-vs.-host disease among recipients of unrelated donor marrow; PCR fingerprinting identified 11 of 53 mismatches not found by restriction fragment-length polymorphism, all of which were related to subtypes of DR4.

Agah R, Charak BS, Chen V, Mazumder A: Adoptive transfer of anti-cytomegalovirus effect of interleukin-2-activated bone marrow: Potential application in transplantation. *Blood* 78:720–727, 1991.

▶ In mice infected with murine cytomegalovirus, the adoptive transfer of interleukin-2+–activated bone marrow exerted a significant antiviral effect in the adoptive recipient. It is possible that the donor graft could be manipulated to help control cytomegalovirus infection in humans.

6 Breast Cancer

Early Detection and Risk Factors

Comparison of Breast Carcinomas Diagnosed in the 1980s With Those Diagnosed in the 1940s to 1960s
Joensuu H, Toikkanen S (Univ Central Hosp of Turku, Turku, Finland)
Br Med J 303:155–158, 1991 6–1

Objective.—According to available statistics, the incidence of breast cancer is increasing, and the survival is improving. These trends may result from earlier detection, improved treatment, or less aggressive tumor behavior. To examine the trends in these prognostic factors, 439 patients with breast cancer diagnosed in 1945–1965, and 370 patients with breast cancer diagnosed in 1980 to 1984 in Turku, Finland, were evaluated in a retrospective comparative cohort study.

Findings.—The age-adjusted incidence of breast cancer increased from approximately 31/100,000 person-years in 1953–1957 to 62/100,000 person-years in 1983–1983. Breast cancer mortality increased from 16.7/100,100 to 17.2/100,000 person-years during the same period. The survival of patients with stage II–IV stage disease improved, whereas the survival of those with stage I disease did not improve during this time period. The average age at diagnosis increased from approximately 56 years in 1945–1955 to 63 years in 1980–1984. The proportion of patients with T0-1 carcinomas increased from 13% to 41%, and the proportion with pN0 carcinomas increased from 43% to 55%. In the 1980–1984 cohort, the carcinomas were more likely to be well differentiated, have lower mitotic counts, have less nuclear polymorphism, have a more defined tumor margin, and have less tumor necrosis, than in the earlier cohort. There was no difference in these variables between the 2 cohorts when tumors of the same size were compared.

Conclusion.—Improved breast cancer survival can be explained at least in part by early detection of increased numbers of small carcinomas with favorable histologic characteristics.

▶ A conscientious effort to detect early breast cancer can make a difference in the mortality of the disease.—D.L. Longo, M.D., F.A.C.P.

Indium-111-Labeled B72.3 Monoclonal Antibody in the Detection and Staging of Breast Cancer: A Phase I Study
Lamki LM, Buzdar AU, Singletary SE, Rosenblum MG, Bhadkamkar V, Esparza L, Podoloff DA, Zukiwski A, Hortobagyi GN, Murray JL (Univ of Texas, Houston)
J Nucl Med 32:1326–1332, 1991 6–2

Objective.—Sixteen patients with biopsy-proved, operable breast cancer underwent imaging studies before mastectomy by using the pancarcinoma monoclonal antibody B72.3. This antibody is an IgG_1 molecule directed against tumor-associated glycoprotein (TAG-72).

Methods.—A dose of 5 mCi of ^{111}In was used to label .2 mg, 2 mg, or 20 mg of antibody by using the site-directed bifunctional diethylenetriaminepentaacetic acid method. Digital, planar, and single photon emission computed tomography images were acquired after 2, 48, 72, and 96 hours whenever possible. Human antimurine antibody (HAMA) responses were estimated at 1, 3, and 6 weeks after infusion of monoclonal antibody.

Results.—All 14 known primary breast lesions were imaged; 2 fibrocystic lesions were negative. Nodal metastases went undetected by scintigraphy in all 7 patients who were affected. A maximum of .004% of the injected dose per gram was taken up by the tumor tissue. The mean activity of tumor to normal breast tissue was 4.3. The plasma activity half-lives ranged from 33 to 41 hours. Positive HAMA tests were obtained in only 2 of 12 patients.

Discussion.—Immunoscintigraphy with ^{111}In-labeled B72.3 antibody can demonstrate primary breast cancers, but it cannot depict involved lymph nodes. It is possible that this insensitivity for cancerous nodes is side dependent.

▶ Although this is an important study, it is, unfortunately, a negative one. The investigators used the monoclonal antibody B72.3 tied with ^{111}In to investigate the detection and staging of breast cancer. The nature of the investigation was phase 1, and the amount of antibody was steadily increased. Patients with diagnosed breast cancer had their primary lesions detected with 100% sensitivity, but none of the lymph nodes (7 of 14 patients) were detected by radioimmunoscintigraphy. The HAMA responses were positive in only 17% of the patients. In the lymph nodes, there is a very low proportional uptake of the total injected isotopic dose using this antibody. Therefore, this technique does not appear to be valuable at the present time in staging axillary disease.—E. Glatstein, M.D.

Familial Breast-Ovarian Cancer Locus on Chromosome 17q12-q23

Narod SA, Feunteun J, Lynch HT, Watson P, Conway T, Lynch J, Lenoir GM (McGill Univ, Montreal; Inst Gustave Roussy, Villejuif, France; Creighton Univ, Omaha; International Agency for Research on Cancer, Lyon, France)

Lancet 338:;82–83, 1991 6–3

Background.—The main risk factor for breast cancer is a positive family history. Research has determined that early onset dominant breast cancer is linked to the D17S74 locus on the long arm of chromosome 17. Five families with a predisposition to breast and ovarian cancer were studied to confirm this result and to determine whether it extends to ovarian cancer.

Methods.—The 5 families included 64 women with ovarian or breast cancer; each family had at least 3 women with breast cancer and 2 with ovarian cancer. Linkage was analyzed using the MLINK program. Peripheral blood lymphocyte DNA was probed with CMM86, and heterogeneity was tested by calculating the log-likelihood separately under 2 hypotheses.

Result.—The largest family had a maximum lod score of 2.72 at a recombination fraction of .07; this corresponded to odds greater than 500 to 1 in favor of linkage to D17S74. Two of the other families also showed evidence of linkage; the other 2 did not.

Conclusions.—The hypothesis that a breast cancer susceptibility locus is assigned to chromosome 17q12-q23 was supported. This region is also associated with some hereditary ovarian cancers. Such mapping is important because the underlying mutations may also occur in nonfamilial cancers.

▶ The data presented in this report provide further evidence in support of the assignment of a familial bresat cancer susceptibility locus to a region on the long arm of chromosome 17 (17q). Furthermore, the findings suggest that this same chromosomal region is also associated with a proportion of hereditary ovarian cancers. Two of the 5 families examined did not show linkage to a marker locus on 17q, indicating that there is genetic heterogeneity with regard to susceptibility to ovarian cancer. Thus, there may be different predisposing genes in different families. Similarly, in breast cancer, the *p53* tumor suppressor gene (located on the short arm of chromosome 17) was recently shown to represent another tumor susceptibility locus (1).

Much work is needed to determine the identity of the predisposing gene on 17q, its role in oncogenesis, and whether the mutations that underlie familial disease may also play a critical role in sporadic breast or ovarian carcinoma. Interestingly, the prohibitin gene (a candidate tumor suppressor gene) has been mapped to the same region of 17q where the familial breast-ovarian cancer gene is located (2); mutations of the prohibitin gene were found in 4 of 23 sporadic breast cancers that either showed loss of heterozygosity on 17q or developed in patients 35 years of age or younger (3). The generality of this finding remains to be determined, particularly as it might relate to familial disease.—J. Testa, Ph.D.

References

1. Malkin D, et al: *Science* 250:1233, 1990.
2. White JJ, et al: *Genomics* 11:228, 1991.
3. Sato T, et al: *Cancer Res* 52:1643, 1992.

Psychological and Behavioral Implications of Abnormal Mammograms

Lerman C, Trock B, Rimer BK, Boyce A, Jepson C, Engstrom PF (Fox Chase Cancer Ctr, Cheltenham, Pa)

Ann Inter Med 114:657–661, 1991 6–4

Introduction.—In large-scale screening programs, as many as 20% of mammograms may be interpreted as abnormal, although most of the women who receive abnormal reports do not have cancer. Thus, there is some concern that women may be reluctant to have regular mammograms because of the anxiety resulting from an initially abnormal report.

Methods.—A group of women who had undergone screening mammograms was evaluated to determine their psychological responses to abnormal findings and their subsequent willingness to continue undergoing annual mammography.

Patients.—Of the 320 women, 121 had normal mammograms, 119 had low-suspicion mammograms, and 68 had high suspicion mammograms. Patients with cancer were excluded from the study sample. The women were interviewed by telephone approximately 3 months after mammography was performed.

Results.—Anxiety about undergoing mammography was reported by 29% of the patients with low-suspicion findings, 24% of those with normal mammograms, and approximately half of those with high-suspicion findings. In addition, 17% of the women with high-suspicion findings had a degree of anxiety that compromised their ability to engage in their daily activities, despite the subsequent exclusion of malignancy. The 3 groups were similar in their rate of adherence to subsequent mammography screening (68% to 78%). Those patients who were most likely to continue to have mammograms were married women with at least a high school education who had undergone 3 or more previous mammograms.

Conclusion.—The psychological stress resulting from an abnormal mammogram does not seem to deter most women from continuing with breast cancer screening. Some concern about breast cancer might serve to heighten a woman's vigilance and motivation.

▶ We spend considerable effort encouraging women to undergo screening mammography, but we pay relatively little attention to the psychological effects of any noncancer abnormality that is detected. These investigators focused on a population of women who had suspicious mammography in which malignancy was subsequently ruled out. Almost half the women with highly suspicious mammograms reported persistent anxiety, compared with approximately 25% of those with either normal mammography or low-suspicion findings. Indeed, 17% of the women with highly suspicious mammography findings reported that their ability to engage in daily activities was compromised despite the negative biopsy findings. Although the adherence to subsequent mammography was not compromised in any of the patients in this particular study, this was a highly motivated group of individuals from a large and active health maintenance organization, and the results may not be so easily generalizable to other populations. Nevertheless, the study does emphasize the importance of continued efforts to promote psychological adjustment and ensure subsequent mammography follow-up.—R.C. Young, M.D., F.A.C.P.

Histopathology and Diagnosis

Ductal Carcinoma *In Situ* With Microinvasion: A Curable Entity Using Surgery Alone Without Need for Adjuvant Therapy

Rosner D, Lane WW, Penetrante R (Roswell Park Cancer Inst, Buffalo, NY)

Cancer 67:1498–1503, 1991 6–5

Background.—There is considerable interest in the use of systemic adjuvant therapy for patients with breast cancer and negative axillary lymph nodes. Ductal carcinoma in situ (DCIS) and DCIS with microinvasion (DCISM) are now commonly found by mammography in an asymptomatic, nonpalpable stage; DCISM may be more aggressive in nature and thus require adjuvant radiation or chemotherapy. The clinical, radiologic, and pathologic features of DCISM and their implications for treatment were studied.

Patients.—During a 12-year period, 408 patients with negative axillary node breast cancer had surgery at the Roswell Park Cancer Institute in Buffalo. Of these, 36 (8.8%) had DCISM. The diagnosis was made solely on the basis of mammographic microcalcifications and/or a radiologic density less than 1.5 cm in 20 of these women. Thirty-three women had modified radical mastectomy, and the other 3 had wide excision with or without axillary dissection. The patients were followed for a mean of 57 months.

Findings.—A total of 67% of the mastectomy specimens showed residual disease after excisional biopsy; 33% were pure DCIS, 18% were frankly invasive, and 15% were DCISM. Half the cases of residual disease and one third of all specimens were multicentric. All patients were free of cancer at follow-up.

Conclusions.—Patients with DCISM are very likely to have cancer remaining after excisional biopsy. Ductal carcinoma in situ with microinvasion appears to be wholly curable by mastectomy alone; adjuvant therapy is unnecessary, regardless of prognostic factors (e.g., tumor size, histologic differentiation, age, or steroid receptor status). There is only a small risk of axillary involvement.

▶ The proper management of DCISM has been hotly debated. Because of the high frequency of residual disease in the breast after excisional biopsy, many physicians have advocated radiation therapy or adjuvant chemo- or hormonal therapy. This retrospective analysis from the Roswell Park Cancer Institute looked at 36 patients with DCISM. The study confirms the high frequency (67%) of residual disease after excisional biopsy. Half of these were multicentric. Nevertheless, these patients were managed with modified radical mastectomy or wide excision with or without axillary node dissection. Some were given radiation therapy or chemo/hormonal treatment, and all were free of disease at 5-year follow-up. Although the study is retrospective and relatively small, it does suggest that surgery alone is a legitimate option for such patients.—R.C. Young, M.D., F.A.C.P.

Expression of the Antimetastatic Gene nm23 in Human Breast Cancer: An Association With Good Prognosis

Hennessy C, Henry JA, May FEB, Westley BR, Angus B, Lennard TWJ (Univ of Newcastle upon Tyne, England)

J Natl Cancer Inst 83:281–285, 1991 6–6

Introduction.—Tumor metastasis is the chief cause of death in patients with solid malignant tumors. The nm23 gene, which is associated with the metastatic potential of murine melanoma, also has been detected in human breast tumors. The expression of nm23 was measured in 71 patients with primary breast cancer, including 67 with ductal carcinoma. Seventeen patients were premenopausal. The state of the lymph nodes was known in 61 cases. Thirty-one tumors expressed high levels of nm23 messenger RNA, and 30 expressed low levels. High levels were found in 69% of node-negative patients and 37% of node-positive patients. The high levels were much more frequent in well-differentiated tumors. Those patients whose tumors expressed high levels of nm23 messenger RNA had longer overall and disease-free survival than did other patients. High levels of expression correlated with longer survival in patients with and without node involvement.

Discussion.–Estimates of the level of expression of nm23 may be a useful adjunct to node sampling in women with breast cancer. The biological function of the nm23 gene is not well understood. It is possible that nm23 protein helps maintain tumor-cell differentiation. Alternately, loss of nm23 expression may result in the cells having a more metastatic phenotype.

▶ The provocative information in this study suggests that the nm23 protein acts as a suppressor of metastases. Increased expression of nm23 in human breast cancer appears to be correlated inversely with the probability of metastases. However, measurement of nm23 expression in the tumor cannot replace pathologic evaluation of the axillary nodes. Of 26 patients with negative nodal status, 8 had low levels of nm23, whereas 13 of the 35 patients with positive lymph nodes had high levels of nm23 messenger RNA. It is possible that nm23 messenger RNA levels are not an independent measure of prognosis, and that larger studies with multivariate analysis are needed. These results suggest that nm23 messenger RNA measurements add additional prognostic information and may identify patients with a poorer prognosis among those who have other, more accepted favorable prognostic factors.—R.F. Ozols, M.D., Ph.D.

Flow Cytometric Analysis of DNA Ploidy and S-Phase Fraction in Breast Cancer Using Cells Obtained by *Ex Vivo* Fine-Needle Aspiration: An Optimal Method for Sample Collection

Eliasen CA, Opitz LM, Vamvakas EC, Espiritu EC, Marsh ER, Roses DF, Harris MN, Feiner HD (New York Univ, New York)

Mod Pathol 4:196–200, 1991 6–7

Objective.—Outcome in breast cancer can be predicted by DNA ploidy and the proliferative index. However, current techniques of cell preparation are labor intensive and time consuming, especially when paraffin-embedded tissue is used. Fine-needle aspiration (FNA) of excised tumors was used to produce adequate single cell suspensions with minimal preparation time.

Methods.—A group of 203 primary invasive breast cancers was sampled by ex vivo FNA at the time of surgical biopsy or mastectomy. An average of 9 passes were made using a 25-gauge needle and syringe. The aspirated cells were spun down, resuspended, and frozen for latter assay. The diploid controls consisted of similarly frozen aliquots of peripheral blood lymphocytes from patients with chronic lymphocytic leukemia. The tumors were analyzed by flow cytometry, and 1 pathologist examined all DNA histograms.

Results.—Adequate cells for analysis were obtained in 96% of the tumors. Ploidy could be determined in 174 tumors; 56% were aneuploid. Ploidy, as well as the mean and median S-phase fractions noted, were comparable to those reported in other studies using various sampling methods.

Conclusions.—Breast cancers can be sampled most easily and quickly for flow cytometric DNA analysis by ex vivo FNA. This technique minimizes preparation time and conserves tumor tissues, allowing the sampling of very small tumors. No prognostic conclusions can yet be made from the data in this study.

▶ Several studies mentioned in previous issues of the YEAR BOOK and in articles included in this edition have emphasized the importance of S-phase fraction in breast cancer prognosis. This study summarizes a novel approach to obtaining this information using samples obtained through FNA. A total of 203 primary invasive breast cancers was sampled by FNA at the time of biopsy or mastectomy; 86% yielded adequate cells for flow cytometry. Of the 174 tumors in which ploidy could be studied, 56% were aneuploid, 44% were diploid, and 11% were indeterminant. These preliminary studies suggest a relatively fast and easy way to obtain samples for flow cytometry using ex vivo FNA at the time of surgery. Although the data is intriguing, ploidy analyses done with aspirated cells has not been evaluated to determine the prognostic implications. One cannot assume that a ploidy analysis done on an aspirated cell population is similar to one more conventionally determined with a greater spectrum of cells analyzed.—R.C. Young, M.D., F.A.C.P.

Primary Management

Timing of Breast Cancer Excision During the Menstrual Cycle Influences Duration of Disease-Free Survival

Senie RT, Rosen PP, Rhodes P, Lesser ML (Ctrs for Disease Control, Atlanta; Mem Sloan-Kettering Cancer Ctr, New York; North Shore Univ Hosp-Cornell Univ Med College, Manhasset, NY)

Ann Intern Med 115:337–342, 1991 6–8

Background.—Some studies have indicated a linkage between survival after breast cancer surgery and position within the menstrual cycle. To further examine this issue, 283 premenopausal patients treated by mastectomy and axillary dissection were followed prospectively to determine the relationship between disease-free survival at 10 years and timing of excision during the menstrual cycle.

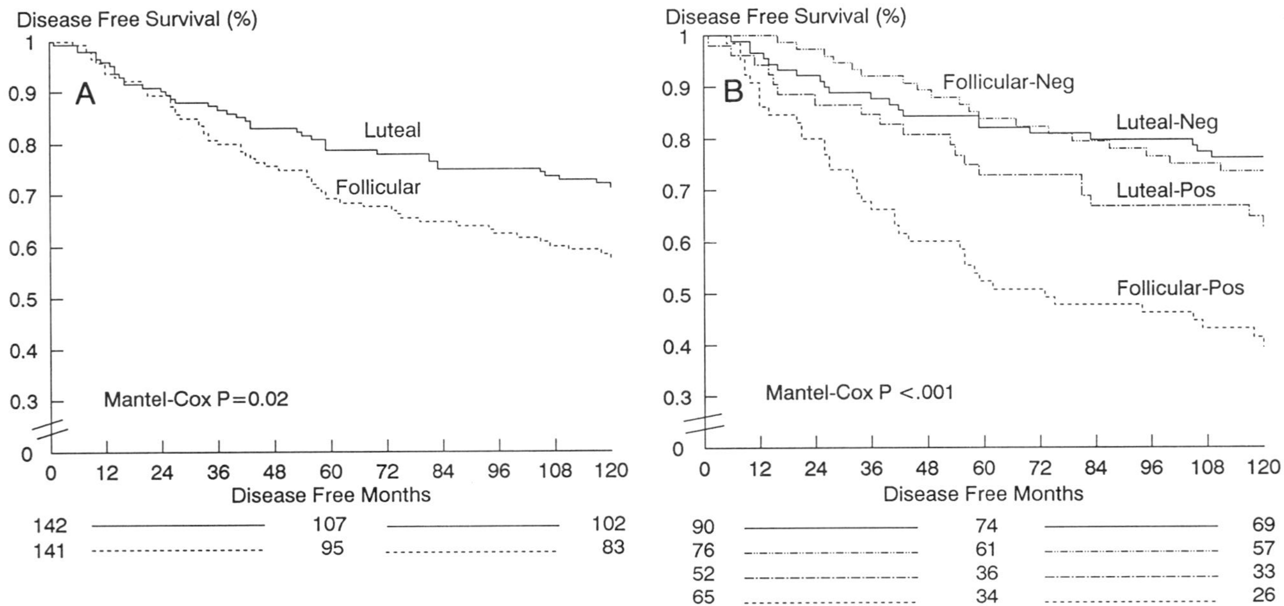

Fig 6–1.—Disease-free survival. **A,** disease-free survival according to menstrual phase at the time the tumor was excised. The number of patients at risk at time 0, at 5 years, and at 10 years is shown for each set of survival curves. Hazard ratio, 1.59 (95% confidence interval (CI), 1.06–2.38). **B,** disease-free survival according to menstrual phase and axillary lymph node status. Negative nodes: hazard ratio, 1.07 (CI, .58–1.99); $P > .2$. Positive nodes: hazard ratio, 1.97 (CI, 1.14–3.41); $P = .02$. (Courtesy of Senie RT, Rosen PP, Rhodes P, et al: *Ann Intern Med* 115:337–342, 1991.)

Results.—The day of ovulation was approximated as being day 14 after the prior menses. Using this approximation, there was a significantly higher risk of recurrence if the tumor was excised during the follicular phase. The recurrence rate was highest for surgery performed between days 7 and 14, and it was lowest for surgery performed between days 20 and 30. Cox regression analysis indicated that the hazard rate of breast cancer recurrence after follicular excision was 1.53 (Fig 6–1). This phase effect was only significant in patients with positive nodes.

Conclusions.—The risk of breast cancer recurrence after tumor excision in premenopausal women may be affected by the stage of the menstrual cycle during which the surgery is peformed. These findings need to be confirmed by a study in which the cycle phase at the time of surgery is biochemically determined.

▶ There has been an enormous amount of media attention focused on the timing of primary breast cancer surgery and the effect of the menstrual cycle on subsequent disease-free survival. This study analyzed 283 premenopausal patients treated with mastectomy and axillary dissection. The results of the study suggest that primary breast cancer surgery done early in the menstrual cycle (days 0–14) is associated with a higher recurrence rate (43%) than surgery performed late in the menstrual cycle (29%). Figure 6–1 illustrates the difference in disease-free survival associated with surgical timing. Some studies have suggested that the timing of surgery affected survival outcome, although several other trials have identified a slightly different window of risk; some were unable to demonstrate any effect of surgical timing on outcome. An editorial by Dr. William McGuire in the same issue of the *Annals of Internal Medicine* suggested that this variation in risk was simply a statistical artifact of multiple testing of patient populations (1). The inconsistency of the published data coupled with the variation in the actual time determined to be prognostically important suggest that there is no specific window of high risk. Until a prospective randomized trial has been completed, there appears to be little evidence that one should alter surgical schedules to reduce risk of breast cancer recurrence.—R.C. Young, M.D., F.A.C.P.

Reference

1. McGuire WL: *Ann Intern Med* 115:401, 1991.

How Important Is Adequate Radiotherapy for the Long-Term Results of Breast-Conserving Treatment?

Kurtz JM, Amalric R, Brandone H, Ayme Y, Spitalier J-M (Univ Hosp, Basel, Switzerland; Academia Méditerranéenne d'Oncologie Clinique, Marseille, France)

Radiother Oncol 20:84–90, 1991 6–9

Background.—In the 1940s, Baclesse showed that protraction of therapy during 3 or 4 months allowed total doses of more than 6,000 R to be

Local Recurrence in the Breast as Function of Total Prescribed Dose to the Tumor Bed

Dose (Gy)	Local recurrence (%)
70 or less	3/15 (20)
71–75	5/11 (46)
76–80	6/47 (14)
More than 80	10/61 (16)
Unknown	0/5

(Courtesy of Kurtz JM, Amalric R, Brandone H, et al: *Radiother Oncol* 20:84–90, 1991.)

administered safely to the intact breast with orthovoltage equipment. Baclesse's fractionation schemes were abandoned in the 1960s, but some patients were treated in this manner after breast-conserving surgery. An unusually high local recurrence rate resulted. The influence of radiotherapy dose parameters on long-term local control was studied in these patients.

Methods.—A group of 134 patients with clinical stage I and II breast cancer was assessed. All were treated by tumorectomy and telecesium therapy in the 1960s.

Results.—Recurrences were more common in patients receiving 75 Gy or less to the tumor bed; those percentages were 31% and 15% at higher doses. Weekly dose rates of less than 8 Gy per week were associated with increased locoregional failure—30% vs. 15% for higher weekly doses. Most locoregional failures occurred in the 53 women with "inadequate" total or weekly radiotherapy doses. The importance of adequate radiotherapy increased both in older patients and in women younger than 40 years of age. The mean interval to recurrence was substantially ;pmger for inadequate radiotherapy, at 111 months vs. 75 months for adequate treatment. Therefore, significant differences in local control became apparent only after 5 years (table).

Conclusions.—The importance of radiotherapy technique in breast-conserving therapy is emphasized. An excessive reduction in the intensity of radiotherapy may lead to an inordinate number of late local failures.

▶ This is a very important paper because the use of lumpectomy and radiation therapy in this series goes back to the 1960s. The follow-up is excellent, and it should be noted that this type of treatment has been standard in France for a long time. The details of radiation therapy have not been well analyzed in the past, and this particular paper suggests that doses that are higher than what we have generally used in the United States will be required to get maximum local control. Once the breast is removed, the risk of local recurrence essentially vanishes—obviously at a very expensive price. There seems to be little question that conservative surgery plus radiation therapy can approach the success rate of radical surgery; however, it may require higher doses than those currently being used in the United States.

The American studies will require intermittent follow-up analyses to whether this trend really holds up. Such studies are very important, because this form of treatment is becoming standard in the United States for most stage I and stage II patients.—E. Glatstein, M.D.

Double-Pedicle TRAM Flap for Unilateral Breast Reconstruction

Wagner DS, Michelow BJ, Hartrampf CR Jr (Akron City Hosp, Akron, Ohio; St Joseph's Hosp, Atlanta, Ga)

Plast Reconstr Surg 88:987–997, 1991 6–10

Indications.—A double-pedicle TRAM flap offers better flap vascularity, venous outflow, and midline crossover blood flow. The risk of partial necrosis is less than that associated with a single-pedicle flap. However, operating time is prolonged, and there is greater abdominal wall morbidity. The double-pedicle flap is indicated when the needed tissue volume exceeds that which can reliably be carried on 1 pedicle or when flap length demands. It also is indicated if the risk of flap necrosis from microvascular dysfunction is increased or an abdominal midline scar is a problem.

Experience.—A double-pedicle TRAM flap was used in 19% of 341 patients undergoing unilateral breast reconstruction. It was used in 60% of the 50 most recent radical mastectomy reconstructions. Three hernias complicated the single-pedicle procedure, whereas 1 occurred in 66 double-pedical TRAM reconstructions. Partial flap loss complicated 6% of the single-pedicle reconstructions and 3% of the double-pedicle cases. Very little abdominal wall morbidity resulted from the double-pedicle procedure, although many patients were unable to do sit-ups.

Conclusion.—A single-pedicle TRAM flap is preferred for unilateral breast reconstruction, but a double-pedicle procedure may be indicated to permit a larger, longer, or safer reconstruction. If fascia is harvested conservatively and the abdominal wall is closed directly, then abdominal wall complications are infrequent.

▶ Despite some possible parochial views of physicians practicing in certain regions of the United States (particularly the Northeast), most patients with breast cancer still undergo amputation of the entire breast in 1 or another fashion as a part of their multimodality treatment for stage I, II, or even III breast cancers (1). Therefore, many women who have either already undergone mastectomy or are facting it in the future should have some pre- or postoperative consideration for reconstruction. Reconstruction is often helpful for cosmetic reasons as well as for full functional rehabilitation. The recent brouhaha over silastic implants puts more of a premium on physicians (particularly nonsurgeons) being aware of the continuing advances in plastic surgical techniques in which autologous patient tissue is used for achieving the goal of full rehabilitation. This technical article by Wagner et al. is an extension of a series of elegant reconstructive techniques by which selected patients who undergo or have undergone mastectomy can be rehabilitated without the perceived or real problems from prosthetic device implantation. Our advice is that a variety of reconstructive approaches should be discussed with all patients as a part of their initial treatment option presentation, particularly with those who, for various reasons, choose not to exercise the option of lumpectomy with or without radiation therapy.—G.D. Steele, Jr., M.D.

Reference

1. Osteen RT, et al: Ca Cancer J Clin 42:39, 1992.

Regional Nodal Failure After Conservative Surgery and Radiotherapy for Early-Stage Breast Carcinoma

Recht A, Pierce SM, Abner A, Vicini F, Osteen RT, Love SM, Silver B, Harris JR (Harvard Med School; Brigham and Women's Hosp; Faulkner Hosp, Boston)

J Clin Oncol 9:988–996, 1991 6–11

Objective.—The risk of regional node failure was examined in a series of 1,624 women with stage I or stage II invasive breast cancer who were treated by conservative surgery and radiotherapy between 1968 and 1985. The patients had a median age of 51 years at the time of diagnosis. The median follow-up was 6½ years.

Management.—Axillary dissection was carried out in nearly three fourths of the patients. Boost doses of radiotherapy were given both interstitially and by external-beam technique. The usual dose to the entire breast was 45–46 Gy. Four hundred patients received adjuvant system treatment, usually in the form of chemotherapy.

Results.—Regional node failure was the first site of treatment failure in 2.3% of cases. The actuarial 5-year survival rate was 2.3%, and the 10-year rate was 3.3%. Axillary failure was infrequent whether or not the regional nodes were irradiated. The same was the case for supraclavicular failure. Infraclavicular and internal mammary node failures were very infrequent. The management of regional node failure was individualized. Eleven of 22 patients with isolated axillary failure were alive without disease when last seen. The complications were somewhat more frequent when the supraclavicular/axillary field was treated.

Recommendations.—Either axillary dissection or axillary radiotherapy is adequate when the axillary nodes are clinically uninvolved; dissection is preferred for its prognostic value. Radiotherapy is not used routinely after adequate dissection if the nodes are negative or if only 1–3 nodes are positive. Whether axillary and supraclavicular irradiation is worthwhile for patients with 4 or more positive nodes remains uncertain.

▶ Local recurrence after conservative surgery and radiotherapy is a major concern. This study from Boston sought to identify those patients who had the highest risk for regional nodal recurrence. Overall, a little more than 2% of the patients relapsed in the axillary nodes. Supraclavicular failure was seen in less than 2% of patients. Even in those patients who had axillary node dissection and 1–3 positive nodes, nodal recurrence was only 2.1%. The data indicates that nodal recurrence is uncommon, even when patients are treated with radiation therapy to the breast alone, as long as adequate axillary nodal dissection is done; less than 3 nodes were positive. Nodal relapse was also uncommon in patients with clinically uninvolved axillae who were treated with breast and nodal radiation without axillary nodal dissection. Nevertheless, when nodal recurrence did occur, only 47% of the patients achieved subsequent regional control with any postrecurrence therapy. Although the incidence of axillary nodal recurrence under these circumstances is low, it is often inadequately controlled if it does occur.—R.C. Young, M.D., F.A.C.P.

Adjuvant Therapy

Systemic Treatment of Early Breast Cancer by Hormonal, Cytotoxic, or Immune Therapy: 133 Randomized Trials Involving 31,000 Recurrences and 24,000 Deaths Among 75,000 Women
Early Breast Cancer Trialists' Collaborative Group
Lancet 339:1–15, 1992 6–12

Background.—A previous overview of randomized trials of tamoxifen and prolonged cytotoxic chemotherapy as adjuvant therapy for early breast cancer showed that each treatment produced moderate but definite improvement in both 5-year survival and recurrence-free survival. A larger worldwide overview of randomized trials addressing any aspect of local or systemic treatment of early breast cancer was reviewed.

Methods.—All available data on mortality and recurrence for all women entered into any randomized trial beginning before 1985 and addressing any aspect of systemic adjuvant therapy for early breast cancer was sought and centrally checked. Analyses of survival and recurrence-free survival involved the "logrank" O-E and its variance V. Data for the analysis included 75,000 women, approximately 90% of all those who were ever randomized. Overall, 32% of the patients had died, and 10% had had a recurrence. A total of 30,000 women had been entered in tamoxifen trials, 3,000 in ovarian ablation trials, 11,000 in polychemotherapy trials, 15,000 in other chemotherapy comparisons, and 6,000 in immunotherapy trials.

Recurrence.—The annual rate of recurrence decreased by 25%, and the annual rate of death decreased by 17% with tamoxifen treatment. The recurrence rate decreased by 26%, and the death rate was reduced by 25% in patients treated by ovarian ablation before 50 years of age. Polychemotherapy decreased the recurrence rate by 28% and the death rate by 16%. No significant decreases were noted with ablation in older patients or with immunotherapy. The risk of contralateral breast cancer was decreased 39%.

Avoidance.—With tamoxifen and polychemotherapy, most of the avoidance of recurrence was noted during the years 0–4, after which the difference was maintained but not increased. However, avoidance of mortality was significant both during and after this time, so that the cumulative differences in survival were greater at 10 than at 5 years. Ovarian ablation produced separately significant reductions in death rate both during and after years 0–9; little information beyond year 10 was available for any of the other treatments.

Treatment Outcome.—Long-term polychemotherapy regimens appeared to have no greater benefits than shorter regimens, but polychemotherapy was superior to singe-agent chemotherapy. No significant differences were noted between the different forms of polychemotherapy or between different doses of tamoxifen. However, long-term tamoxifen, given as long as 5 years, was better than shorter tamoxifen regimens. In patients aged 70 years and older, tamoxifen demonstrated efficacy, but no evaluations were available for chemotherapy. In patients aged 50–69 years, the combination of chemotherapy and tamoxifen was better for recurrence and mortality than chemotherapy alone; it was also better for recurrence than tamoxifen alone. In younger patients, chemotherapy and ovarian ablation appeared to be comparable in effectiveness, and the combination may have been even better. Combined chemo-endocrine treatment in middle-aged patients gave 30% to 40% reductions in proportional risk. These advantages were similar in patients with node-positive and node-negative disease. However, women with node-positive cancer had nearly twice the absolute improvement in 10-year survival than that of women with node negative cancer.

Conclusions.—A review of the greatest amount of randomized evidence ever assembled for evaluation of the long-term outcome of cancer treatment showed that polychemotherapy and endocrine therapy have highly significant effects on 10-year outcome in women with early breast cancer. The benefits remain moderate in size, and subgroup analyses may be useful in determining patient treatment. Future research into these moderate differences in survival will require not only large numbers of properly randomized subjects but collaboration between investigators.

▶ This analysis hit the press and the media with great fanfare. To be sure, the analysis is one of the largest ever done, including 133 randomized trials involving 75,000 women. The analysis confirms many observations made earlier: (1) a significant decrease in recurrence and mortality for patients treated with tamoxifen; (2) a similar decrease in recurrence and mortality rate at 10-year follow-up for younger patients treated with ovarian ablation; and (3) a significant improvement in disease-free survival and survival for combination chemotherapy in node-positive patients. Six months of adjuvant chemotherapy appears to have an equivalent effect to longer periods of treatment (e.g., 12 months). Combination chemotherapy is significantly better than single-agent chemotherapy, but there are no striking differences between various combinations. Neither ovarian ablation after the age of 50 nor immunotherapy was associated with a significant improvement in disease-free survival or survival. The benefit of both chemotherapy and tamoxifen was primarily seen in the first 4 years after surgery. For patients between the ages of 50 and 70, disease-free survival and survival are better with combination therapy plus tamoxifen than with chemotherapy alone; this combination therapy also is better than tamoxifen alone for disease-free survival. For premenopausal women younger than the age of

50 years of age, the effect of chemotherapy appears to be similar to that achieved by ovarian ablation.

Despite this enormously detailed analysis, it surprises me how little new information emerges from the data. Certainly, the effects of tamoxifen in postmenopausal patients and the survival impact of combination chemotherapy on node-positive disease was well established. Some of the subtleties, such as the failure to document a substantial difference with various combinations or the lack of a dose response effect for tamoxifen, are not as well established but are hardly surprising. The study confirms that tamoxifen is associated with a significant decrease in breast cancer in the contralateral breast, thereby supporting the concept of the Tamoxifen Breast Cancer Prevention Trial. However, similar data was established previously from the analysis of the National Surgical Adjuvant Breast Project trials. The take-home message from this very well analyzed and complete study is that dramatic differences are often discernible from single trials, whereas subtle differences may only be detected through meta-analysis. Nevertheless, it is the dramatic effects rather than the subtle ones that alter medical practice.—R.C. Young, M.D., F.A.C.P.

Adjuvant Cyclophosphamide, Methotrexate, and Fluorouracil in Patients With Axillary Node-Positive Breast Cancer: An Update of the Guy's Manchester Trial

Richards MA, O'Reilly SM, Howell A, George WD, Fentiman IS, Chaudary MA, Crowther D, Rubens RD (Guy's Hosp, London; Christie Hosp, Manchester, England; Holt Radium Inst, Manchester, England; West Infirmary, Glasgow, Scotland)

J Clin Oncol 8:2032–2039, 1990 6–13

Backgrounds.—In patients with early breast cancer, adjuvant chemotherapy can improve survival, but there is uncertainty about its efficacy in postmenopausal patients. It has been suggested that the effect in premenopausal patients may result in part from ovarian suppression. The influence of adjuvant chemotherapy treatment in different subgroups was reported after a median follow-up of 8 years.

Methods.—During a 19-year period, 391 patients with operable breast cancer and positive axillary lymph nodes were entered into the study. There were 202 premenopausal and 189 postmenopausal patients. After total mastectomy and axillary clearance, 193 patients were randomized to receive cyclophosphamide, methotrexate, and fluorouracil (CMF), and 198 received no adjuvant therapy. Both treatment and menopausal status groups were well balanced for size of primary tumor and number of involved axillary nodes.

Results.—At 5 years, treatment with CMF improved survival to a difference of 10% overall (Fig 6–2). However, this benefit was confined to premenopausal patients. At 8 years, both relapse-free survival (RFS) and survival remained significantly prolonged in premenopausal patients who received CMF (Fig 6–3). The improvement in RFS was seen in premenopausal patients with both steroid receptor-positive and steroid receptor-

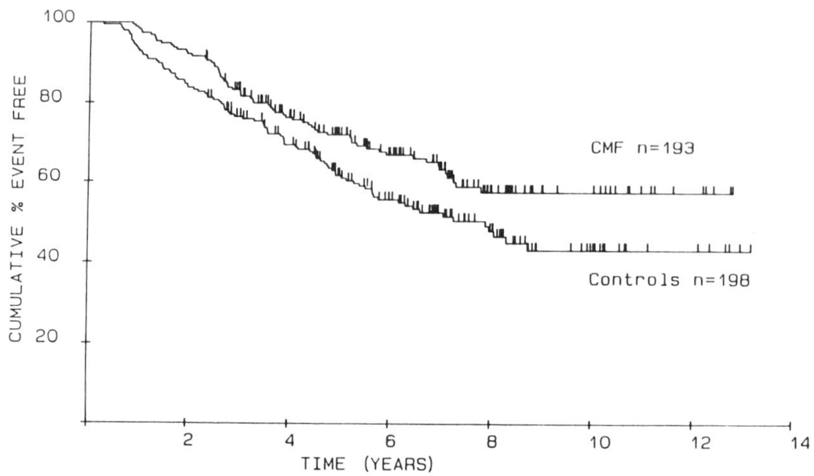

Fig 6–2.—Survival of all patients: controls vs. those who received CMF. (Courtesy of Richards MA, O'Reilly SM, Howell A, et al: *J Clin Oncol* 8:2032–2039, 1990.)

negative tumors and in subgroups of premenopausal patients defined by the number of involved axillary nodes. Relapse-free survival was also improved in premenopausal patients in whom permanent amenorrhea developed. It developed in almost all patients older than age 40 years. Among younger patients, outcome was not affected by the development of amenorrhea. Neither controls, nor CMF postmenopausal patients, nor any subgroup of these patients, showed any difference in outcome.

Conclusions.—In premenopausal patients, CMF reduces both locoregional recurrence and distant metastasis. Receptor status is no longer significant in determining the efficacy of CMF.

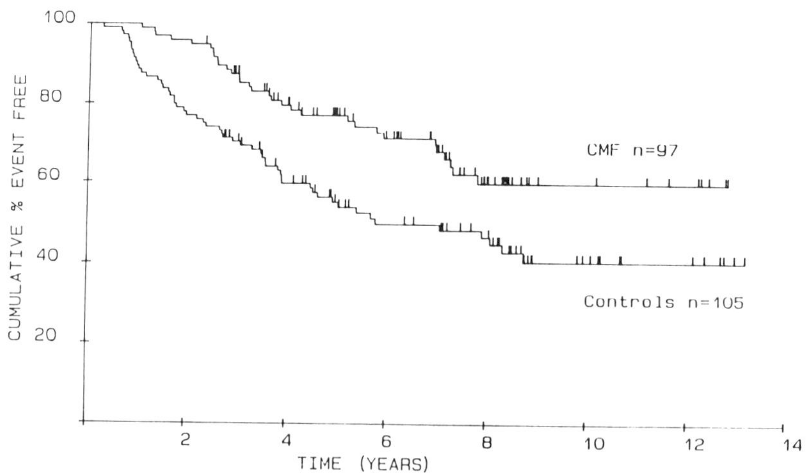

Fig 6–3.—Survival of premenopausal patients: controls vs. those who received CMF. (Courtesy of Richards MA, O'Reilly SM, Howell A, et al: *J Clin Oncol* 8:2032–2039, 1990.)

▶ Since the first report of the benefit of adjuvant chemotherapy in node positive breast cancer was done by Bonnadonna (1), there has been a relative absence of confirmatory trials with a "no treatment" arm. There has also been an understandable reluctance to perform such trials. This study is a long-term follow-up on a Guys/Manchester trial comparing CMF with no therapy in node-positive breast cancer. As Figures 6–2 and 6–3 demonstrate, there is a highly statistically significant 10-year survival difference in favor of CMF for all patients—particularly for premenopausal patients. Nevertheless, for postmenopausal patients, there is an insignificant survival difference between CMF and no therapy. This study also looked at the influence of hormone receptor status on outcome and was unable to demonstrate a difference in prognosis associated with receptor positivity. As in virtually all other studies, there was a highly significant difference in relapse-free survival at 5 years according to the number of positive nodes. For 1–3 nodes, there was a 76% 5-year survival with CMF vs. a 52% 5-year survival with 4 or more positive nodes. This trial solidly confirms the observations on CMF published earlier by Bonnadonna. Adjuvant chemotherapy should be a part of the postsurgical management of virtually all premenopausal patients with node-positive breast cancer.—R.C. Young, M.D., F.A.C.P.

Reference

1. Bonnadonna G, et al: *Breast Cancer Res Treatment* 5:95, 1985.

Efficacy and Cost-Effectiveness of Adjuvant Chemotherapy in Women With Node-Negative Breast Cancer: A Decision-Analysis Model

Hillner BE, Smith TJ (Virginia Commonwealth Univ, Richmond)

N Engl J Med 324:160–168, 1991 6–14

Background.—Recent recommendations of the National Cancer Institute have been interpreted as suggesting that adjuvant chemotherapy should be given to all women with node-negative breast cancer. This is a controversial recommendation, because it would involve treatment of many patients who would not have a recurrence. A decision-analysis model was used to explore the effectiveness of adjuvant therapy in women with node-negative breast cancer at different levels of recurrence risk.

Methods.—The model involved 2 groups: 45-year-old premenopausal women and 60-year-old postmenopausal women. The cost-effectiveness of chemotherapy was studied by calculating life expectancy as adjusted for quality of life. The various scenarios evaluated included improved disease-free survival for 5 years (with a lesser effect on overall survival), lifelong benefit from chemotherapy, and benefit in disease-free survival but no change in overall survival by year 10. A 30% reduction in the relative risk of recurrence for 5 years was assumed.

Results.—Baseline analysis found an average lifetime benefit from chemotherapy of 5.1 quality-months at a cost of $15,400 per quality-year for the 45-year-old woman. For the 60-year old woman, the average lifetime benefit was 4 quality-months at a cost of $18,800 per quality-year. In both groups, the benefit of chemotherapy varied from 1.4–14 quality-months under the more and less optimistic scenarios. Sensitivity analysis suggested that chemotherapy would be beneficial if the annual probability of recurrence was greater than .4%.

Conclusions.—The average woman will have a substantial increase in quality-adjusted life expectancy with chemotherapy; the cost is comparable to that of other accepted therapies. If changes in long-term survival are less than those in disease-free survival, the benefit decreases markedly. Refinements in risk stratification and explicit evaluations of patients' risk preferences may maximize the benefit of chemotherapy when used selectively.

▶ Earlier clinical trials have focused primarily on the impact of adjuvant chemotherapy on disease-free survival and survival. Recently, this country's constantly increasing health care costs have caused more and more focus on the cost effectiveness of intervention therapies through so-called cost-effectiveness or outcomes research. This study uses a decision analysis model to look at the cost effectiveness of chemotherapy in various groups of women with node-negative breast cancer. The analysis suggests that chemotherapy substantially increases quality-adjusted life expectancy, with a cost consistent with many other widely accepted therapies. The authors estimate the financial cost of gaining an additional quality-year of life to be approximately $15,400 for the premenopausal group and $18,800 for the postmenopausal group. Although our society has not yet defined acceptable levels of expense, we are certain to see more and more such analyses in an effort to look seriously at the cost of providing health care in this country.—R.C. Young, M.D., F.A.C.P.

Node-Negative Breast Cancer: Prognostic Subgroups Defined by Tumor Size and Flow Cytometry

O'Reilly SM, Camplejohn RS, Barnes DM, Millis RR, Rubens RD, Richards MA (Guy's Hosp, London; St Thomas' Hosp, London)

J Clin Oncol 8:2040–2046, 1990 6–15

Background.—It is easiest to justify the use of adjuvant systemic therapy for women with node-negative breast cancer in those who are at highest risk of relapse. However, no single feature of the primary tumor is sufficient to discriminate between high- and low-risk groups. The findings at DNA flow cytometry were combined with other prognostic factors in an attempt to identify more precisely those patients at high and low risk of relapse.

Methods.—The DNA flow cytometry test was done on 169 sections from patients with axillary node-negative breast cancer and palpable primary tumors. Relapse-free survival (RFS) was measured from the date of primary treatment to the date of first relapse and survival from date of

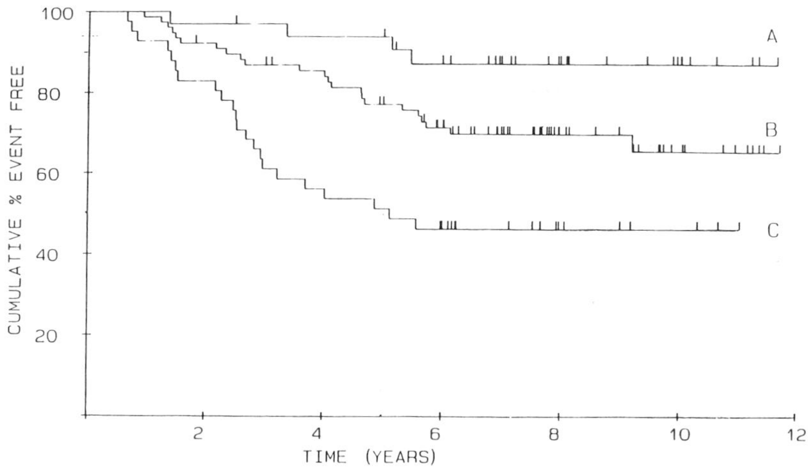

Fig 6–4.—Relapse-free survival. *A,* tumor 1 cm or less, 33 patients; *B,* tumor greater than 1 cm with low SPF, 76 patients; *C,* tumor greater than 1 cm with high SPF, 41 patients. (Courtesy of O'Reilly SM, Camplejohn RS, Barnes DM, et al: *J Clin Oncol* 8:2040–2046, 1990.)

primary treatment to death. The factors investigated were tumor size, histologic grade, estrogen receptor (ER) status, tumor ploidy, and S-phase fraction (SPF).

Results.—Relapse-free survival was significantly better in patients with tumors that measured 1 cm or less; 96% of these patients were relapse free at 5 years. Among patients with larger tumors, tumor ploidy, ER status, and progesterone receptor status could not predict RFS. The prognosis was significantly better in patients who had grade 1 or 2 infiltrating ductal tumors than in those with grade 3 tumors. The prognostic factor that gave the widest separation between subgroups, however, was SPF. The 5-year RFS was 78% for those patients whose tumors were larger than 1 cm and who had an SPF of 10% or less, compared with 52% for those with an SPF greater than 10%.

Conclusions.—In patients with node-negative breast cancer, 3 prognostic groups can be identified by combining tumor size and SPF (Fig 6–4). Relapse-free survival is best for patients with small tumors and worst for those with larger tumors and an SPF of greater than 10%. These findings may help in selecting the patients that are best suited for adjuvant therapy.

▶ Many efforts have been made to define subsets of patients with node-negative breast cancer who have poor prognostic outcomes and who, thus, are candidates for adjuvant therapy. This study evaluated 169 patients with node-negative breast cancer for tumor size, histologic grade, estrogen receptor status, tumor ploidy, and S-phase fraction. The study found tumor size and S-phase fraction to identify 3 prognostic groups as illustrated in Figure 6–4. Patients with tumors less than 1 cm in diameter comprise group A; those with tumors greater than 1 cm in diameter but with low S-phase fraction form group B, and patients with tumors greater than 1 cm plus high S-phase fraction form group C. Group A patients had a 96% relapse-free survival; group B, 78% relapse-free survival; and group C, 52% relapse-free survival. Patients with small lesions (as defined in group A) would not benefit significantly from adjuvant therapy. In contrast, those in group C clearly should receive adjuvant therapy. A 5-year survival rate of 78% in group B probably justifies the use of additional therapy. Although S-phase fraction does contribute something to this analysis, it is still striking how prominent size is in determining outcome in node-negative breast cancer.—R.C. Young, M.D., F.A.C.P.

Correlation Between c-*erb*B-2 Amplification and Risk of Recurrent Disease in Node-Negative Breast Cancer

Paterson MC, Dietrich KD, Danyluk J, Paterson AHG, Lees AW, Jamil N, Hanson J, Jenkins H, Krause BE, McBlain WA, Slamon DJ, Fourney RM (Cross Cancer Inst; Misericordia Hosp; Univ of Alberta, Edmonton, Alta, Canada; Univ of California, Los Angeles)

Cancer Res 51:556–567, 1991 6–16

Background.—The possibility of a link between alterations in the proto-oncogene c-*erb*B-2 and poor prognosis for breast cancer has often been tested. Such a prognostic factor would be a valuable indicator of high-risk breast cancer, especially in women with negative axillary lymph nodes; however, studies of the predictive value of c-*erb*B-2 overexpression have given conflicting results. The ability of amplification of this and other proto-oncogenes to predict outcome in node-negative breast cancer was assessed in a case-control study.

Methods.—A group of 704 patients with histologically negative axillary lymph nodes was identified from the Northern Alberta Breast Cancer Registry, a comprehensive population-based registry that includes approximately 7,800 patients with breast cancer. The study sample was followed for 5–16 years. A total of 115 women had had recurrent disease; these patients were matched to 115 controls who had not relapsed for primary tumor size, menopausal status, estrogen receptor status, anniversary year of treatment, and age. Slot-blot hybridization was used to analyze proto-oncogene copy number in tumor DNA; the proto-oncogenes studied, in addition to c-*erb*B-2, were c-*erb*A, c-*myc*, *int*-2, and *hst*-1.

Results.—With a cutoff gene copy number of 3, 21 case and 6 control samples had as much as a 22-fold elevation in c-*erb*B-2 genomic equivalents. Thus, 18% of the cases had excessive copies of c-*erb*B-2 compared with only 5% of the controls; this finding was a significant marker of poor prognosis and disease-free interval in particular. This marker was independent of most commonly used prognostic factors and had greater predictive power as well. However, the sensitivity of c-*erb*B-2 measurement was low, with a positive predictive value for recurrence of 70% when more than 6 gene copies were seen. Probing for the other 4 proto-oncogenes suggested that they were amplified in only 2% to 3% of the patients, even in the high-risk group.

Conclusion.—Because amplification of c-*erb*B-2 may play a role in the pathogenesis of some forms of node-negative breast cancer, it may be useful in identifying a subset of high-risk patients. As this proto-oncogene encodes a putative growth factor receptor, the predisposing factor may be amplification of the unaltered gene via increased protein kinase activity. Low sensitivity would be the main drawback to routine use of c-*erb*B-2 as a prognostic marker.

▶ The presence of amplified copies of the c-*erb*B-2 (HER-2/*neu*) oncogene has been demonstrated in some studies to confer a poor prognosis on patients with node-negative breast cancer. Unfortunately, the observation has been an inconsistent finding, and investigators have sought additional data to resolve the controversy. This case-control study looked at 704 patients with node-negative disease who were identified through a population-based registry in northern Alberta. A total of 18% of the patients with node-negative cancer was determined to have excess copies of c-*erb*B-2. This was associated with a statistically significantly poorer prognosis. However, it could only be identified in a minority of cases, and the low sensitivity argues against its routine use as a prognostic marker. Similar conclusions were made from a study from the San Antonio Group (1), which included 362 patients (including 177 with node-negative disease). Although overall amplification of HER-2/*neu* was seen in 33% of the patients, amplification did not correlate with either disease-free or overall survival, in either univariant or multivariant analyses. This was particularly true in patients with node-negative breast cancer. Both these studies suggest that although HER-2/*neu* (c-*erb*B-2) amplification may be biologically important in breast cancer, it is unlikely to be a useful prognostic factor predicting clinical outcome.—R.C. Young, M.D., F.A.C.P.

Reference

1. Clark GM, McGuire WL: *Cancer Res* 51:944, 1991.

Should All Patients With Node-Negative Breast Cancer Receive Adjuvant Therapy? Identifying Additional Subsets of Low-Risk Patients Who Are Highly Curable by Surgery Alone

Rosner D, Lane WW (State Univ of New York at Buffalo; Roswell Park Cancer Inst, Buffalo, New York)

Cancer 68:1482–1494, 1991 6–17

Background.—Some new way is needed to determine which patients with axillary node-negative (ANN) breast cancer are at high risk of recurrence and thus should have adjuvant therapy. Using cost-effective and readily available clinical and pathologic factors, patients with ANN breast cancer were studied to identify low-risk patients.

Methods.—The study sample consisted of 408 women treated by surgery alone during an 11-year period. The median patient age was 56.9 years, with two thirds of the patients older than 50 years of age. The ini-

Disease-Free Rates for Subgroups at Low Risk of Recurrence

	No. of patients (%)†	Disease-free rate ‡	*P* value
Size (≤ 1 cm)	113 (28)	95 ± 5	
Well and moderately differentiated	48 (12)	100–6	0.068
Poor and anaplastic	59 (15)	91 ± 8	
Up to age 50	36 (9)	90 ± 11	0.089
Older than age 50	77 (19)	99 ± 3	
Poor and anaplastic up to age 50	24 (6)	85 ± 16	0.27
Poor and anaplastic older than age 50	35 (9)	97 ± 6	
Size (1.1–2.0 cm)	125 (31)	86 ± 8	
Well and moderately differentiated	44 (11)	91 ± 9	0.13
Poor and anaplastic	77 (19)	79 ± 14	
Up to age 50	36 (9)	74 ± 24	0.56
Older than age 50	89 (22)	91 ± 6	
Well and moderate up to age 50	8 (2)	83 ± 30	0.61
Well and moderate older than age 50	36 (9)	94 ± 8	
DCISM	36 (9)	100–13	
Not included in other good-prognosis groups	22 (5)		

Abbreviation: DCISM, ductal carcinoma in situ with microscopic invasion.
†Percent of total population.
‡Plus 95% confidence interval.
(Courtesy of Rosner D, Lane WW: *Cancer* 68:1482–1494, 1991.)

tial diagnosis was infiltrating duct carcinoma in 62%. A total of 73% of the patients had modified radical mastectomy, and 27% had wide excision. The prognostic factors investigated were tumor size, histologic differentiation, and age. Survivors were followed for a median of 52 months; follow-up was 95% complete.

Results.—Four patient subsets had a 7-year relapse rate of 6% or better. The first subset included 12% of the patients with well- or moderately differentiated tumors measuring 1 cm or less in size. Their disease-free rate (DFR) was 100%. The second subset included 9% of the patients with poorly differentiated or anaplastic tumors measuring 1 cm or less. In such patients older than 50 years of age, DFR was 97% (table). Another 9% of the patients had well or moderately differentiated tumors measuring 1.1–2 cm; those older than 50 years of age had a DFR of 94%. Finally, 9% of the patients had ductal carcinoma in situ with microscopic invasion, with a DFR of 100%. Most of these patients, who comprised 5% of the patient population, could not be included in any of the other subsets. In the 37% of patients with tumors larger than 2 cm, the DFR was 74%; for patients with tumors as large as 2 cm who were not included in the low-risk categories, the DFR ranged from 79% to 85%.

Conclusions.—Four subsets of patients at low risk of recurrent breast cancer who did not require adjuvant chemotherapy were identified. These patients comprise approximately one third of the entire population of patients with node-negative breast cancer. Those patients with tumors greater than 2 cm in size should have adjuvant therapy. For patients in the "gray area," second-generation prognostic factors should be obtained.

▶ Which patients with node-negative breast cancer don't require adjuvant therapy? The answer to this question is critical in optimal breast cancer management, and it affects a large number of women. Obviously, if long survival is possible with surgery alone, then those patients should be spared the inconvenience, toxicities, cost, and worry of adjuvant treatments—even relatively simple ones. A long-term follow-up of more than 400 patients with node-negative breast cancer from the Roswell Park Cancer Institute provides insight into the types of subsets with excellent prognoses after surgery alone. Patients with tumors of 1 cm or less and well or moderately differentiated histology (12% of the total) were included in 1 of these subsets. All of these women survived with surgery alone. A second group of women (9% of the total) had tumors less than or equal to 1 cm in size, but they had poorly differentiated or anaplastic histology. Those older than 50 years of age had a 97% DFR with surgery alone. The third group included postmenopausal women with tumors 1.1–2 cm in diameter with well- or moderately differentiated histology (9% of the total). These women had DFR of 94%. Patients with ductal carcinoma in situ with microscopic invasion had a 100% DFR.

As the table illustrates, these groups of patients have an extremely low risk of recurrence without adjuvant therapy, and they can be justifiably managed with surgery alone. Although some of the subsets are small and the physician might not be comfortable without adjuvant treatment, a group of approximately 35% of patients with node-negative breast cancer had an estimated 7-year DFR of 94% or better. In our haste to improve survival in breast cancer, we should carefully consider such data, which identifies patients who do well with surgery alone.—R.C. Young, M.D., F.A.C.P.

Fatal Myocardial Infarction in the Scottish Adjuvant Tamoxifen Trial

McDonald CC, Stewart HJ (Scottish Cancer Trials Office, Edinburgh)

Br Med J 303:435–437, 1991 6–18

Introduction.—Tamoxifen is the primary endocrine treatment for breast cancer; optimal results are obtained when it is given for more than 2 years. This raises questions about the long-term treatment effects. Data from a trial of adjuvant tamoxifen were analyzed to assess the incidence of fatal myocardial infarction in women receiving long-term tamoxifen.

Methods.—The randomized trial included 1,070 postmenopausal women with operable breast cancer. Treatment was either with adjuvant tamoxifen, given for 5 years or until relapse in 539 patients, or tamoxifen, given for at least 6 weeks on the confirmation of a first recurrence in 531 patients. A group of 176 women continued tamoxifen treatment for longer than 5 years, either after rerandomization or electively. The hospital records of all women who died were carefully examined to establish the cause of death with the greatest possible certainty.

Findings.—There were 451 deaths, 200 in the adjuvant arm and 251 in the observation arm. In the adjuvant arm, 44 patients were free of cancer when they died; 10 of the 44 (median age, 71 years) died of myocardial infarction. Their median duration of tamoxifen treatment was 29 months. In the observation group, 61 patients had no evidence of systemic cancer; 25 of the 61 died of myocardial infarction. Only 4 of these women had ever been exposed to tamoxifen. Thus, women who received adjuvant tamoxifen therapy were significantly less likely to die of myocardial infarction.

Conclusions.—Long-term tamoxifen therapy—given for at least 5 years as adjuvant treatment for breast cancer—appears to have an estrogen-like cardioprotective effect in postmenopausal women. Whether tamoxifen has a similar effect on the incidence of nonfatal myocardial infarction is currently being studied.

▶ This year marks the start of a 16,000-patient tamoxifen breast cancer prevention trial. The use of this drug in healthy patients who are at high risk of the disease developing has highlighted the importance of tamoxifen's side effects, both positive and negative. In general, tamoxifen is extremely well tolerated, with modest side effects that include hot flashes and menopause-like symptoms, liver function abnormalities, vascular thromboses, an increase in endometrial cancer and, rarely, potential retinopathy. This study highlights some of the potentially beneficial side effects of tamoxifen, including a suggested cardiovascular benefit. The study analyzes more than 1,000 postmenopausal patients with breast cancer who were given adjuvant tamoxifen to prevent recurrence. Analyzing the group for all causes of death, the study documents a significant reduction in fatal myocardial infarction in the group treated with tamoxifen. Although the number of myocardial infarctions in each group was relatively small (25 on the observation arm and 10 on the adjuvant arm), this retrospective study does suggest that tamoxifen may well reduce serious cardiovascular complications in postmenopausal women, independent of any potential effect on reducing the incidence of breast cancer.—R.C. Young, M.D., F.A.C.P.

Venous and Arterial Thrombosis in Patients Who Received Adjuvant Therapy for Breast Cancer

Saphner T, Tormey DC, Gray R (Univ of Wisconsin, Madison; Harvard School of Public Health, Boston)

J Clin Oncol 9:286–294, 1991 6–19

Introduction.—Previous studies have suggested that tamoxifen with or without chemotherapy may contribute to thrombotic complications in patients with breast cancer and melanoma. The records of patients enrolled in 7 consecutive Eastern Cooperative Oncology Group (ECOG) studies of adjuvant treatment for breast cancer were reviewed to estimate both the frequency of venous and arterial thrombi and the contribution of chemotherapy and tamoxifen to these complications.

Observation.—The records of 2,673 patients were analyzed. All protocols were opened and closed between 1977 and 1987. The frequency of both venous and arterial thrombosis combined was 5.4% among patients who received adjuvant therapy and 1.6% among patients who were observed. The premenopausal women who received chemotherapy and tamoxifen had significantly more venous complications than those patients who were given chemotherapy without tamoxifen. Postmenopausal women who were given tamoxifen and chemotherapy had significantly more venous thrombi than those who received tamoxifen alone or who were only observed. Premenopausal women in the tamoxifen and chemotherapy group had a 1.6% frequency of arterial thrombosis, significantly greater than that in the group given chemotherapy alone. However, the frequency of arterial thrombosis among postmenopausal women was not significantly correlated with adjuvant therapy.

Discussion.—The combination of chemotherapy and tamoxifen is associated with more venous and arterial thromboembolic complications than chemotherapy alone in premenopausal women. It is also associated with more venous thrombi than tamoxifen alone in postmenopausal women.

▶ Although tamoxifen is relatively well tolerated, there have been reports of increased vascular complications associated with its use. The Eastern Cooperative Oncology Group reviewed the records of more than 2,600 patients who were given a variety of adjuvant chemo-hormonal therapy treatments to identify any increased thrombotic events. This study documents a statistically significant increase in the frequency of thrombosis in those patients treated with adjuvant therapy (5.4% vs. 1.6%). Premenopausal women who received both chemotherapy and tamoxifen had more venous thrombosis than those receiving chemotherapy alone. Postmenopausal patients who received chemotherapy and tamoxifen had significantly more venous thrombi than those who received tamoxifen alone. In addition, premenopausal patients who received both tamoxifen and chemotherapy had more arterial thromboses than those receiving chemotherapy alone. Although the incidence of these complications is not high and the mortality rate is quite low, it is a well-described complication of combined-modality adjuvant treatment. Although combined-modality therapy was implicated most often, this data provides a cautionary note for the tamoxifen breast cancer prevention trial in healthy women.—R.C. Young, M.D., F.A.C.P.

Advanced Disease

Combination Hormonal Therapy With Tamoxifen Plus Fluoxymesterone *Versus* Tamoxifen Alone in Postmenopausal Women With Metastatic Breast Cancer: An Updated Analysis

Ingle JN, Twito DI, Schaid DJ, Cullinan SA, Krook JE, Mailliard JA, Tschetter LK, Long HJ, Gerstner JG, Windschitl HE, Levitt R, Pfeifle DM (Mayo Clinic and Found, Rochester, Minn; Billings Clinic, Billings, Mont; Illinois Oncology Research Assoc, Peoria; Duluth Clinic, Duluth, Minn; Creighton Univ, Omaha, et al)

Cancer 67:886–891, 1991 6–20

Background.—The hormonal agent of choice for postmenopausal women with metastatic breast cancer is tamoxifen (TAM); fluoxymesterone (FLU) also has antitumor activity. A previous study suggested that the combination of these 2 agents was superior to TAM alone, but the

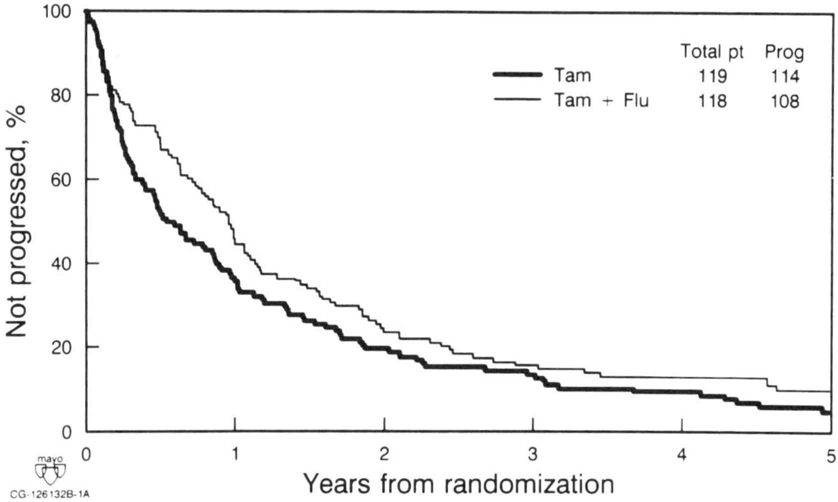

Fig 6–5.—The time to disease progression for patients treated with tamoxifen alone or in tamoxifen combination with fluoxymesterone. (Courtesy of Ingle JN, Twito DI, Schaid DJ, et al: *Cancer* 67:886–891, 1991.)

advantage was not strong enough to recommend routine clinical use of the combination. The study was updated with 2.5 years of additional follow-up.

Methods.—The study sample comprised 249 postmenopausal women with metastatic breast cancer. All had a measurable or evaluable indicator lesion. The patients were stratified and randomized to receive TAM alone or TAM and FLU at doses of 10 mg orally twice a day. Those patients with no response to TAM alone received FLU. A total of 238 women, (median age, 67 years) was included in the present analysis.

Findings.–Forty-two percent of the TAM group and 54% of the TAM plus FLU group had an objective response. The median interval to progression of disease was 6.5 months for the TAM group, compared with 11.6 months for the TAM plus FLU group (Fig 6–5). The median duration of response was 15.6 months for both groups, and survivals were similar. A group of 97 patients had an estrogen receptor value of 10 fmol or greater and were aged 65 years or older; in this group, TAM plus FLU significantly improved the response rate and time to progression. The median survival was 27.8 months for TAM and 42.9 months for TAM plus FLU, which approached significance.

Conclusions.—The combination of TAM and FLU appeared to be superior to TAM alone in the treatment of metastatic breast cancer in elderly women with estrogen receptor status of 10 fmol or greater. A prospective randomized trial would be needed to confirm this finding. A comparative trial to evaluate the addition of FLU to TAM in the adjuvant setting has been begun.

▶ Hormone therapy in patients with advanced breast cancer is generally given sequentially, with changes in therapy introduced only at the time of disease recurrence. These investigators did a randomized comparison of tamoxifen alone with tamoxifen plus fluoxymesterone in postmenopausal women with metastatic disease. Although there was no significant difference in objective responses, the time to disease progression was better for the combination therapy (11.6 vs. 6.5 months). In patients older than 65 years with estrogen-receptor–positive status, there was a highly significant difference in response rate and time to progression; there also was a marginal survival advantage for the combination. The study suggests that, for elderly patients with metastatic breast cancer with estrogen-receptor–positive status, the combination of hormones is the preferred initial therapy.—R.C. Young, M.D., F.A.C.P.

Additional Reading

Mansi JL, Easton D, Berger U, et al: Bone marrow micrometastases in primary breast cancer: Prognostic significance after 6 years' follow-up. *Eur J Cancer* 27:1552–1555, 1991.

▶ Detection of bone marrow micrometases using monoclonal antibodies predicts for early relapse and decreased survival.

Weidner N, Semple JP, Welch WR, et al: Tumor angiogenesis and metastasis—correlation in invasive breast carcinoma. *N Engl J Med* 324:1–8, 1991.

▶ Neovascularization in invasive breast cancer may be an independent predictor of metastatic disease.

Schapira DV, Kumar NB, Lyman GH, et al: Obesity and body fat distribution and breast cancer prognosis. *Cancer* 67:523–528, 1991.

▶ Obese postmenopausal women with breast cancer tend to have more axillary node involvement than their leaner counterparts.

Gelber RD, Goldhirsch A, Cavalli F: Quality-of-life-adjusted evaluation of adjuvant therapies for operable breast cancer. *Ann Intern Med* 114:621–628, 1991.

▶ Six or seven months of adjuvant chemotherapy or chemo-/hormonal therapy improved both quantity and quality of life for patients with node positive breast cancer.

Haffty BG, Fischer D, Rose M, et al: Prognostic factors for local recurrence in the conservatively treated breast cancer patient: A cautious interpretation of the data. *J Clin Oncol* 9:997–1003, 1991.

▶ Adjuvant systemic therapy reduces the recurrence rate of ipsilateral breast cancer in patients treated with conservative surgery and radiation therapy.

Aaltomaa S, Lipponen P, Eskelinen M, et al: Prognostic factors in axillary lymph node-negative (pN−) breast carcinomas. *Eur J Cancer* 27:1555–1559, 1991.

▶ This study suggests that mitotic activity index and nuclear morphometry are better predictors of recurrence in node-negative disease than conventional histologic grading.

Malfetano JH: Tamoxifen-associated endometrial carcinoma in postmenopausal breast cancer patients. *Gynecol Oncol* 39:82–84, 1990.

▶ Seven new cases of endometrial carcinoma developing in postmenopausal women receiving tamoxifen therapy for breast cancer are reported.

Love RR, Cameron L, Connel BL, et al: Symptoms associated with tamoxifen treatment in postmenopausal women. *Arch Intern Med* 151:1842–1847, 1991.

▶ Tamoxifen recipients reported moderate or severe vasomotor symptoms as often as 17% more frequently than placebo subjects; they reported gynecologic symptoms as often as 4% more frequently. Persistent vasomotor, gynecologic, or other major side effects were reported by 48% of the patients receiving tamoxifen vs. 21% of the placebo subjects.

Bentley CR, Davies G, Aclimandos WA: Tamoxifen retinopathy: A rare but serious complication. *Br Med J* 304:495–6, 1992.

▶ A case of ocular toxicity from tamoxifen is reported.

Love RR, Mazess RB, Barden HS: Effects of tamoxifen on bone mineral density in postmenopausal women with breast cancer. *N Engl J Med* 326:852–856, 1992.

▶ Tamoxifen is associated with preservation of the bone mineral density of the lumbar spine but not the radial bone.

Mueller CB, Lesperance ML: NSABP trials of adjuvant chemothrapy for breast cancer. *Ann Surg* 214:206–212, 1991.

▶ A contrarian's view of the National Surgical Adjuvant Breast Project data on the impact of adjuvant chemotherapy on breast cancer.

Mittra I, MacRae KD: A meta-analysis of reported correlations between prognostic factors in breast cancer: Does axillary lymph node metastasis represent biology or chronology? *Eur J Cancer* 27:1574–1583, 1991.

▶ These authors suggest that the prognostic influence of node status and tumor size cannot be explained by the biology of breast cancer, and that it is, in fact, reflective of the chronological age of the disease.

Buzdar AU, Kau S-W, Hortobagyi GN, et al: Clinical course of patients with breast cancer with ten or more positive nodes who were treated with doxorubicin-containing adjuvant therapy. *Cancer* 69:448–452, 1992.

▶ Of the patients with 10 or more nodes positive who were treated with Adriamycin containing adjuvant chemotherapy, 41% and 37% were free of disease at 5 and 7 years, respectively.

7 Lung Cancer

Etiology

Neuropeptide Signal Transduction in Lung Cancer: Clinical Implications of Bradykinin Sensitivity and Overall Heterogeneity

Bunn PA Jr, Chan D, Dienhart DC, Tolley R, Tagawa M, Jewett PB (Univ of Colorado, Denver)

Cancer Res 52:24–31, 1992 7–1

Introduction.—Some of the neuropeptides produced by small-cell lung cancers (SCLC), including gastrin-releasing peptide (GRP), appear to be mitogenic for human SCLC lines in vitro and in vivo. However, interference with the GRP pathway alone does not appear to have antitumor effects in most cases. The effect of 7 peptide classes on signal transduction and growth in human lung and breast cancer cell lines was studied to define the role of neuropeptides in the biology of lung cancers.

Methods.—Flow cytometry was used to measure the calcium response of individual cells to a number of peptides, either alone or in combination. Growth was assessed by [^{3}H]thymidine, 3-(4,5-dimethylthiazol-2-yl)-2,5-diphenyltetrazolium bromide, and soft agarose colony assays.

Results.—A calcium response to at least 1 peptide was demonstrated by all lung cancer cells, with classic SCLC lines being most responsive. The variant SCLC lines were less responsive, and the non-SCLC lines were least responsive. The breast cancer cell lines demonstrated little to no response. Among the individual neuropeptides, calcium response and the pattern of response varied greatly. The peptide to which most lines responded was bradykinin. Calcium release was greater with peptide combinations, but not in a quantitatively additive manner. For each peptide, there was a refractory period specific to that peptide class. The neuropeptide had little or no stimulating effect on growth, and the effects observed were not correlated with calcium signal transduction.

Conclusions.—Lung cancer cells are widely sensitive to neuropeptides, but in a very heterogeneous manner. It seems unlikely that interference with any single neuropeptide will have a major role in lung cancer therapy. The heterogeneity of peptide response should be considered in the design of future strategies.

▶ Ligand binding by 3 classes of transmembrane receptor is known to stimulate cell proliferation: (1) receptor tyrosine kinases (e.g., epidermal growth factor and platelet-derived growth factor receptors; (2) hematopoietic growth factors (e.g., interleukin-2, IL2, GMCSF); and (3) G-protein–coupled receptors with 7 transmembrane domains (e.g., bombesin, serotonin) (1). Because of the similarity between tyrosine kinase receptors and the oncogenes of acutely transforming retroviruses, this group was molecularly defined early; the molecular abnormalities of its members have been found in human cancers (e.g., amplification and rearrangement of the epidermal growth factor in glioblastomas; *erb*B-2 amplification in breast cancer; and rearrangement of the HGF receptor and bek in stomach cancers). The possibility that G-protein–coupled receptors might play a role in neoplasia by participating in autocrine loops was originally suggested by the observations that bombesin—like peptides—are secreted by SCLC and can stimulate the growth of these cells. It was also suggested that antibodies to bombesin inhibits cell proliferation.

This paper describes the effect of a wide variety of neuropeptides on calcium flux in a variety of lung cancer cell lines. The major finding is that there is great variability in response to these neuropeptides among different SCLC cell lines. This, combined with the finding that the growth stimulatory effects of these neuropeptides did not correlate with the calcium signal transduction, indicates that the role of these peptides in SCLC is complex, and that therapies based on interference with any single peptide interaction are not likely to succeed. As members of this class of receptors are defined molecularly, their role in neoplasia will become better understood. It is likely that molecular abnormalities will be found in tumors.—G. Kruh, M.D., Ph.D.

Reference

1. Aaronson SA: *Science* 254:1146, 1991.

Small-Cell Lung Cancer

Is There Ever a Role for Salvage Operations in Limited Small-Cell Lung Cancer?

Shepherd FA, Ginsberg R, Patterson GA, Feld R, Goss PE, Pearson FG, Todd TJR, Winton T, Rubinger M, Johansen E (Univ of Toronto)

J Thorac Cardiovasc Surg 101:196–200, 1991 7–2

Introduction.— Although combined chemotherapy and radiotherapy induce tumor regression in most patients with small-cell lung cancer, the impact on survival has been minimal, and less than 20% of patients with limited disease survive for 2 years. After treatment failure or relapse, survival time is extremely short. A third of the patients have recurrences only at the primary site.

Methods.—Surgical resection was attempted in 28 patients with limited small-cell lung cancer who did not have complete remission with standard treatment or who had only local recurrence after treatment in an attempt to prolong survival. All patients had undergone chemotherapy, and 13 had undergone preoperative radiotherapy to the primary site and mediastinum.

Results.—After complete remission, 8 patients underwent surgery for relapse. Five had not responded to treatment, 3 had a slight response followed by progression during chemotherapy, and 12 who had a partial response also had residual masses of greater than 3 cm. Pneumonectomy was necessary in 12 patients, and lobectomy was necessary in 15. In 1 patient, the disease was unresectable, 2 had bulky residual masses after surgery, and 3 had microscopic residual disease. The median survival was 105 weeks from the date of diagnosis and 74 weeks from the date of operation. The 5-year survival rate was projected to be 23%. The 2 patients with residual masses died with local progression. Distant metastatic disease developed in 17 other patients. One patient died without recurrent disease at 6 years, and 8 were alive 2–5 years after diagnosis. Of these patients, 7 needed lobectomy only; 4 had stage I, 2 had stage II, and 2 had stage III disease; 5 had pure small-cell lung cancer; and 3 had mixed small-cell and non-small-cell tumors. All patients with pathologic stage I disease were alive, compared with 1 of 10 patients with stage II and 2 of 14 with stage III disease.

Conclusion.—Relapse or failure to respond to chemotherapy may be a result of non-small-cell lung cancer or a mixed tumor. A second biopsy is recommended to determine the cell type of localized resistant or recurrent small-cell lung cancer. Although few patients will fall into this favorable subgroup, they should be identified, because curative therapy may be possible.

▶ After a couple of decades in which surgery has been out of favor in the management of small-cell carcinoma of the lung, there has been a recent resurgence of interest in using surgery for patients with limited-stage small-cell lung cancer. This is a good study of *carefully selected* patients showing that 20% to 25% of the patients may be cured by a surgical resection after either an incomplete response to initial treatment or a local relapse. The key to management is patient selection, both from a standpoint of pulmonary function and from the standpoint of extent of disease. It is essential to note in this study that they are talking about either N1 disease or T3N0. Although they also have included some "early" N2 disease (I interpret this to mean microscopically positive nodes that are not suspected clinically in the mediastinum), they have excluded patients with bulky mediastinal adenopathy, supra clavicular nodes, or pleural effusions. There is little question in my mind that there is a role for surgical resection in very carefully selected patients. The more extensive the nodal disease, the less sense it makes. I believe one can agree that, with the kinds of patients that Shepherd et al. selected, there is still a significant degree of salvage to be achieved.—E. Glatstein, M.D.

Surgical Treatment for Limited Small-Cell Lung Cancer: The University of Toronto Lung Oncology Group Experience

Shepherd FA, Ginsberg RJ, Feld R, Evans WK, Johansen E (Toronto Gen Hosp; Mount Sinai Hosp, Toronto; Princess Margaret Hosp, Toronto; Univ of Toronto)
J Thorac Cardiovasc Surg 101:385–393, 1991 7–3

Backgrounds.—Interest in surgical treatment for some patients with small-cell lung cancer (SCLC) has been revived with the finding that T1 N0 tumors have a projected 5-year survival rate of 60%. Although 80%

of patients may respond to chemotherapy, less than 15% will be alive at 2 years. A series of 119 patients who underwent combined therapy for SCLC, including surgery, was investigated.

Patients.—Patients were treated during a 10-year period. Surgery was done first in 79 patients (58 men and 21 women; median age, 63 years). Adjuvant chemotherapy was used in 67 of these patients. Chemotherapy was done first in 40 patients (27 men and 13 women; median age, 59 years). Of these, 94% had at least a partial response before surgery. Preoperatively, there were 69 stage I, 27 stage II, and 23 stage III tumors. Lobectomy was done in 88 cases, pneumonectomy in 26, and no resection in 5. On postoperative pathologic examination, SCLC only was found in 95 cases, non-small-cell lung cancer in 3, mixed findings in 17, and no residual tumor in 4. Postoperatively, there were 35 stage I, 36 stage II, and 48 stage IIIa tumors.

Outcome.—The overall median survival was 111 weeks, and the projected 5-year survival was 39%, with no difference between those who had chemotherapy before and after surgery. Median survival was not reached for patients with stage I disease, compared with 82 weeks for stage II and 83 weeks for stage III disease. The projected 5-year survivals were 51%, 28%, and 19%. Of the 12 patients who received no chemotherapy, 7 were alive as long as 4 years. Sixty-seven patients died, 11 with no evidence of disease. There were only 10 cases of relapse in the primary site alone, 7 at primary and distant sites, and 39 in distant sites only.

Conclusions.—In patients with SCLC, resection appears to improve control at the primary site. Combination therapy can achieve long-term survival and cure in many patients with stage I disease. In patients with stage II and IIIa type SCLC, survival is similar to that in patients with surgically treated stage IIIa non-small-cell lung carcinoma.

▶ The most interesting aspect of the Toronto Lung Oncology Group experience in limited SCLC is not what the study proves but, rather, what it reflects as the current vogue of multimodality treatment approaches. Quite succinctly, the article proves nothing. What it reflects is a rekindling of interest in surgery for limited SCLC. As to whether surgery makes a difference, this remains hypothetical. As to whether the combination of treatment makes a difference (defined here as projected 5-year survival statistics), this also remains hypothetical; however, it may be more secure than the implication that surgery, done either before or after chemotherapy, protects against local disease recurrence. The long-term needs include a greater array of remission induction, second-line or maintenance systemic therapies of increased effectiveness, and better monitors of early diagnosis that would be applicable in a surveillance-type approach.—G.D. Steele, Jr., M.D.

Thoracic Radiotherapy Variables: Influence on Local Control in Small Cell Lung Cancer Limited Disease

Turrisi AT III, Glover DJ (Univ of Michigan, Ann Arbor; Univ of Pennsylvania)
Int J Radiat Oncol Biol Phys 19:1473–1479, 1990 7–4

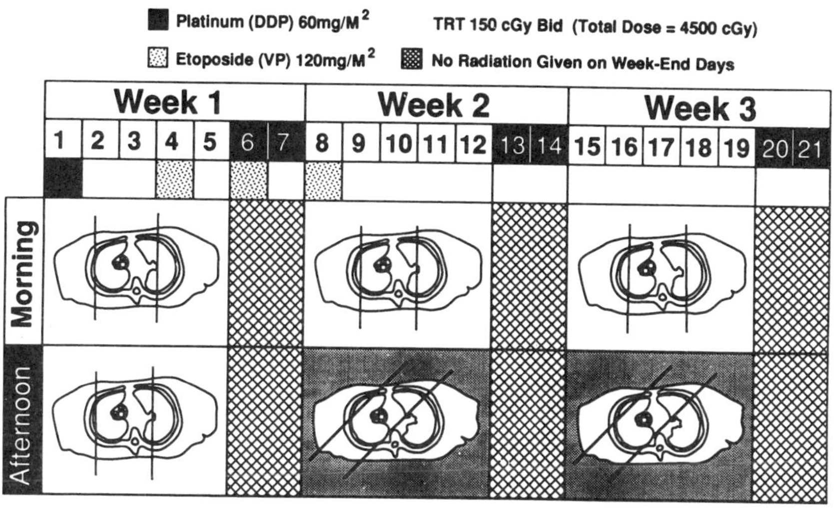

Fig 7–1.—Induction schema. During week 1, both sessions are treated AP/PA. During weeks 2 and 3, the afternoon session is angled to avoid the spinal cord. At day 22, another identical cycle of chemotherapy was added at week 6. Response was then assessed, followed by 6 cycles of chemotherapy maintenance. Prophylactic cranial irradiation completed therapy, usually at week 24. (Courtesy of Turrisi AT III, Glover DJ: *Int J Radiat Oncol Biol Phys* 19:1473–1479, 1990.)

Introduction.—Local control remains a challenge in small-cell lung cancer. The local failure rate varies from 60% to 100% with chemotherapy alone, and the addition of external beam radiothrapy has a local failure rate of approximately 30%. In an effort to define methods that would improve local control of limited small-cell lung cancer (LSCLC), a twice-daily radiotherapy regimen used concurrently with platinum-etoposide chemotherapy was designed.

Treatment.—Platinum (60 mg/m^2) was infused intravenously on days 1 and 22, and etoposide (120 mg/m^2) was infused on days 4, 6, and 8, and days 25, 27, and 29 with concurrent twice-daily 150 cGy, for a total dose of 4,500 cGy (Fig 7–1). For chest radiotherapy, the target volume, using thoracic CT as a guide, was defined as the primary tumor plus a 1–1.5 cm margin of normal lung and mediastinal lymph nodes at least 1.5-cm cephalo-caudad margin. The supraclavicular fossa was included only infrequently, and the contralateral hilum was not included at all. Angled fields were used in the afternoon sessions to minimize the dose to the spinal cord.

Outcome.—Thirty-two consecutive patients with LSCLC were treated using this concurrent chemoradiotherapy regimen with twice-daily radiotherapy. Complete response was achieved in 29 of 31 (94%) evaluable patients, including all 27 patients with pure small cell and 2 of 4 patients with variant histology; the difference was significant. Furthermore, local failure occurred in all 4 patients with variant histology, whereas the only pure small-cell local failure occurred in a patient who received only 3 radiotherapy fractions because of toxicity. The CT scans were inaccurate prognostic indicators. During 16–57 months of follow-up, 5 patients

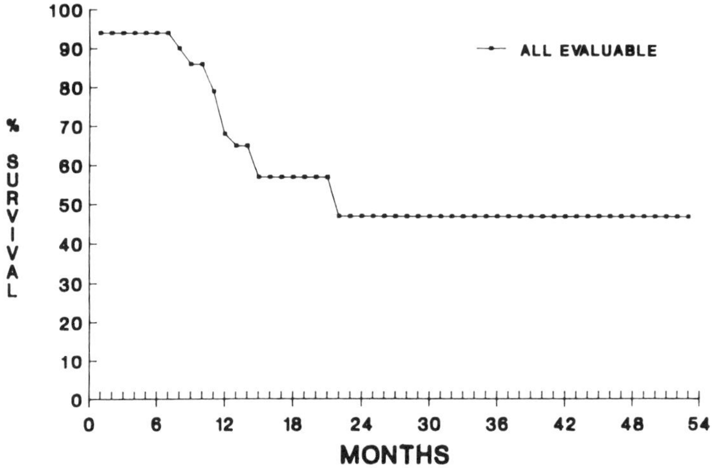

Fig 7–2.—Small-cell lung cancer disease-free survival for all 32 patients. The minimum follow-up was 15 months, and the median follow-up was 43 months. Berkson-Gage method. (Courtesy of Turrisi AT III, Glover DJ: *Int J Radiat Oncol Biol Phys* 19:1473–1479, 1990.)

died of unrelated causes, 15 died of the disease, and 12 remained alive and disease-free (Fig 7–2).

Conclusion.—With concurrent chemoradiotherapy and twice-daily radiotherapy for the treatment of LSCLC, variant histology is more predictive of local control than the physical factors of dose or volume.

▶ This is an excellent series on LSCLC treated in a combined-modality fashion with a high degree of local success, especially if there are no variant histologies. The data from this study are truly remarkable, and they give us a real target to shoot for in terms of optimizing our treatment. This is the best series of LSCLC ever reported.—E. Glatstein, M.D.

Reduction by Granulocyte Colony-Stimulating Factor of Fever and Neutropenia Induced by Chemotherapy in Patients With Small-Cell Lung Cancer

Crawford J, Ozer H, Stoller R, Johnson D, Lyman G, Tabbara I, Kris M, Grous J, Picozzi, Rausch G, Smith R, Gradishar W, Yahanda A, Vincent M, Steart M, Glaspy J (Duke Univ and Durham VA Med Ctr, Durham, NC; Univ of North Carolina, Chapel Hill; Univ of Pittsburgh; Vanderbilt Univ, Nashville, Tenn; et al)
New Engl J Med 325:164–170, 1991 7–5

Background.—Fever with neutropenia is a life-threatening complication in patients with cancer undergoing chemotherapy. Mortality remains approximately 10% among patients with documented infection. A randomized clinical trial was designed to test whether recombinant methionyl granulocyte colony-stimulating factor (G-CSF) can reduce chemotherapy-realted neutropenia in patients with cancer.

Methods.—A group of 211 patients with small-cell lung cancer was randomly assigned to receive either recombinant methionyl G-CSF or placebo. Treatment with G-CSF or placebo began on day 4 and continued through day 17 of a 21-day cycle of cyclophosphamide, doxorubicin, and etoposide. Treatment safety was evaluated in 207 of the 211 patients, and efficacy was evaluated in 199 patients.

Findings.—A total of 40% of the G-CSF group had at least 1 episode of fever with neutropenia, compared with 77% of the placebo group. During the 6 cycles of chemotherapy, the median duration of grade IV neutropenia was 6 days with placebo and 1 day with G-CSF. The G-CSF reduced the number of days of treatment, the number of days of hospitalization, and the incidence of confirmed infections by approximately 50% compared with placebo. Of the patients, 20% receiving G-CSF continued to experience mild-to-moderate medullary bone pain.

Conclusions.—As an adjunct to chemotherapy in patients with small-cell lung cancer, G-CSF is well tolerated. Granulocyte colony-stimulating factor reduced the incidence of fever with neutropenia and culture-confirmed infections; the incidence, duration, and severity of grade IV neutropenia; the total number of days of treatment with intravenous antibiotics; and the days of hospitalization by approximately half compared with placebo.

▶ Hemopoietic growth factors have burst on the clinical scene and are now in widespread use. The ability of these growth factors to stimulate the recovering or compromised bone marrow is associated with accelerated marrow recovery and, in many studies, a reduction in infectious complications. This randomized double-blind trial of G-CSF in patients receiving chemotherapy for small-cell lung cancer demonstrates a significant decrease in serious neutropenia, a reduction in the total number of days requiring intravenous antibiotics, and a reduction in hospitalization. Although these observations are important, the central question of whether such growth factor treatment improves therapeutic outcome or survival is still unresolved. The study does suggest that modest increases in dose intensity are feasible using growth factor therapy. Whether the magnitude of dose intensity increases (2–4×) are sufficient to make a significant therapeutic impact is problematic. The availability of hemopoietic growth factors does represent an advance in our ability to reduce treatment-related morbidity. However, whether it will impact significantly on cancer survival remains an open question.—R.C. Young, M.D., F.A.C.P.

Non-Small-Cell Lung Cancer

Radiation Therapy Following Resection of Non-Small Cell Bronchogenic Carcinoma

Slater JD, Ellerbroek NA, Barkley HT Jr, Mountain C, Oswald MJ, Roth JA, Peters LJ (Univ of Texas, Houston)

Int J Radiat Oncol Biol Phys 20:945–951, 1991 7–6

Introduction.—Although postoperative radiotherapy has reduced local recurrence rates in patients with lung carcinoma, its effect on long-term

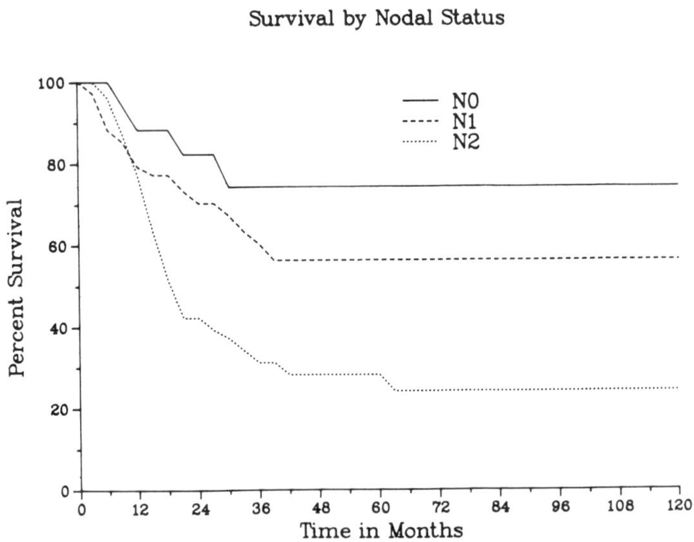

Fig 7–3.—Survival of patients according to nodal status. (Courtesy of Slater JD, Ellerbroek NA, Barkley HT Jr, et al: *Int J Radiat Oncol Biol Phys* 20:945–951, 1991.)

survival remains controversial. The results of postoperative radiotherapy on local disease control and survival in patients with lung cancer were reviewed.

Methods.—In 1970–1982, 102 patients underwent radiotherapy after attempted curative resection of bronchogenic carcinoma. The pathologic

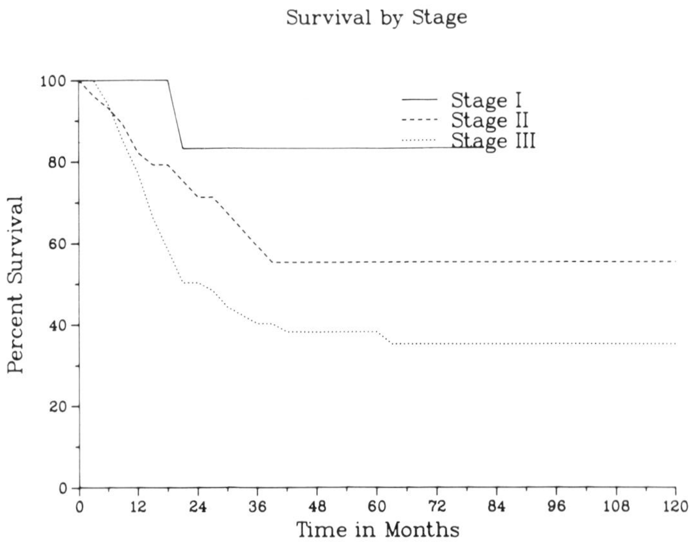

Fig 7–4.—Survival of patients according to disease stage. (Courtesy of Slater JD, Ellerbroek NA, Barkley HT Jr, et al: *Int J Radiat Oncol Biol Phys* 20:945–951, 1991.)

TABLE 1.—Incidence of Distant Metastasis and Stage of Disease

Stage	Distant metastases*
I	1/7 (14%)
II	9/24 (38%)
III	32/57 (56%)
T1†	3/8 (30%)
T2	30/57 (53%)
T3	9/20 (45%)
N0	3/16 (19%)
N1	10/30 (33%)
N2	29/42 (69%)

*Excludes 14 patients whose cause of death was not known.
†Excludes 1 patient with TX primary stage.
(Courtesy of Slater JD, Ellerbroek NA, Barkley HT Jr, et al: *Int J Radiat Oncol Biol Phys* 20:945–951, 1991.)

disease stage was I in 8 patients, II in 29, and III in 65. The survivors were followed for at least 3 years.

Results.—The 5-year actuarial survival rate was 83% for patients with stage I, 55% for those with stage II, and 38% for those with stage III disease. This rate was 74% for patients with N0, 56% for those with N1, and 28% for those with N2 disease (Fig 7–3). The difference in survival based on T stage or tumor histology was not significant (Fig 7–4). There was gross residual disease after operation in 9 patients and microscopic residual disease in 19. The 5-year actuarial survival rate for 12 patients without nodal disease but with known gross or microscopic residual tumor after surgery was 78%. The most significant factor affecting the frequency of metastatic relapse was the pathologic status of the hilar and mediastinal lymph nodes; distant metastases developed in 19% of patients with N0, 33% of those with N1, and 69% of those with N2 disease (Table 1). The overall rate of recurrence intrathoracically was 16%,

TABLE 2.—Tumor Histology and Sites of Recurrence

Histology	Local	Distant	Local and distant
Squamous cell			
n = 51	6	19	2
Adenocarcinoma			
n = 34	1	14	5
Other			
n = 3	0	2	0
Total = 50/88	7	35	7

Abbreviation: n, total number.
(Courtesy of Slater JD, Ellerbroek NA, Barkley HT Jr, et al: *Int J Radiat Oncol Biol Phys* 20:945–951, 1991.)

confirming that postoperative radiotherapy is effective in preventing local relapse, even in patients with proved nodal involvement (Table 2).

Conclusions.—Even when excision appears to be complete, surgical resection of lung cancer is associated with significant local and distant recurrence. Radiotherapy can reduce local recurrence in patients with minimal residual disease or hilar or mediastinal lymph node metastases. The impact of adjuvant radiotherapy on survival cannot be determined from these findings. Further study is needed, preferably well-designed prospective investigations.

▶ Because of the Lung Cancer Study Group's negative study on the effects of postoperative radiotherapy on complete resected stage II and III cancer of the lung (1), many individuals concluded that that there is no role for postoperative radiotherapy after an attempted curative resection of bronchogenic lung cancer.

The reader must be aware that the Lung Cancer Study Group excluded patients who had positive nodes at the upper margin of the resection. That is to say, unless the uppermost nodes were negative at the time of an extensive mediastinal resection of the nodes (a very atypical procedure), the patient was excluded. What the Lung Cancer Study Group has published is really a subset of stage II and III patients, rather than a representative cross section. The authors report a retrospective group of patients who are much more realistic in terms of the surgery that was performed. The results in stages I, II, and III are really quite good with postoperative radiotherapy, and the data include the nodal status as well. It is interesting to note that, of the subset of patients without nodal disease but *with* known gross or microscopic residual tumor after an incomplete resection, the 5-year actual rate of survival was 78% after postoperative radiation therapy.

The authors state that the impact of adjuvant radiotherapy on survival cannot be determined from these data, and that there is a need for well-designed prospective studies. I certainly agree. However, for those who quote from the Lung Cancer Study Group data without carefully reading the paper, I would hesitate to throw out the proverbial baby with the bath water.—E. Glatstein, M.D.

Reference

1. Lung Cancer Study Group: *N Engl J Med* 315:1377, 1986.

8 Genitourinary Cancers

Testis

Two-Drug Therapy in Patients With Metastatic Germ Cell Tumors

Bajorin DF, Geller NL, Weisen SF, Bosl GJ (Mem Sloan-Kettering Cancer Ctr, New York; Cornell Unit, New York)
Cancer 67:28–32, 1991 8–1

Introduction.—A mathematical model was developed to predict the likelihood of a complete response (CR) in patients with germ-cell tumors (GCT). The model identified patients with a high probability of CR, thereby allowing use of less toxic chemotherapy. Patients were randomized to receive either a 5-drug regimen or a 2-drug regimen of cisplatin and etoposide. Early results show equivalent survival and response rates and substantially less toxicity in the patients receiving the 2-drug therapy. In this study, 82 patients with good-risk GCT were evaluated for late relapse.

Methods.—Etoposide and cisplatin were administered at 3–4 week intervals. Surgical resection of residual disease sites was performed after induction therapy. Responses were classified as a complete response or incomplete response (IR).

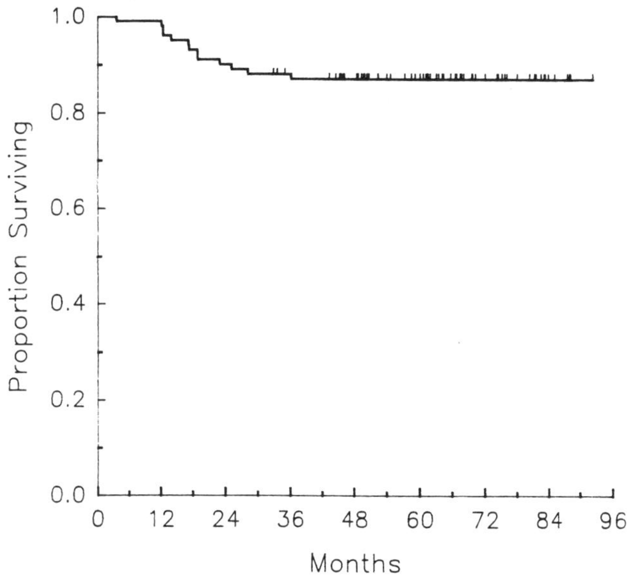

Fig 8–1.—Survival distribution of 82 patients treated with etoposide and cisplatin according to the Kaplan-Meier method. (Courtesy of Bajorin DF, Geller NL, Weisen SF, et al: *Cancer* 67:28–32, 1991.)

Results.—In 76 of 82 patients, a CR was achieved; in 6, an IR was achieved (Fig 8–1). Of the patients with CR, 72 had a response to chemotherapy alone, and 56% had surgical excision of residual abnormalities. Although 9 patients had a relapse at 6–17.5 months, no relapses occurred after 17.5 months. During a median follow-up of 63 months, 71 patients remained free of disease.

Conclusion.—The use of 2-drug therapy with etoposide and cisplatin for treatment of GCT is effective, with a high proportion of CR and long-term remission. This dose and schedule can be considered standard therapy for all patients with seminoma and patients with nonseminomatous GCT who have good risk. Late relapses were not observed during a median follow-up of 5 years. The excellent duration of response may be a result of the dose of etoposide, the lack of dose modification for myelosuppression, and the surgical resection of all residual disease after completion of chemotherapy.

▶ The necessity of adding bleomycin to cisplatin plus etoposide (EP) for the treatment of favorable-prognosis GCT has been questioned in several clinical trials. In a patient population expected to have long-term survival, the elimination of a drug that can produce Raynaud's phenomenon, pulmonary fibrosis, and even death without sacrificing efficacy is an obvious goal. Four cycles of EP produce excellent results (as described in this study), and the authors suggest that, in this dose and schedule, bleomycin is not necessary. It has also been demonstrated (1) that there is no need to use 4 cycles of bleomycin plus EP (BEP) in good-risk patients, because 3 cycles produce equivalent results with less toxicity. However, in a recent randomized trial of 3 cycles of EP vs. BEP, there was a higher rate of recurrence in patients not receiving bleomycin (2). It appears, therefore, that 3 cycles of BEP produce the same results as 4 cycles of EP in favorable-prognosis nonseminomatous GCT. Both approaches are well tolerated and can be considered equivalent therapy in this group of patients.—R.F. Ozols, M.D., Ph.D.

References

1. Einhorn LH, et al: *J Clin Oncol* 7:387, 1989.
2. Loehrer PJ, et al: *Proc Amer Soc Clin Oncol* 10:169, 1991.

Randomized Study of Cisplatin Dose Intensity in Poor-Risk Germ Cell Tumors: A Southeastern Cancer Study Group and Southwest Oncology Group Protocol

Nichols CR, Williams SD, Loehrer PJ, Greco FA, Crawford ED, Weetlaufer J, Miller ME, Bartolucci A, Schacter L, Einhorn LH (Indiana Univ, Indianapolis; Indianapolis VA Hosp; Vanderbilt Univ, Nashville; Univ of Colorado, Denver; Southeastern Cancer Study Group, Birmingham, Ala; et al)

J Clin Oncol 9:1163–1172, 1991 8–2

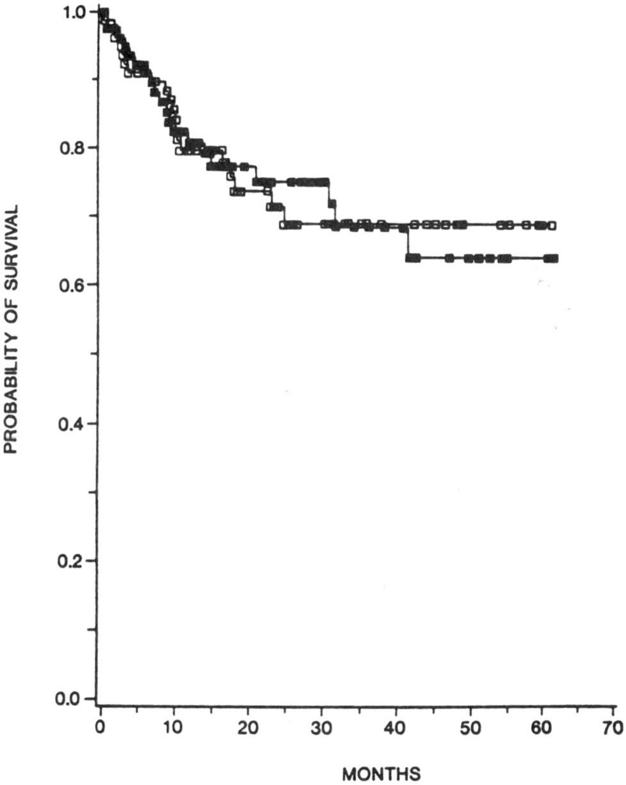

Fig 8–2.—Overall survival: *closed squares* indicate high-dose therapy; *open squares,* standard therapy; P = .977. (Courtesy of Nichols CR, Williams SD, Loehrer PJ, et al: *J Clin Oncol* 9:1163–1172, 1991.)

Introduction.—Using intensified doses of conventional chemotherapeutic agents is an alternative to adding new drugs. The value of using more intense cisplatin therapy was examined in 159 patients with advanced germ-cell cancers representing all histologic subtypes and primary sites.

Methods.—In addition to etoposide and bleomycin, patients received either standard-dose cisplatin (20 mg/m^2/day for 5 days) or a dose of 40 mg/m^2/day for 5 days. All but 6 patients were evaluable for response and toxicity.

Results.—A complete response was achieved with chemotherapy alone in 45% of the high-dose patients and 47% of the standard-dose patients. Relapse was more frequent in the standard-dose patients. Survival did not differ significantly during a median follow-up of 2 years (Fig 8–2). High-dose patients had significantly more ototoxicity, neurotoxicity, and gastrointestinal toxicity. Hematologic toxicity also was more frequent with high-dose cisplatin therapy. Three high-dose patients and 1 standard-dose patient died of treatment-related complications.

Conclusion.—These findings raise questions about the value of exceeding the full standard dose of cisplatin. Excessive toxicity has resulted with no commensurate therapeutic benefit.

▶ A 1988 prospective randomized trial from the National Cancer Institute demonstrated that PVeBV [double-dose cisplatin (200 mg/m^2), velban, bleomycin, and VP-16] was superior to what was then standard therapy with PVeB [standard-dose cisplatin (100 mg/m^2), velban, and bleomycin] (1). It was demonstrated subsequently that BEP [bleomycin, VP-16 (etoposide), and cisplatin] was superior to PVeB, with regard to both efficacy and toxicity (2). This current study fails to find any increased benefit from double-dose cisplatin compared with standard-dose cisplatin when used together with VP-16 and bleomycin. The results suggest that the primary reason that PVeBV was superior to PVeB in the National Cancer Institute trial was the presence of VP-16—not the increased dose of cisplatin. This does not mean that the dose of cisplatin is not critical. Other randomized trials have demonstrated that a dose of 125 mg of cisplatin per m^2 was superior to 75 mg of cisplatin per m^2 per cycle. Consequently, full-dose cisplatin (100 mg/m^2) should be used together with VP-16 and bleomycin in the treatment of poor-risk patients with germ-cell cancer. This study also suggests that improvement in the survival of patients with germ-cell tumor who are at poor risk will require more than increasing the dose of a currently active agent. Even high-dose chemotherapy with autologous bone marrow transplantation, which leads to a two- to threefold increase in the actual platinum dose, is unlikely to increase the cure rate substantially in this group of patients.—R.F. Ozols, M.D., Ph.D.

References

1. Ozols RF, et al: *J Clin Oncol* 6:1031, 1988.
2. Williams SD, et al: *N Engl J Med* 316:1435, 1987.

Prostate

Long-Term Follow-up Results After Expectant Management of Stage A1 Prostatic Cancer

Zhang G, Wasserman NF, Sidi AA, Reinberg Y, Reddy PK (Univ of Minnesota, Minneapolis; VA Med Ctr, Minneapolis)
J Urol 146:99–103, 1991 8–3

Introduction.—It is generally believed that stage A1 adenocarcinoma of the prostate carries a low risk for disease progression and may be managed expectantly. However, recent evidence suggests that stage A1 prostatic cancer may not be as innocuous as was once thought. The risk of disease progression after long-term follow-up was assessed retrospectively in patients who were managed expectantly after diagnosis.

Patients.—The study population consisted of 132 men, aged 49–85 years at diagnosis, with stage A1 prostatic adenocarcinoma. Diagnosis was made by transurethral resection with histopathologic tissue examination in all patients. The follow-up ranged from 5–23 years, with a mean of 8.2 years. The follow-up examinations that were performed every 6–12 months included digital rectal examination, determination of the serum level of prostatic acid phosphatase and, recently, determination of the serum prostate-specific antigen. The policy of annual bone scans was later changed to performing bone scans only in those patients with suspected disease progression.

Results.—During the follow-up period, 52 patients had a second staging transurethral prostatic resection, and 14 of them had residual foci of well-differentiated cancer. Two of the 14 underwent early radical prostatectomy, and 12 were not treated further at the time. Three of the 12 (25%), as well as 3 of 38 patients (8%) in whom no residual disease was found at second resection, had locally progressive disease. Three of 44 patients who underwent transrectal ultrasonography of the prostate and ultrasound-guided biopsy had progressive disease. Another 4 patients had either locally or systemically progressive disease. Thus, 13 of the 132 patients (10%) had locally or systemically progressive disease after long-term follow-up. The interval between diagnosis and detection of disease progression ranged from 6 months to 20 years. Ten patients underwent definitive treatment, 2 received palliative treatment, and 1 was not treated. Six of the 10 patients who underwent definitive treatment are alive without evidence of disease.

Conclusion.—The detection of residual cancer at second staging transurethal resection of the prostate is associated with a high probability of disease progression. However, negative findings at second staging resection may not preclude the possibility of disease progression. Although expectant management of stage A1 disease is warranted, regular and long-term follow-up is mandatory.

▶ This study confirms that, although patients with stage A1 prostate cancer have a low progression rate, careful follow-up is nevertheless indicated. A rather restrictive definition of stage A1 was used in this study: 5% tumor volume and less than Gleason's grade 4. Other studies have used the same volume of tumor and a higher Gleason's grade to select patients with stage A1 prostate cancer for aggressive treatment. Even in the more favorable group of patients in this study, the recurrence rate was substantial (10%). A more troubling finding was that, of the patients who had recurrence after expectant monitoring, half had disease that was no longer confined to the prostate. It remains to be determined whether monitoring with newer modalities (serum prostate specific antigen and transrectal ultrasonography) will detect recurrences while they are still confined to the prostate and are highly curable. What is certain is that patients with stage A1 disease cannot be simply reassured that they need not worry about recurrence of their disease.—R.F. Ozols, M.D., Ph.D.

The Effect of Local Control on Metastatic Dissemination in Carcinoma of the Prostate: Long-Term Results in Patients Treated With ^{125}I Implantation

Fuks Z, Leibel SA, Wallner KE, Begg CB, Fair WR, Anderson LL, Hilaris BS, Whitmore WF (Mem Sloan-Kettering Cancer Ctr, New York)

Int J Radiat Oncol Biol Phys 21:537–547, 1991 8–4

Introduction.—The significance of local residual prostatic cancer after surgery or radiotherapy in patients with early-stage disease has been a concern. The effect of locally recurring tumor on the occurrence of metastatic disease was examined in 679 patients with stage B-C/N0 prostatic carcinoma. The patients, seen between 1970 and 1985, were followed for a median of 97 months. All the patients had negative lymph nodes confirmed at the time of ^{125}I implantation.

Observations.—Patients who were at risk 15 years after initial treatment had a distant metastasis-free survival (DMFS) rate of 37%. Although local failure was the factor most closely related to DMFS, stage, tumor grade, and implant volume were also independent predictors. The relative risk of metastatic spread was fourfold higher after local failure than when local relapse was not observed, regardless of stage, grade, or implant dose. A group of 268 patients with locally recurrent disease who did not receive hormonal therapy initially had a median local relapse-free survival of 51 months and a median DMFS rate of 71 months. Distant metastases were evident sooner in patients with local control than in those with local relapse.

Implications.—In patients with early-stage prostatic cancer, local relapse after definitive treatment is closely associated with the chance that distant metastasis will eventually develop. Early, complete elimination of the primary tumor is necessary for a long-term cure.

▶ This is an extremely important paper that purports to show that patients with prostate cancer whose tumors are controlled locally have a lesser propensity for metastatic spread than patients whose tumors are uncontrolled. Although this is probably true, it is implied that the improvement in local control would therefore yield better survival. This implication is probably not true, at least not to any major degree. We have seen controlled studies in breast cancer, lung cancer, and rectal cancer, all of which show that postoperative radiotherapy makes an enormous difference in local control but really has very little impact on survival. The present analysis by Fuks et al. is interesting because the patients had lymph node dissection that was negative, a potentially important distinction from previous controlled clinical trials that were virtually always restricted to greater dissemination associated with local failure. I believe it is wrong to assume that there will be survival gain, because there are multiple reasons competing for death in this group of patients, and a patient can die only once. Some deaths are the result of complications of cancer, some are caused by complications of treatment, and some are simply a result of the aging population that is included in this group. In any event, the implication that survival gains will be affected by major improvements in local control has not yet been substantiated. Perhaps this could be shown by meta-analysis of larger numbers of patients; however, I personally have little trust in that type of manipulation.

This study is interesting because there is no simple survival curve that shows that the patients who had local control actually had better survival than the patients who did not have local control. It has made me think considerably about the subject, and I believe that this is fundamentally analogous to the traditional pattern of analysis-by-response, which medical oncologists have fortunately outgrown. Any time you define groups by the function of their treatment and then compare their survivals, a fundamental fallacy has been introduced. That local failure begets metastatic disease is not being challenged here, only the implication that there will be major survival gains resulting from the improvements that can be achieved in local control. Neither this paper, nor any other of which I am aware, established this fact. It remains to be demonstrated.

There are a couple of other points in the analysis that make the data somewhat soft. First of all, there are no autopsy data and few biopsies. The basic definition of local failure is clinical growth, and the local definition for local control is the absence of such growth. Thus, local control as a group is as a relatively unreliable outcome, at least in these patients. In addition, there is an inherent bias in how a local control is scored; once overt metastastic disease has been manifested in a patient, there is a great tendency in the clinic to follow his/her local tumor much less rigorously than one found in a patient without metastatic disease. This is a psychological issue for the doctor, but going over the charts retrospectively may give incorrect results.— E. Glatstein, M.D.

Carcinoma of the Prostate: MR Images Obtained With Body Coils Do Not Accurately Reflect Tumor Volume

Quint LE, Van Erp JS, Bland PH, Mandell SH, Del Buono EA, Grossman HB, Glazer GM, Gikas PW (Univ of MIchigan, Ann Arbor)

ARJ 156:511–516, 1991 8–5

Introduction.—The spread of tumor through the prostatic capsule is not reliably, directly demonstrated by MRI using a body coil. However,

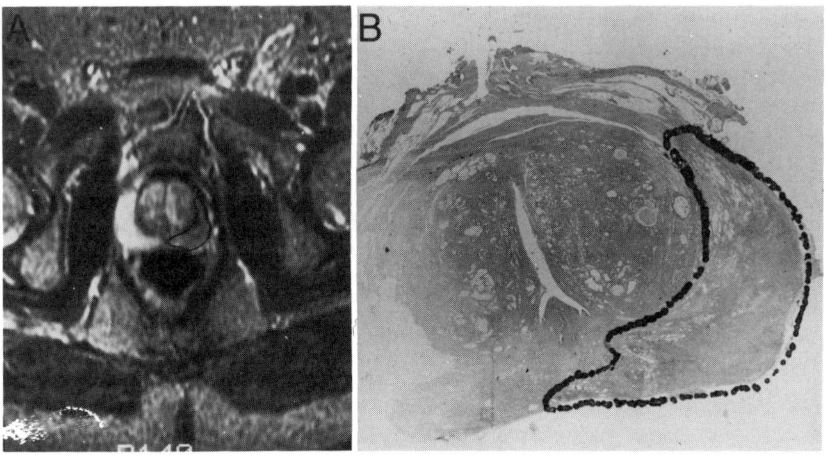

Fig 8–3.—A and B, the volume of the lesion in the left posterior peripheral region of the prostate was underestimated on MRI (A) by only 5% of the volume determined from pathologic examination of the specimen (B). Capsular penetration was present at microscopic examination. (Courtesy of Quint LE, Van Erp JS, Bland PH, et al: *AJR* 156:511–516, 1991.)

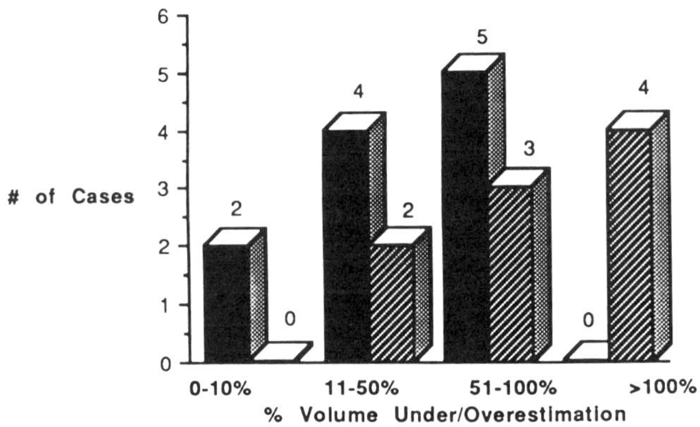

Fig 8–4.—Bar graph showing the degree of under- *(solid bar)* or overestimation *(hatched bar)* of tumor volumes on MRI in 20 patients. (Courtesy of Quint LE, Van Erp JS, Bland PH, et al: *AJR* 156:511–516, 1991.)

as tumor volume increases, it becomes more likely that the cancer has spread beyond the capsule. The accuracy of indirect diagnosis of capsular penetration was evaluated by estimating prostatic tumor volume in 26 patients from a study of MRI and endorectal sonography in staging prostatic cancer. All patients had radical prostatectomy within 3 weeks of the MRI examination.

Methods.—The MRI scans were reviewed in a blinded fashion, and the lesion was manually outlined on the T2-weighted image. These images were correlated visually with the outlined whole-mount surgical specimens. The voxel summation technique was used to calculated total volumes for each lesion.

Results.—Of the 31 lesions diagnosed prospectively on MRI scans, 20 corresponded to malignant lesions seen on microscopic examination. Of the matched lesions, 12 were mostly or entirely within the capsule, and 8 involved both the peripheral and central regions of the gland. The MRI scans underestimated tumor volume in 11 patients and overestimated it in 9. Overestimation tended to occur with small and underestimation with large tumors, and only 2 estimations came within 10% of the actual volume (Fig 8–3 and 8–4). There was a significant overlap between lesions with and without capsular penetration, and the differing histologic findings contributed to inaccuracies of measurement.

Conclusions.—The prostatic tumor volumes estimated by MRI using a body coil and determined from pathologic specimens are not well correlated. Advances in MRI technology may improve its accuracy in this setting. Knowledge of the size of the lesion is important in predicting its behavior.

▶ This paper evaluates the use of MRI in prostate cancer, with special attention given to the direct tumor spread beyond the prostatic capsule. As the authors demonstrate, the images are quite good, but not good enough. The size estimates of neoplasm are not very accurate. They show that there is much that remains to be done in the area of tumor imaging for prostate cancer. Fortunately for the study, their gold standard was pathologic examination.—E. Glatstein, M.D.

Prostate Specific Antigen Levels After Definitive Irradiation for Carcinoma of the Prostate

Schellhammer PF, Schlossberg SM, El-Mahdi AM, Wright GL, Brassil DN (Eastern Virginia Med School, Norfolk)

J Urol 145:1008–1011, 1991 8–6

Introduction.—Prostate-specific antigen (PSA) is a glycoprotein produced only by the prostate. The detectable serum PSA levels after prostatectomy may indicate incomplete removal of the structure, residual local extraprostatic disease, or metastatic disease.

Study Design.—The levels of PSA were estimated in 78 patients considered to be free of disease clinically 3 years or more after completion of radiotherapy for prostatic cancer. Both PSA and prostatic acid phosphatase were determined by radioimmuoassay.

Findings.—Prostate-specific antigen was undetectable in only 3% of patients before treatment. Of the 78 study patients, 38% had undetectable serum PSA (.5 ng/mL or less), and the same proportion had normal levels (4 ng/mL or less). All stages and grades of carcinoma were represented in these groups. Similar proportions of the 24 patients with negative biopsy specimens had undetectable, normal, and increased levels of PSA.

Discussion.—Prostate-specific antigen may be more sensitive than prosttic acid phosphtase in detecting prostatic cancer, but its value as a marker of radiation failure is uncertain. Although it is undetectable in some treated patients, it is not clear whether this reflects suppression of marker production alone or ablation of the cancer tissue producing the marker.

▶ After radical prostatectomy, an increased serum PSA level is often an indication for additional therapy. Increased PSA levels after surgery will predict for recurrence in almost 100% of patients, whereas an undetectable level of PSA is associated with a recurrence rate of approximately 10%. In previous studies, pelvic irradiation given to patients with an increased post-prostatectomy serum PSA resulted in undetectable levels in approximately 35% to 40% of patients. Increased or detectable PSA levels after definitive radiotherapy have not been associated with the same degree of accuracy for predicting recurrence that has been found after prostatectomy. Detectable levels of PSA after radiation may be a result of residual local radioresistant disease, distant metastases, or benign prostatic tissue remnants that can produce antigen. Consequently, an elevated PSA level after radiotherapy may not indicate an early treatment failure. It will be important to prospectively monitor PSA levels after curative radiation to determine whether ultimate failure is associated with detectable serum levels after treatment.—R.F. Ozols, M.D., Ph.D.

Prostate Specific Antigen and Prostatic Acid Phosphatase for Monitoring Therapy of Carcinoma of the Prostate

Dupont A, Cusan L, Gomez J-L, Thibeault M-M, Tremblay M, Labrie F (CHUL Research Ctr, Quebec; Laval Univ, Quebec)

J Urol 146:1064–1068, 1991 8–7

Introduction.—Prostate-specific antigen (PSA) and prostatic acid phosphatase (PAP) are useful in monitoring patients with established prostate carcinoma. After prostatectomy, persistent PSA and PAP indicate more advanced disease, whereas after radiation or endocrine therapy, increasing levels suggest recurrent disease.

Methods.—The effectiveness of these markers, as analyzed by 2 different methods, was evaluated in 871 patients treated with hormonal combination therapy for prostate cancer during an 85-year period. Of the patients, 95 had stage C and 776 had stage D2 disease. The average follow-up period was 26 months. The effectiveness of the 2 serum markers in predicting recurrent disease was evaluated using 2 statistical methods at the time of progression and at 6 and 12 months before clinical relapse. The optimized cutoff values were 2 μg/L for serum PAP and 4 μg/L for PSA levels.

Results.—At the time of progression, the sensitivity was 61.1% for PAP and 86.7% for PSA. The specificity was 79.6% for PAP and 92.4% for PSA. According to receiver-operating characteristic analysis, PSA had the greater accuracy (89.2% vs. 92.4%). The positive predictive value was 89.6% for PAP and 81.4% for PSA; however PSA had a negative predictive value of 92.4% compared with 79.6% for PAP.

Conclusion.—In patients with stage C and D prostate cancer who have undergone combination endocrine therapy, evaluating serum PSA levels is superior to evaluating serum PAP levels in predicting recurrent disease. The PAP measurement makes no significant addition to the measurement of PSA alone. Accuracy is highest at a threshold decision of 4 μg/L for PSA, whereas the corresponding upper normal limit for PAP should be less than 2 μg/L.

▶ There is little doubt that an increasing serum PSA level after prostatectomy is an extremely accurate test for ultimate treatment failure. This current study confirms the clinical usefulness of PSA measurements in this situation. It was of particular interest that measurement of serum PAP did not provide any additional clinical utility to the PSA level. The frequent clinical practice of obtaining both tests while monitoring patients after treatment should be reconsidered. It also must be remembered that PSA levels can be normal at the time of disease progression (13% in this series). Treatment decisions should not be made solely on the basis of a single serum test. Serial monitoring of tumor markers coupled with radiologic tests, and clinical signs and symptoms remain the most appropriate manner of follow-up.—R.F. Ozols, M.D., Ph.D.

Prostate-Specific Antigen Levels From Completely Sectioned, Clinically Benign, Whole Prostates

Brawn PN, Speights VO, Kuhl D, Riggs N, Spiekerman AM, McCord RG, Coffield KS, Stewart DT, Lind ML (VA Med Ctr, Temple, Tex; Texas A & M Univ, Temple; Central Florida Regional Hosp, Sanford; Univ of Texas, Dallas)

Cancer 68:1592–1599, 1991 8–8

Introduction.—The serum level of prostate-specific antigen (PSA) is widely used in managing patients with prostatic cancer, making it important to define the conditions under which it becomes elevated. Clinically benign, whole prostate glands and pelvic lymph nodes were obtained from 105 patients at autopsy. All patients also had premortem serum specimens available for estimation of PSA.

Correlations.—Twenty-eight of the 105 patients had prostatic cancers with a volume of less than 1 mL, and 9 had larger cancers. The PSA was increased (more than 4 ng/mL) in 5 of 8 patients with an untrimmed prostatic weight of 80 g or more but no cancer, in both patients with small cancers in a gland of this weight, and in the 1 patient with a larger tumor. Among the 94 patients with a prostatic weight of less than 80 g, 10 of 60 without prostatic cancer had elevated levels of PSA, as did 2 of 26 with small cancers and all 8 with larger cancers.

Implications.—Patients with an increased level of PSA and a clinically benign untrimmed prostate gland that weighs less than 80 g are at substantial risk of harboring a cancer larger than 1 mL. The risk increases with the degree of PSA increase.

▶ The use of the PSA as a screening agent is rapidly gaining popularity in the United States. This paper points out some of the potential problems in an autopsy study. It suggests that elevated levels of PSA can occur in large prostates, even without carcinoma of the prostate. Small carcinomas (less than 1 mL) appear not to increase the PSA level to a detectable level, whereas larger carcinomas do. The development of this assay is now causing a reevaluation of carcinoma of the prostate, because the diagnosis is now being made before the lesion is detectable clinically. One can reliably anticipate that the diagnosis of carcinoma of the prostate will be made more frequently now than it has been in the past and that, hopefully, it will detect the earlier stage more frequently than has been detected in the past.

In a related paper by Russell et al. (1), the treatment levels of PSA appear to be an independent prognostic factor for patients with prostate cancer treated with primary radiotherapy. The failure of PSA to return to normal range within 1 year of completion of radiotherapy indentified a group of patients at very high risk for tumor recurrence.—E. Glatstein, M.D.

Reference

1. Russell KJ, et al: *J Urol* 146:1046, 1991.

Impact of Anatomical Radical Prostatectomy on Urinary Continence

Steiner MS, Morton RA, Walsh PC (Johns Hopkins Med Insts, Baltimore)

J Urol 145:512–515, 1991 8–9

Background.—Total urinary incontinence can result as a complication of radical prostatectomy, although various sugical modifications have been used. During the past decade, an anatomical approach to the operation has been developed. The impact of anatomical radical prostatectomy on urinary continence was investigated.

Methods.—A total of 600 consecutive males underwent radical retropubic prostatectomy done by a single surgeon between April 1982 and July 1988. The 600 patients ranged in age from 34 to 76 years old. All had an evaluation every 3 months for the first year, then yearly thereafter; such follow-up data were available on 593 patients.

Results.—One year or more after prostatectomy, 547 patients (92%) of the 593 demonstrated complete urinary control, whereas 46 (8%) had stress urinary incontinence. No patient had total urinary incontinence. Only 2 individuals (.3%) had stress incontinence that required the use of an artificial urinary sphincter. None of the following factors—age, nerve-sparing, postoperative potency, prior transurethral resection of the prostate, pathologic stage of the cancer, prostate weight, and minor modifications of the surgical procedure—influenced the outcome for the development of urinary incontinence in this patient population.

Implications.—These results suggest that anatomical parameters (not the preservation of the autonomic innervation of the patient) may act to improve urinary control related to the use of an anatomical radical prostatectomy. Recently, the striated urethral sphincter has been incorporated into the anastomosis made in the operation and has resulted in a quicker recovery of urinary continence in these patients. A longer follow-up of this patient population is planned.

▶ Numerous new areas of interest focus on diagnosis and treatment of prostatic cancer. First, the recent application of PSA screening in combination with rectal ultrasound in national study settings will eventually allow a much better understanding of the natural history of prostatic cancer. Secondly, the therapeutic implications of early diagnosis of encapsulated prostatic cancers will need to be investigated formally. Third, all of the biological interest in the cellular regulation of benign and transformed prostatic tissue is paralleled by a continued significant modification in the surgical techniques used for the treatment of locally invasive prostatic cancer. Walsh has looked—and continues to look—closely at the anatomical considerations of cancer surgery for prostate cancer to minimize sexual and urinary ill consequences without sacrifice of cure. This article represents a continued commitment by the Hopkins group to tailor their operations for maximal benefit to the patient and minimum toxicity. It is important to remember that the potential for improvement in cancer treatment lies as much in the elegant analysis of our surgery as it does in many of the cell biological and molecular biological investigations that will ultimately determine the etiology of prevalent solid tumors.—G.D. Steele, Jr., M.D.

Zoladex Versus Orchiectomy in Treatment of Advanced Prostate Cancer: A Randomized Trial

Soloway MS, for the Zoladex Prostate Study Group (Univ of Tennessee, Memphis)

Urology 37:46–51, 1991 8–10

Introduction.—The disadvantages of orchiectomy and diethylstilbestrol (DES) therapy in the treatment of advanced prostatic cancer have prompted a search for alternative therapies. Goserelin acetate (Zoladex) is a long-acting, biodegradable, sustained-release depot preparation belonging to the new therapeutic class of luteinizing hormone-releasing hormone agonist analogues, which are being investigated for use in the treatment of advanced prostate cancer. Goserelin and orchiectomy were compared in a prospective, randomized, multicenter study.

Patients.—The study was done in 164 previously untreated men with a histologically confirmed diagnosis of stage D2 prostate cancer; 81 were randomized to receive goserelin and 83 underwent orchiectomy. Goserelin was administered every 28 days by subcutaneous injection of a 3.6-mg sustained-release depot dose. Response was assessed at 4, 8, and 12 weeks and every 12 weeks thereafter. Those patients with less than 3 months' life expectancy were excluded from the study.

Results.—Sixty-six goserelin-treated patients (81%) and 65 orchiectomy-treated patients (78%) had either a complete response, a partial response, or stable disease at 12 weeks. Nine goserelin-treated patients (11%) and 8 orchiectomy patients (10%) had disease progression. The remaining 16 patients were not evaluable. The median serum levels of testosterone were reduced to castrate levels within 4 weeks and remained supprssed for as long as 60 weeks with either treatment. The median serum levels of acid phosphatase were also similar. There were 29 treat-

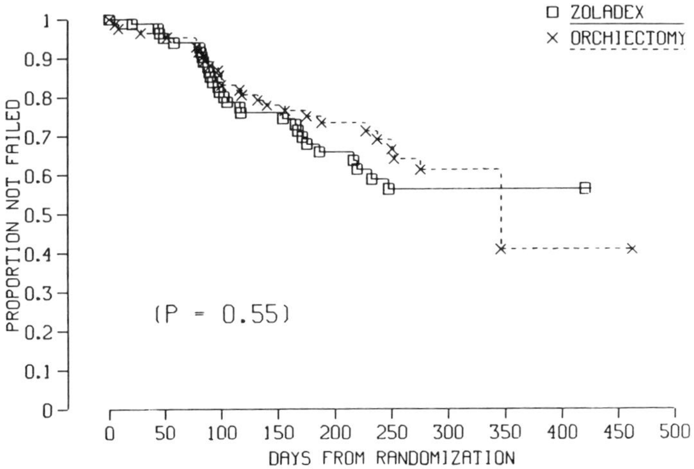

Fig 8–5.—Distribution of time to treatment failure in patients randomized to Zoladex or orchiectomy. (Courtesy of Soloway MS, Smith JA Jr, Chodak G, et al: *Urology* 37:46–51, 1991.)

ment failures with goserelin and 28 with orchiectomy. Time to treatment failure did not differ significantly between the 2 groups (Fig 8–5). The side effects, including hot flashes, pain, and urinary symptoms, were also similar. The median follow-up for all patients was 210 days.

Conclusion.—Goserelin and orchiectomy are equally effective for the treatment of stage D2 prostate cancer. Both treatment modalities have an acceptable safety profile. The effect of goserelin on survival remains to be determined.

▶ There currently is no clear-cut evidence that any form of hormonal therapy for metastatic prostate cancer is superior to orchiectomy. In this randomized trial, orchiectomy and treatment with a long-acting sustained-release luteinizing hormone-releasing hormone agonist led to identical levels of serum testosterone and produced the same response rates and disease-free survival. The major factor for selection of hormonal therapy for stage D2 prostate is basically an issue of toxicity. Orchiectomy and goserelin produced similar toxicities that were attributable to a decrease in androgen levels. However, this trial has not reported on more subjective criteria, such as the effect on sexuality and body image after orchiectomy compared with goserelin. Because total androgen-blockade, orchiectomy, and luteinizing hormone-releasing hormone agonists all have the same antitumor effect, selection of therapy is primarily the patient's individual choice.—R.F. Ozols, M.D., Ph.D.

Bladder

Prognostic Factors in Invasive Bladder Carcinoma in a Prospective Trial of Preoperative Adjuvant Chemotherapy and Radiotherapy

Fung CY, Shipley WU, Young RH, Griffin PP, Convery KM, Kaufman DS, Althausen AF, Heney NM, Prout GR Jr (Massachusetts Gen Hosp; Harvard Med School, Boston)

J Clin Oncol 9:1533–1542, 1991 8–11

Background.—Neoadjuvant chemotherapy is being investigated as a way to reduce the rate of distant metastasis and improve survival in patients with muscle-invasive bladder carcinoma. Because there have been no studies of the prognostic factors in patients undergoing neoadjuvant chemotherapy and radiation therapy, clinical and pathologic factors were analyzed in 40 such patients.

Patients and Treatment.—The study sample comprised 24 men and 16 women with localized muscle-invasive bladder carcinoma (mean age, 65.2 years). A total of 34 tumors was stage T2 or T3. All patients participated in a prospective study of bladder-preserving treatment, consisting of transurethral resection; neoadjuvant chemotherapy with methotrexate, cisplatin, and vinblastine; and radiotherapy, 4,000 cGy, and concurrent cisplatin. If there was a complete response, radiation with cisplatin, 6,480 cGy, was given. If residual disease occurred, then cystectomy was recommended.

Findings.—Distant metastases occurred in no patient with a T2 tumor, 39% of those with T3–T4 tumors, 6% of those with tumors less than 5 cm, and 59% of those with tumors 5 cm or more. Recurrence was greater in those with tumor-associated carcinoma in situ than in those without. The significant predictors of complete response were stage T2 and absence of carcinoma in situ. Outcomes were similar for papillary and solid tumors. Carcinoma in situ predicted local recurrence. Distant metastasis was predicted by tumor size, response to chemoradiotherapy, and vascular invasion. There were 8 local bladder tumor recurrences; 6 of these were superficial. No patient with a T2 tumor had a distant metastsis at 3 years. The 3-year actuarial survival rate was 89% for patients with T2 stage tumors and 50% for patients with T3–T4 tumors; these results were encouraging compared with those of historical controls.

Conclusion.—Preliminary results suggest that this chemoradiotherapy method may have beneficial effects in the treatment of muscle-invasive bladder carcinoma. Longer follow-up is needed to confirm the prognostic findings. The real value of neoadjuvant chemotherapy needs confirmation by randomized trials.

▶ The standard treatment for advanced localized bladder cancer has been radical surgery, radical radiotherapy, or combined-modality treatment. In the past 2 decades, improved surgical and radiotherapeutic techniques have been developed, yet the 5-year survival rates have remained the same (50% or less), with death resulting most frequently from distant metastases. The goal of preoperative chemotherapy is to decrease the probability of distant metastases and also to decrease the morbidity of procedures aimed at local control, i.e., an attempt to avoid cystectomy. The preliminary results of the aggressive chemoradiation approach described in this study provide a measure of optimism that this is a reachable goal in bladder cancer. Not only was the complete response rate high [62% (25 of 40) patients had intact bladders], but the analysis of prognostic factors indicated that the biology of the disease may have been altered. Of particular promise was the 89% 3-year survival rate and the rate of 0% distant metastasis for patients with stage T2 tumors.—R.F. Ozols, M.D., Ph.D.

A Randomized Trial of Intravesical Doxorubicin and Immunotherapy With Bacille Calmette-Guérin for Transitional-Cell Carcinoma of the Bladder

Lamm DL, Blumenstein BA, Crawford ED, Montie JE, Scardino P, Grossman HB, Stanisic TH, Smith JA Jr, Sullivan J, Sarosdy MF, Crissman JD, Coltman CA (West Virginia Univ, Morgantown; Southwest Oncology Group Statistical Ctr, Seattle; Univ of Colorado, Denver; Vanderbilt Med Ctr, Nashville; Baylor College of Medicine, Houston; et al)

N Engl J Med 325:1205–1209, 1991 8–12

Background.—Some recent controlled trials have indicated that bacille Calmette-Guérin (BCG) therapy is better than standard intravesical chemotherapy for carcinoma in situ of the bladder. Other studies have had different results, and some have included patients at low risk of tumor recurrence. A randomized multicenter study was conducted to address the relative merits of these 2 therapies.

Methods.—The subjects were 262 patients with carcinoma in situ or rapidly recurrent stage Ta or T1 transitional-cell bladder carcinoma. The patients were stratified according to the presence or absence of carcinoma in situ and previous chemotherapy and were then randomized to receive either chemotherapy or immunotherapy. Immunotherapy consisted of BCG, 40 mg, most of which was instilled intravesically; a small amount given percutaneously. Chemotherapy consisted of doxorubicin. Biopsy and urine cytologic analysis were done to confirm a complete response to treatment of carcinoma in situ.

Results.—Among patients who had Ta and T1 tumors and no carcinoma in situ, the estimated 5-year disease-free survival rates were 17% in the doxorubicin group and 37% in the BCG group. Treatment failure (cessation of treatment resulting from persistence, recurrence, or progression of disease) occurred after a median of 10.4 months with doxorubicin and after 22.5 months with BCG. Patients with carcinoma in situ who received doxorubicin had a 34% estimated probability of complete response; compared with 70% for those receiving BCG. In this group, median times to treatment failure were 5.1 months with doxorubicin and 39 months with BCG. In patients with carcinoma in situ, the 5-year disease-free survival was 18% with doxorubicin and 45% with BCG (Fig 8–6). There were more systemic toxic effects and local irritative symptoms with BCG, but most were not severe.

Conclusions.—In patients with superficial bladder cancer, immunotherapy with BCG appears to improve protection against recurrence compared with intravesical doxorubicin. The treatment can be given safely and effectively. Use of BCG may be the best intravesical treatment of bladder carcinoma in situ.

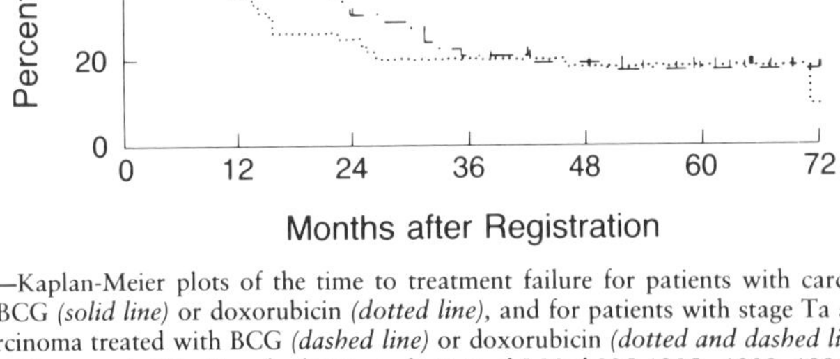

Fig 8–6.—Kaplan-Meier plots of the time to treatment failure for patients with carcinoma in situ treated with BCG *(solid line)* or doxorubicin *(dotted line)*, and for patients with stage Ta and T1 transitional-cell carcinoma treated with BCG *(dashed line)* or doxorubicin *(dotted and dashed line)*. (Courtesy of Lamm DL, Blumenstein BA, Crawford ED, et al: *N Engl J Med* 325:1205–1209, 1991.)

▶ Even though prospective randomized trials demonstrated that intravesical BCG was superior to surgery alone in the treatment of superficial bladder cancer, reservations were frequently expressed about its general applicability, primarily in relation to concerns about toxicity. This prospective randomized study was conducted by the Southwest Oncology Group, and it unequivocally establishes that BCG can be safely administered in a cooperative group setting. Furthermore, BCG was more effective than doxorubicin in preventing recurrences. There were no major differences in toxicity, making intravesical BCG the treatment of choice for rapidly recurrent (stage Ta or T1) or in situ transitional-cell carcinoma of the bladder.—R.F. Ozols, M.D., Ph.D.

Curative Radiotherapy Following Chemotherapy for Invasive Bladder Carcinoma: A Preliminary Report

Farah R, Chodak GW, Vogelzang NJ, Awan AM, Quiet CA, Moormeier J, Schoenberg H, Weichselbaum RR (Univ of Chicago Hospitals)

Int J Radiat Oncol Biol Phys 20:413–417, 1991 8–13

Background.—Patients with invasive bladder carcinoma treated with radical cystectomy have a 5-year survival of only 28% to 50%, and operative treatment may lead to major postoperative complications and sexual dysfunction. Radical cystectomy and adjuvant radiotherapy yield equivalent survival to radical radiotherapy alone. Trials were initiated combining chemotherapy with radiotherapy to enhance local control, sterilize micrometastases, and increase survival while avoiding the complications of surgical procedures. It was found that patients treated with transurethral resection, cisplatinum, and curative radiotherapy had improvement in local response rates compared with radiation therapy alone.

Patients.—Twenty-five patients had invasive transitional-cell carcinoma of the bladder at stage T_2, T_3, or T_4. All patients received combined-modality therapy using 4 cycles of methotrexate, vinblastine, adriamycin, and cisplatin (MVAC) chemotherapy followed by surgery or radiation therapy (RT).

Results.—Sixteen of the 25 patients had complete or partial response to MVAC. Eleven responders with T_2 or T_3 disease were alive after curative RT, and 7 had normal bladder function. Two patients with T_4 disease died of the disease despite RT. Three patients required salvage cystectomy for local recurrence, and 1 patient had cystectomy for bladder stones. There were no late intestinal or bladder complications related to chemotherapy or radiotherapy treatment, except for 1 bladder stone formation.

Conclusions.—A treatment plan of MVAC chemotherapy followed by radiotherapy is possibly superior to radiotherapy alone for muscle-invading transitional-cell carcinoma of the bladder. Patients with stage T_2 or T_3 disease who have a complete or partial response to MVAC appear to be excellent candidates for a bladder-sparing treatment.

▶ This is an interesting preliminary paper dealing with the complex subject of bladder cancer. Combined-modality efforts are being put forth everywhere, and investigators are just beginning to learn how to integrate chemotherapy, radiation therapy, and surgery. The point of this series is that it would appear that a large proportion of patients who have invasive bladder cancer with a typically grim prognosis can expect to retain their bladder without necessarily going through a cystectomy. In many ways, developments on this front would be analogous to the developments in breast cancer, where conservative treatment preserving organ function appears to be comparable in outcome with radical surgical procedures.—E. Glatstein, M.D.

Additional Reading

Zagars GK, Sherman NE, et al: Prostate-specific antigen and external beam radiation therapy in prostate cancer. *Cancer* 67:412–420, 1991.

▶ The levels of PSA after external beam radiation therapy remained detectable in the sera of all patients with localized prostate cancer. In some patients, increasing levels of PSA were detected within 6 months of treatment; however, a correlation with clinical relapse has not been established.

Davies AH, Cranston D, et al: Effect of blood transfusion on survival after radiotherapy as treatment for carcinoma of the prostate. *Ann R Coll Surg Engl* 73:116–118, 1991.

▶ Recurrence of tumor was 72% compared with 21% in patients with prostate cancer who required transfusions at transurethral resection compared with nontransfused patients. (P = <.1).

Wozniak AJ, Samson MK, et al: A randomized trial of cisplatin, vinblastine, and bleomycin versus vinblastine, cisplatin, and etoposide in the treatment of advanced germ cell tumors of the testis: A Southwest Oncology Group study. *J Clin Oncol* 9:70–76, 1991.

▶ Bleomycin was omitted from a 3-drug regimen (vinblastine, cisplatin and VP-16) for testicular cancer without adverse effects.

Motzer RJ, Geller NL, et al: Salvage chemotherapy for patients with germ cell tumors. *Cancer* 67:1305–1310, 1991.

▶ Those patients with testicular cancer who never achieve a complete response have only a 9% survival to salvage therapy, compared with a 36% survival for patients treated with salvage therapy after relapse from a complete remission.

Chodak GW, Vogelzang NJ, et al: Independent prognostic factors in aptients with metastatic (stage D2) prostate cancer. *JAMA* 265:618–621, 1991.

▶ Patients with absence of bone pain, low serum alkaline phosphatase level (<115 IU); high serum testosterone (>8.6 nmol/L), and an Eastern Cooperative Oncology Group performance status of 0 or 1 had a 2-year survival rate of 84% compared with 8% for patients with none of the factors favorable for survival ($P < .0001$).

Harstrick A, Schmoll H-J, et al: Cisplatin, etoposide, and ifosfamide salvage therapy for refractory or relapsing germ cell carcinoma. *J Clin Oncol* 9:1549–1555, 1991.

▶ Salvage therapy with VIP [VP-16, ifosfamide and cisplatin] in testicular cancer produced a 33% rate of complete response and a 90% relapse rate. Only those patients who had a prior response to induction therapy had a chance for cure with VIP.

9 Gynecologic Cancers

Ovary

Human Müllerian Inhibiting Substance Inhibits Tumor Growth In Vitro and In Vivo

Chin T, Parry RL, Donahoe PK (Taipei Veterans Gen Hosp, Taipei, Taiwan; Nat Naval Med Ctr, Bethesda, Md, Harvard Med School, Boston)

Cancer Res 51:2101–2101, 1991 9–1

Background.—Müllerian inhibiting substance (MIS) leads to regression of the müllerian duct in the male fetus. Bovine MIS reportedly inhibits the growth of some gynecologic tumors, but this effect was elicited using natural MIS. Since then, the bovine and human MIS genes have been cloned, and the human protein has been expressed in Chinese hamster ovary cells.

Methods.—Recombinant human MIS (rhMIS) was produced in transfected Chinese hamster ovary cells and highly purified by immunoaffinity chromatography. Introduction of a salt wash before elution of MIS removed a growth-stimulating factor or factors derived from the hamster ovary cells.

Observations.—Immunopurified rhMIS inhibited the growth of A431 vulvar epidermoid carcinoma, HT-3 cervical carcinoma, HEC-1-A endometrial adenocarcinoma, NIH:OVCAR-3 ovarian adenocarcinoma, and OM431 ocular melanoma human cell lines in colony inhibition assays. The preparation failed, however, to alter the growth of Hep 3B hepatocellular carcinoma and RT4 transitional-cell bladder papilloma. The growth of A431 and OM431 cells also was inhibited by rhMIS using an in vivo subrenal capsule assay in irradiated mice.

Conclusions.—The growth of some human tumor-cell lines is inhibited in vitro and in vivo by rhMIS. Systemic MIS has caused no obvious toxicity in animals.

▶ It is interesting to consider that the human body may possess factors with the capacity to inhibit malignant tumor growth. The role of MIS in regression of the müllerian duct in the male fetus has suggested that this molecule might have such utility in the treatment of tumors from female organs that originate in the müllerian duct. These tumors include those from the ovaries, fallopian tubes, uterus, cervix, and upper vagina. This paper demonstrates modest inhibitory effects on the growth of such tumor classes in vitro and in vivo. The data suggest that MIS is a cytostatic rather than a cytotoxic agent. The paper further shows that some earlier data indicating that MIS had a minimal effect in such tumors likely resulted from the co-purification of a growth stimulatory factor along with MIS. This factor partially reversed the cytostatic effects of MIS.—T.C. Hamilton, Ph.D.

Cellular DNA Content as a New Prognostic Tool in Patients With Borderline Tumors of the Ovary

Kaern J, Trope C, Kjorstad KE, Abeler V, Pettersen EO (Norwegian Radium Hosp, Oslo)

Gynecol Oncol 38:452–457, 1990 9–2

Introduction.—Patients with borderline tumors of the ovary generally have an excellent prognosis. Flow cytometry of cellular DNA content may provide an additional parameter to identify borderline tumors with truly malignant potential. A new prognostic tool for borderline ovarian tumors was developed.

Methods.—Histologic sections from 370 patients with borderline tumors treated in 1970–1982 were reviewed. Histologic typing was performed on all specimens. Flow cytometric measurement of DNA content was performed on specimens from 34 patients who either had a relapse or died of their disease. It was also done on specimens from 30 living patients without known recurrence. Follow-up ranged from 84 to 218 months.

Results.—The overall disease-free survival rate was 89.8%, higher for serous compared with mucinous tumors (Fig 9–1). In the patients who died or had a recurrence, there were 15 diploid and 19 aneuploid tumors and 10 serous and 24 mucinous tumors. Overall, 66% of the tumors were diploid and 34% were aneuploid; 15% of the serous tumors were aneuploid, compared with 47% of the mucinous tumors.

Conclusions.—Measurement of DNA may be a useful adjunct to conventional histopathologic diagnosis of borderline ovarian tumors. Data on ploidy, together with histopathologic and clinical parameters, may help identify patients for whom conservative treatment is justified.

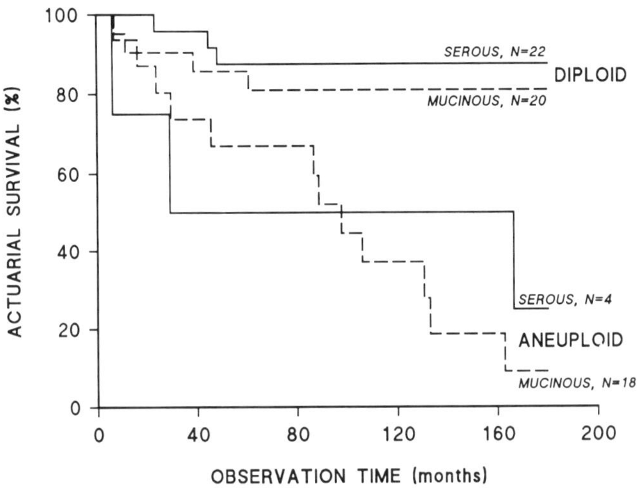

Fig 9–1.—Actuarial 15-year survival in 64 diploid and aneuploid tumors. (Courtesy of Kaern J, Trope C, Kjorstad KE, et al: *Gynecol Oncol* 38:452–457, 1990.)

▶ Borderline tumors of the ovary, also known as tumors of low malignant potential, have an excellent overall prognosis. Even in patients with disseminated (stage III) disease, the 5-year survival rates are approximately 75%. This important study must be confirmed in a larger patient population. The initial results suggest that cellular DNA content may be an important prognostic factor in identifying the subset of patients with borderline tumors of the ovary who have an unfavorable prognosis. If larger retrospective studies of DNA content confirm these results, then a prospective trial of adjuvant chemotherapy in aneuploid borderline tumors is indicated. Currently, there is no evidence that any form of equivalent therapy is useful in borderline tumors.—R.F. Ozols, M.D., Ph.D.

Laparoscopic Excision of Ovarian Neoplasms Subsequently Found To Be Malignant

Maiman M, Seltzer V, Boyce J (State Univ of New York, Brooklyn; Albert Einstein College of Medicine, Jamaica, NY)

Obstet Gynecol 77:563–565, 1991 9–3

Introduction.–Operative laparoscopic surgery in the management of ovarian cysts has become popular in the past few years, despite the fact that no studies have been done to compare the efficacy of laparoscopy with laparotomy for this indication. The laparoscopic excision of ovarian neoplasms that are later found to be malignant is of particular concern.

Survey Design.—Gynecologic oncologists were surveyed to assess the characteristics of neoplasms, the subsequent histopathology, and the completeness and timing of surgery in cases of ovarian lesions found to be malignant after laparoscopic excision was attempted. A total of 156 gynecologic oncologists returned the 13-question survey on the laparoscopic management of ovarian neoplasms that later proved to be malignant. The survey response rate was 42%.

Findings.—Nineteen percent of the responders (29) had treated 42 cases of ovarian malignancy. In 38% of the cases, the laparoscopic procedure was aborted, with or without aspiration of the cyst. Partial or complete excisions were attempted in 33% and 29% of the cases, respectively. The masses were less than 8 cm in 67% of the cases, cystic in 62%, unilocular in 48%, and unilateral in 91%. All 4 benign characteristics were noted in 31% of the cases that later proved to be malignant. Three of the 4 characteristics were present in 24%. Laparotomy was done concurrently with laparoscopy in 17%, at an average of 4.8 weeks after laparoscopy in 71%, and not at all in 12%. Of the patients, 57% had invasive epithelial malignancies and 29% had tumors of low malignant potential. At least half of the patients had stage II–IV tumors.

Discussion.—Attempted laparoscopic excision of adnexal masses that are later found to be malignant is not uncommon. The presence of the so-called benign characteristics does not mean the mass is not malignant. Attempts at partial or complete excision and delays in subsequent definitive surgery are also common. The stage of disease in such cases is frequently high. All histologic types of malignancy are encountered. The practice of operative laparoscopic surgery for ovarian cysts should be carefully assessed, and strict guidelines should be developed to insure optimal care.

▶ Laparoscopic excision of "everything in sight" appears to be one of the fastest growing new techniques in medical practice. In certain settings, laparoscopic surgery *can* simplify surgical intervention, reduce the duration of hospitalization, and substantially reduce morbidity. However, there are likely to be situations in which this technique is suboptimal. This study looked at operative laparoscopic surgery in the management of ovarian cysts. It emphasized some potentially serious problems with the procedure in patients who are subsequently found to have ovarian cancer. In 42 cases of ovarian cancer that were initially evaluated with laparoscopy, aspiration of cysts, subtotal resections, and spilled tumor contents were common. The tumor markers in these patients were rarely sent before evaluation, and frozen section diagnosis was requested in a minority of cases. Although one anticipates that laparoscopy staging techniques will improve when used for gynecologic cancer, this preliminary experience suggests that many of the classic principles of proper tumor surgery are being applied inadequately. Frighteningly, 12% of the patients in this study had no subsequent surgical management after the disease was diagnosed by laparoscopy. The authors correctly advocate careful preoperative evaluation with CA-125 and sonography, and they urge that the use of laparoscopy in this setting be confined to patients at low risk for an ovarian malignancy.—R.C. Young, M.D., F.A.C.P.

Primary Surgical Therapy of Ovarian Cancer: How Much and When

Potter ME, Partridge EE, Hatch KD, Soong S-J, Austin JM, Shingleton HM
(Univ of Alabama, Birmingham)

Gynecol Oncol 40:195–200, 1991 9–4

Introduction.—Since Griffith first related the volume of disease left at the completion of primary operation for ovarian cancer to patient survival, maximal operative intervention has been advocated. However, improved patient survival with extensive debulking, including peritoneal stripping and bowel resection, has not yet been demonstrated. The impact of the timing and extent of operation, the operative findings, and the effects of subsequent chemotherapy on survival were investigated in patients with invasive epithelial ovarian cancer.

Methods.—During a 10-year period, 328 women were treated for ovarian tumors; of these, 302 had invasive epithelial malignancies. Operative summaries were used both to estimate the volume of residual disease and the number of disease foci present at the completion of the primary operation, and to assess the extent of surgical resection performed.

Results.—Despite extensive debulking efforts, patients who had bowel resections to achieve no residual disease fared no better than those who still has residual disease at the completion of operation and did not undergo bowel resection. Of the patients, 43% were operated on by gynecologic oncologists and 57% were treated by nongynecologic oncologists. However, surgical specialty did not have any significant impact on survival and did not affect the volume of residual disease present at the completion of primary surgery. Those patients with stage III and IV disease were given platinum-based chemotherapy, Alkeran, or other combination chemotherapy; however, the type of chemotherapy did not influence survival. Of the 21 patients with stage III or IV disease who underwent reoperation for what was thought to be unresectable carcinoma, 9 had immediate reoperation and debulking followed by chemotherapy, and 12 had chemotherapy first and then debulking. Both groups had similar survival.

Conclusion.—Although diligent attempts (short of bowel resection) to remove the bulk of the tumor metastases may influence survival, extensive debulking procedures have demonstrated no improved survival, even if the volume of residual disease is reduced by only 1 cm.

▶ One of the constant debates in management of ovarian cancer is how extensive a surgical procedure should be undertaken if cure with surgery alone is not possible. These investigators compared the long-term survival of patients who underwent extensive debulking procedures (such as peritoneal stripping or bowel resection) with long-term survival in patients who received more modest debulking. The patients were subsequently treated with appropriate combination chemotherapy regimens. This retrospective study was unable to document a significant survival benefit of extensive surgical debulking; however, it is impossible to determine whether extensive debulking was required because of a biologically more aggressive tumor. The authors also looked at the utility of having patients who were believed to be unresectable at the time of initial referral undergo reoperation. Although initial chemotherapy did allow many patients to have successful surgery, the operation after initial therapy did not improve long-term survival.—R.C. Young, M.D., F.A.C.P.

Chemotherapy in Advanced Ovarian Cancer: An Overview of Randomised Clinical Trials

Stewart LA, for the Advanced Ovarian Cancer Trialists Group (Cambridge, England)

BMJ 303:884–893, 1991 9–5

Objective.—Many chemotherapy regimens have been used for advanced ovarian cancer, including cisplatin plus cyclophosphamide and single-agent platinum; some institutions are using carboplatin instead of cisplatin. None of the individual trials has been large enough to detect survival differences of realistic magnitude. Updated patient data from all available randomized trials were used in a quantitative overview of the role of platinum and combination chemotherapy in the treatment of advanced ovarian cancer.

Methods.—The analysis included 8,139 patients from 45 different trials, published and unpublished. Studies had to address 1 of 5 compari-

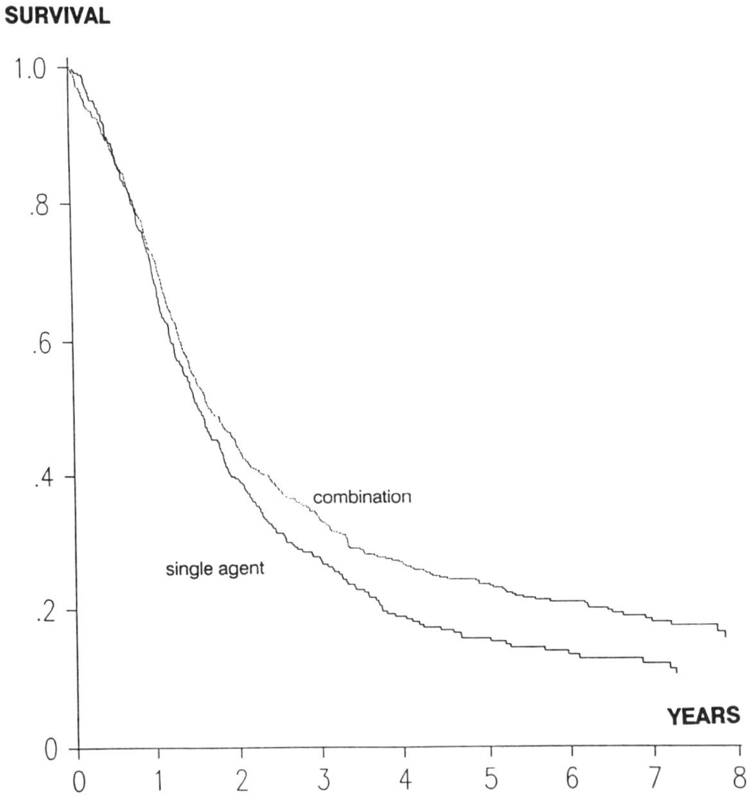

Single-agent platinum								
360	**246**	**125**	**73**	**47**	**35**	**24**	**16**	**9**
Platinum combination								
563	**397**	**230**	**156**	**116**	**95**	**69**	**38**	**14**

Numbers at Risk

Fig 9–2.—The survival curves for comparison IV (single agent platinum vs. platinum combination). (Courtesy of Stewart LA, for the Advanced Ovarian Cancer Trialists Group: *BMJ* 303:884–893, 1991.)

sons between different forms of chemotherapy. Most patient data were updated, allowing median follow-ups of 3–10 years.

Results.—Although no firm conclusions could be reached, platinum-based treatments appeared to offer a better chance of survival than nonplatinum-based treatments, with an overall relative risk .93. At the same dose, platinum in combination appeared superior to platinum alone, with an overall relative risk of .85 (Fig 9–2). No difference in effectiveness was noted between cisplatin and carboplatin (overall relative risk, 1.05).

Conclusions.—An overview of clinical trials of chemotherapy for advanced ovarian cancer offers an important hypotheses as to how incremental gains in survival may be achieved. Past studies have been too small to detect benefits of this degree. A new international trial comparing cisplatin, doxorubicin, and cyclophosphamide, in which it is planned to accrue 2,000 patients, has begun.

▶ This study summarizes the results of a large meta-analysis of 45 different ovarian cancer chemotherapy trials including more than 8,000 patients. A number of conclusions were made on the basis of the analysis: (1) platinum-based chemotherapy is more effective than nonplatinum-based regimens, (2) platinum in combination is better than single-agent platinum; and (3) cisplatinum and carboplatin are equally effective. Although the differences in outcome for each of these 3 groups were not dramatic, the large number of patients analyzed allowed the detection of these small differences. What is surprising and somewhat perplexing is that the authors have proposed a trial that appears to ignore, in part, the conclusions of their own meta-analysis. Their analysis suggests that platinum in combination is better than single-agent platinum, but their proposed trial randomizes patients to either CAP or single-agent carboplatin. Why this trial design should emerge from their analysis is problematic. Although I am inclined to believe the overall conclusions of their study, the fact that they do not appear to be using the conclusions to guide subsequent trial design makes me wonder.—R.C. Young, M.D., F.A.C.P.

Long-Term Survival in Ovarian Cancer: Mature Data from The Netherlands Joint Study Group for Ovarian Cancer

Neijt JP, ten Bokkel Huinink WW, ven der Burg MEL, van Oosterom AT, Willemse PHB, Vermorken JB, van Lindert ACM, Heintz APM, Aartsen E, van Lent M, Trimbos JB, de Meijer AJ (Utrecht Univ Hosp, The Netherlands; Netherlands Cancer Inst, Amsterdam; Daniël den Hoed Kliniek, Rotterdam, The Netherlands; Univ Hosp, Antwerp, Belgium; Groningen Univ Hosp, The Netherlands, et al)

Eur J Cancer 27:1367–1372, 1991 9–6

Background.—There have been few reports on long-term survival in patients with advanced ovarian cancer. Two studies of advanced epithelial ovarian cancer, begun in 1979 and 1981, included 377 patients.

Methods.—Subjects in the first study were randomized to receive hexamethylmelamine, cyclophosphamde, methotrexate, and 5-fluorouracil (Hexa-CAF), or cyclophosphamide, hexamethylmelamine, doxorubicin, and cisplatin for 5 days (CHAP-5). In the second study, patients received either CHAP-5 or cyclophosphamide and cisplatin on 1 day (CP). In the first study, patients who failed to respond to Hexa-CAF were given a cisplatin-containing regimen. The patients in the first study were followed for a median of 9.5 years, and those in the second study were followed for 7.7 years.

Results.—The 10-year survival rates were 9% for patients initially treated with Hexa-CAF and 21% for those treated with CHAP-5. The 8-

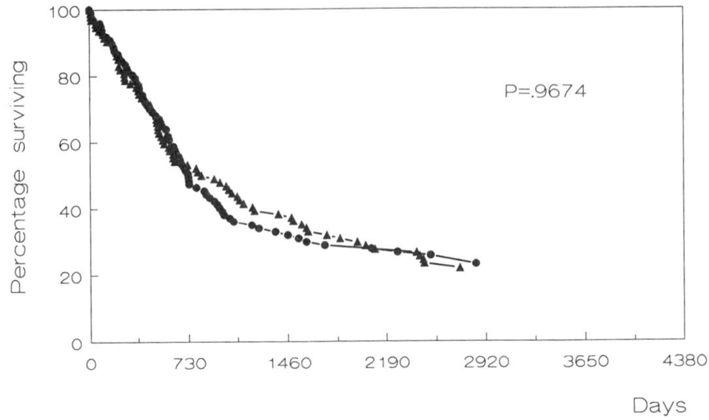

Fig 9–3.—Survival after treatment with CHAP-5 or CP. *Triangles* represent CHAP-5 treatment (94 patients entered; 73 died); *circles* represent CP treatment (97 patients entered; 73 died). (Courtesy of Neijt JP, ten Bokkel Huinink WW, ven der Burg MEL, et al: *Eur J Cancer* 27:1367–1372, 1991.)

year survival rates were 21% for patients treated with CHAP-5 and 23% for those treated with CP (Fig 9–3). Of those patients in the Hexa-CAF group who were still alive, 50% had had progressive disease treated successfully with cisplatin. In both studies, of the patients who achieved complete remission, approximately 60% were alive at 5 years and 40% at 10 years. Of the patients who had microscopic disease at second-look surgery, 35% survived for 5 years. At 5 years, almost half the patients with grade I tumors were still alive; at 10 years 30% were alive. For the other grades, these survivals were halved.

Conclusions.—Cisplatin-containing chemotherapy regimens can increase the 5- and 10-year survival rates from advanced ovarian cancer by more than 10%. Cisplatin appears to be the best regimen for the treatment of these cancers.

▶ Although combination chemotherapy has been used to treat advanced ovarian cancer for more than 2 decades, there has been relatively little data on the long-term survival of patients so treated. This study from the Netherlands Joint Study Group for Ovarian Cancer provides important information on the long-term success of such therapies. The study shows that the 5- and 10-year survivals of patients treated with platinum-based combinations exceed those of nonplatinum-based combinations. The studies further show that use of cyclophosphamide and cisplatinum is as effective as combinations including additional agents, (i.e., CHAP-5). Most importantly, this study documents that 21% of the patients who had advanced ovarian cancer treated with platinum-based combinations were alive at 10-year follow-up. Similar data is presented on the 2-drug combination of cyclophosphamide and cisplatin. This study provides solid evidence that advanced ovarian cancer is curable in approximately 20% of patients undergoing existing therapies.—R.C. Young, M.D., F.A.C.P.

Moving?

I'd like to receive my ***Year Book of Oncology*** without interruption.

Please note the following change of address, effective: ______________________

Name: ______________________

New Address: ______________________

____

City: ______________________ State: __________ Zip: __________

Old Address: ______________________

____

City: ______________________ State: __________ Zip: __________

Reservation Card

Yes, I would like my own copy of the ***Year Book of Oncology***. Please begin my subscription with the current edition according to the terms described below.* I understand that I will have 30 days to examine each annual edition. If satisfied, I will pay just $59.95 plus sales tax, postage and handling (price subject to change without notice).

Name: ______________________

Address: ______________________

City: ______________________ State: __________ Zip: __________

Method of Payment

❑ Visa ❑ Mastercard ❑ AmEx ❑ Bill me ❑ Check (in US dollars, payable to Mosby-Year Book, Inc.)

Card number ______________________ Exp date __________

Signature ______________________

LS-0907

*Your *Year Book* Service Guarantee:

When you subscribe to the ***Year Book***, we'll send you an advance notice of future volumes about two months before they publish. This automatic notice system is designed to take up as little of your time as possible. If you do not want the ***Year Book***, the advance notice makes it quick and easy for you to let us know your decision; and you will always have at least 20 days to decide. If we don't hear from you, we'll send you the new volume as soon as it's available. And, of course, the ***Year Book*** is yours to examine free of charge for 30 days (postage, handling and applicable sales tax are added to each shipment).

NO POSTAGE
NECESSARY
IF MAILED
IN THE
UNITED STATES

BUSINESS REPLY MAIL
FIRST CLASS MAIL PERMIT No. 762 CHICAGO, IL

POSTAGE WILL BE PAID BY ADDRESSEE

Chris Hughes
Mosby-Year Book, Inc.
200 N. LaSalle Street
Suite 2600
Chicago, IL 60601-9981

NO POSTAGE
NECESSARY
IF MAILED
IN THE
UNITED STATES

BUSINESS REPLY MAIL
FIRST CLASS MAIL PERMIT No. 762 CHICAGO, IL

POSTAGE WILL BE PAID BY ADDRESSEE

Chris Hughes
Mosby-Year Book, Inc.
200 N. LaSalle Street
Suite 2600
Chicago, IL 60601-9981

Prognostic Factors for Recurrence Following Negative Second-Look Laparotomy in Ovarian Cancer Patients Treated With Platinum-Based Chemotherapy

Rubin SC, Hoskins WJ, Saigo PE, Chapman D, Hakes TB, Markman M, Reichman B, Almadrones L, Lewis JL Jr (Mem Sloan-Kettering Cancer Ctr, New York)

Gynecol Oncol 42:137–141, 1991 9–7

Background.—There have been several studies of the risk of recurrent ovarian cancer in patients who have had a negative second-look laparotomy after chemotherapy. However, theses studies have generally included patients who underwent both platinum and nonplatinum chemotherapy regimens and only short follow-up. The risk factors for recurrence and long-term outcome were determined in 91 patients, all of whom were treated with platinum chemotherapy.

Patients.—The patients (mean age at diagnosis, 57 years) all had a negative second-look laparotomy after a mean of 6.3 cycles of platinum chemotherapy. Ten patients had stage I, 18 had stage II, 57 had stage III, and 6 had stage IV disease. At negative second-look laparotomy, a mean of 12 biopsy specimens were taken and 52% of the patients had lymph node biopsies. The mean follow-up was 54.6 months from the time of second-look laparotomy.

Findings.—Recurrence was seen in 44% of the patients, outside the peritoneal cavity in almost 40% of the cases. The mean interval to recurrence was 24 months. Significant associations were found between the risk of recurrence and tumor stage, histologic grade, and the amount of tumor remaining after the first operation. Ten percent of stage I, 28% of stage II, 54% of stage III, and 50% of stage IV tumors recurred. By grade, 22% of grade 1, 39% of grade 2, and 56% of grade 3 tumors recurred. The risk of recurrence was unrelated to the number of cycles of platinum, the number of biopsy specimens taken at second-look laparotomy, or number of months until second look.

Conclusions.—The risk of recurrent ovarian cancer is significant in patients who have a negative second-look laparotomy after platinum chemotherapy. This is especially true during the first 3 years. Consolidation therapy against both intraperitoneal and extraperitoneal disease should be considered for these patients.

▶ One of the frustrating things about ovarian cancer is that even those patients who are rendered completely free of disease with surgery and induction chemotherapy and are documented by a second-look laparotomy to be free of disease have a significant risk for recurrence. This study from the Memorial Sloan-Kettering Cancer Center assessed 91 patients rendered free of disease with platinum-based chemotherapy and sought to determine the risk factors associated with recurrence. Stage, histologic grade, and the amount of tumor remaining after initial operation were significant prognostic findings. These 3 prognostic factors allow one to define a group of patients with a high risk of subsequent recurrence. Although stage I patients were unlikely to recur after a negative second-look laparotomy, patients with stages II, III, and IV had a 48% risk of recurrence. Grade 1 tumors recurred in only 27% of patients, compared with a 60% recurrence rate for grade 3 tumors; those patients with residual tumor of less than .5 cm had a recurrence rate of 32% compared with a 61% recurrence rate for patients with larger volume residual disease. Of interest, 40% of the recurrences in the patients were in extraperitoneal locations. The authors suggest that any additional therapy undergoing further study in such patients should address the high risk of extraperitoneal relapse.—R.C. Young, M.D., F.A.C.P.

Responses to Second-Line Cisplatin-Based Intraperitoneal Therapy in Ovarian Cancer: Influence of a Prior Response to Intravenous Cisplatin

Markman M, Reichman B, Hakes T, Jones W, Lewis JL Jr, Rubin S, Almadrones L, Hoskins W (Mem Sloan-Kettering Cancer Ctr, New York)

J Clin Oncol 9:1801–1805, 1991 9–8

Background.—There have been several trials of intraperitoneal (IP) administration of antineoplastic agents in patients with advanced ovarian cancer; the most extensively tested agent by this route has been cisplatin. Phase II trials have suggested that IP delivery of cisplatin can achieve objective responses—and even complete responses—in patients with persistent, small-volume disease after primary intravenously administered cisplatin therapy. Eighty-nine patients were studied to assess the influence of a prior response to systemic cisplatin on the activity of second-line IP administration of cisplatin.

Methods.—The patients were drawn from 2 phase II trials of cisplatin-based IP-administered therapy for persistent or recurrent ovarian cancer. One group received etoposide, and the other received cytarabine in addition to cisplatin; all had received frontline systemic cisplatin-based therapy. Differences in the response rates among the various patient groups were assessed.

Results.—A total of 58% of the patients had responded previously to intravenously administered cisplatin. This group had a 56% overall response rate to second-line IP-administered cisplatin-based therapy and a 33% complete response rate. For patients who had not previously responded to cisplatin, the response rates were 11% and 3%, respectively. Thirty-six patients had responded to systemic cisplatin and had tumors measuring less than 1 cm at the start of IP-administered therapy; this group had a 42% rate of complete response compared with 7% in patients with similar sized tumors who had not responded to systemic cisplatin.

Conclusions.—Patients with ovarian cancer who respond to systemic cisplatin-based therapy have a better chance of responding to second-line IP-delivered cisplatin therapy. The response rates are particularly good in patients with small tumors. Alternative therapies should be considered for patients with cisplatin-resistant tumors.

▶ Intraperitoneal therapy for ovarian cancer has now been studied for more than 15 years. A wide variety of chemotherapeutic agents can be placed directly into the peritoneal cavity in very high concentrations. Objective responses have been seen in approximately one third of patients who began therapy with minimal residual disease; however, there is limited evidence for benefit in patients with bulky tumor. Much of the earlier data was based on studies that had not previously defined the extent of drug resistance present in the patients treated subsequently. This study shows that the probability of subsequent response can be related to the sensitivity of the patient's tumor to cisplatin. Although a 42% remission rate was observed in patients receiving intraperitoneal platinum who had previously been platinum sensitive, only a 7% complete remission rate was seen in patients who had previously failed to respond to systemic cisplatin. Those patients who are truly platinum-resistant are unlikely to respond to intraperitoneal platinum, even with the marked increase in dose intensity associated with intraperitoneal use.—R.C. Young, M.D., F.A.C.P.

Chemotherapy of Advanced Dysgerminoma: Trials of the Gynecologic Oncology Group

Williams SD, Blessing JA, Hatch KD, Homesley HD (Indiana Univ, Indianapolis; Indianapolis VA Med Ctr; Roswell Park Cancer Inst, Buffalo, NY; Univ of Arizona, Tucson; Wake Forest Univ, Winston Salem, NC)

J Clin Oncol 9:1950–1955, 1991 9–9

Background.—There are few data on chemotherapy for advanced ovarian dysgerminoma. Patients with dysgerminoma from 2 studies of advanced ovarian disease were analyzed to determine response to chemotherapy, second-look information, survival, and prognostic factors.

Methods.—During a 5-year period, 24 patients with incompletely resected ovarian dysgerminoma were treated according to 1 of 2 Gynecologic Oncology Group protocols at 17 institutions. Both protocols included cisplatin, bleomycin, and either vinblastine or etoposide; the latter protocol also included consolidation chemotherapy with vincristine, dactinomycin, and cyclophosphamide. Twenty patients were considered evaluable, with a median follow-up of 26 months.

Results.—Of 11 patients with clinically measurable disease, 10 responded completely. Of the 14 second-look laparotomies that were done, all were negative. Nineteen patients are alive and free of disease, and the other patient died of recurrent disease. The toxic effects were the same as those seen in patients with other tumors, including alopecia, nausea, and vomiting, and leukopenia.

Conclusions.—Advanced dysgerminoma may be effectively treated with cisplatin-based chemotherapy. Toxicity is acceptable. In patients with complete resection, adjuvant chemotherapy should be given rather than radiation therapy.

▶ Germ-cell tumor of the ovary has become one of the more curable solid tumors. In the 1991 YEAR BOOK, we reviewed an experience of the M.D. Anderson Hospital using platinum-based combination chemotherapy in the treatment of a wide variety of malignant germ-cell tumors. Ovarian dysgerminoma has long been treated with irradiation because it is the most radiation sensitive of all the germ-cell tumors. Cure of many patients with dysgerminoma has been possible using standard field radiation therapy, often with relatively low doses (2,000–2,500 cGy). Nevertheless, there are women who are seen with advanced dysgerminoma that cannot be treated easily with radiation therapy, and these patients have been treated with chemotherapy. The remarkable curative effect of such treatment in patients with advanced disease has stimulated a careful study of platinum-based chemotherapy in a larger group of patients with ovarian dysgerminoma. This study summarizes the Gynecologic Oncology Group's experience with 20 patients with incompletely resected ovarian dysgerminoma. Using primarily platinum-based chemotherapy (BEP-cisplatinum, etoposide, and bleomycin), 19 of the 20 patients are free of disease at more than 2 years of follow-up. The toxicity from these treatments is similar to that experienced with platinum-based combinations. Many of these women can be treated with limited surgical intervention to preserve fertility. On the basis of these results, it is my view that platinum-based chemotherapy should replace postoperative radiation in the treatment of ovarian dysgerminomas requiring adjuvant therapy.—R.C. Young, M.D., F.A.C.P.

Endometrium

▶ ↓ The widespread use of unopposed estrogens in postmenopausal women has been clearly associated with an increase in the occurrence of endometrial cancer. In an effort to reduce this risk, many physicians have used cyclic estrogen-progesterone treatments for postmenopausal women. Several earlier studies have suggested that this combination might prevent the increase in endometrial cancers seen in these postmenopausal women. This case-control study reaches similar conclusions. Women that used unopposed estrogen for more than 3 years had a fivefold increase in the risk of endometrial cancer. However, those who used progesterones for a least 6 months had no increase in risk. The risk of endometrial cancer apparently was influenced by the number of days per month that progesterones were used. An increased risk of endometrial cancer risk was seen if fewer than 10 days per month were used; but no increased risk was seen in women who took progesterones for 10 or more days of per month. This observation is of importance, because many cyclic estrogen-progesterone regimens use less than 10 days of progesterone treatment.—R.C. Young, M.D, F.A.C.P.

Progestagen Supplementation of Exogenous Oestrogens and Risk of Endometrial Cancer

Voigt LF, Weiss NS, Chu J, Daling JR, McKnight B, van Belle G (Fred Hutchingson Cancer Research Ctr, Seattle; Univ of Washington, Seattle)

Lancet 338:274–277, 1991 9–10

Background.—The increased risk of endometrial cancer from estrogen administration has led many physicians to recommend concurrent use of a progestogen, which counters endometrial proliferation. Few data, however, are available on the effect of exogenous

Risk of Endometrial Cancer Associated With Use of Estrogens for at Least 3 Years and Progesterones

—	No (%) of cases*	No (%) of controls	OR (95% CI)†
No hormone	78 (72)	132 (85)	..
Oestrogen only	43 (19)	11 (7)	5·7 (2·5–12·8)
Any progestagen‡	13 (9)	13 (8)	1·6 (0·6–3·9)
< 10 days/month	7 (6)	4 (3)	2·4 (0·6–9·3)
Time between reference and last use:			
≤1 yr	4 (3)	3 (2)	
>1 yr	3 (3)	1 (1)	
≥10 days/month	6 (4)	9 (6)	1·1 (0·4–3·6)
Time between reference and last use:			
≤1 yr	5 (3)	6 (4)	
>1 yr	1 (1)	3 (2)	

*Percentages standardized to age distribution of controls.
†Adjusted for age (continuous), parity (continuous), and Quetelet's index (continuous).
‡All progestogen use was for 6 months or longer.
(Courtesy of Voigt LF, Weiss NS, Chu J, et al: *Lancet* 338:274–277, 1991.

progestogen used as a supplement to noncontraceptive estrogen.

Methods.—This population-based case-control study included 158 incident cases of endometrial cancer diagnosed in women aged 40–64 years during the period 1985–1987. The patient were interviewed in person by trained personnel, and controls were recruited by random telephone dialing.

Observations.—Women who had used exogenous estrogen (but not progestogen) at any time had a threefold greater risk of having endometrial cancer than those who had never used either hormone. The risk increased after 3 years of estrogen use and increased subsequently. Estrogen users who had also used a progestogen for at least 4 months had a relative risk of only 1.3. The relative risk was .9 for women using a progestogen 10 or more days a month. Women who used a progestogen as well as estrogen for longer than 3 years had a relative risk that was less than 2 (table). When a progestogen was used at least 10 days a month, there was no excess risk relative to nonusers.

Conclusion.—The risk of endometrial cancer associated with unopposed estrogen use is substantially reduced by concomitant use of a progestogen for 10 or more days a month.

Relationship Between Surgical-Pathological Risk Factors and Outcome in Clinical Stage I and II Carcinoma of the Endometrium: A Gynecologic Outcome Group Study

Morrow CP, Bundy BN, Kurman RJ, Creasman WT, Heller P, Homesley HD, Graham JE (Univ of Southern California, Los Angeles; Roswell Park Mem Inst, Buffalo, NY; Johns Hopkins Med Inst, Baltimore; Med Univ of South Carolina, Charleston; Univ of Pennsylvania, Philadelphia, et al)

Gynecol Oncol 40:55–65, 1991 9–11

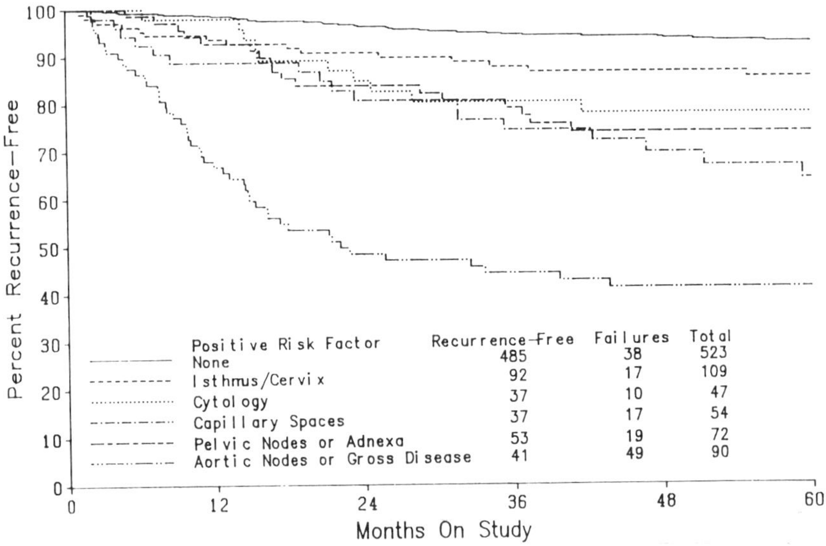

Fig 9–4.—Recurrence-free interval by ranking of selected risk factors. (Courtesy of Morrow CP, Bundy BN, Kurman RJ, et al: *Gynecol Oncol* 40:55–65, 1991.

Introduction.—In 1975, the Gynecologic Oncology Group sponsored a multicenter pilot study of surgica-pathologic staging of early endometrial carcinoma. The results were important enough to begin a groupwide study to obtain a much larger database that could support more detailed analysis of the many surgical-pathologic factors correlated with risk for clinically occult metastases and prognosis.

Methods.—The relationship between the surgical-pathologic risk factors and outcome in clinical stages I and II carcinoma was investigated. Of the 1,180 women who were studied in 1977–1983, data on 895 who had endometroid or adenosquamous carcinoma were evaluable. Proportional hazards modeling of time to recurrence was performed.

Results.—For women without metastasis as determined by surgical-pathologic staging, the best determinant of recurrence was grade 3 histology. Of the 48 women with histologically proved aortic node metastasis, 47 had grossly positive pelvic nodes, grossly positive adnexal metastasis, and/or myometrial invasion in the outer one third. Pelvic radiation was administered to 48% of patients, and vaginal brachytherapy alone was administered to 10.2% after surgery; 42% received no adjuvant radiation treatment. None of the 3 recurrences in the vaginal implant group were vaginal or pelvic. Of the 95 recurrences in the pelvic radiotherapy group, 7.4% were vaginal and 16.8% were pelvic. Of the recurrences in the group that received no radiation treatment, 18.2% were vaginal and 31.8% were pelvic. The 5-year recurrence-free intervals for women with negative surgical-pathologic risk factors was 92.7%; with involvement of the isthmus or cervix, 69.8% with positive pelvic cytology, 56%; with vascular space invasion, 55%; with pelvic node or adnexal metastases, 57.8%; and with aortic node spread or gross laparotomy findings,

41.2% (Fig 9–4). The relapse rate among patients who were cervix positive or cervix negative and had grade 3 lesions and deep myinvasion did not differ significantly.

Conclusion.—The proportion of vaginal and pelvic failures suggests that the use of adjuvant radiation treatment for patients with more than one third myoinvasion and grade 2 or 3 tumor may be beneficial. Malignant cytology appears to be a serious adverse finding, especially in the risk for regional or distant and abdominal failure.

▶ This large surgical staging study by the Gynecologic Oncology Group evaluated more than 1,000 women with endometrial carcinoma and sought to determine the important surgical pathologic risk factors in stage I and II disease. Patients with no evidence of extrauterine disease, no cervical invasion, and no capillary space involvement were at low risk for recurrence. The presence of aortic node metastases was seen to convey a poor prognosis, but those patients with pelvic node metastases in the absence of any other adverse factors had excellent survival. On the basis of the local and regional failure rates, the authors suggest that patients with more than one third myometrial invasion or grade 2 and 3 tumors are at sufficiently high risk for recurrence that they should receive adjuvant radiation therapy. Although they observed a high relapse rate in those patients with positive peritoneal cytology, those patients often had other adverse risk factors, including deep myometrial invasion and high grade. Nevertheless, their data does indicate that positive cytology is associated with an increased risk of abdominal recurrences as well as regional and distant recurrences.—R.C. Young, M.D., F.A.C.P.

MR Imaging Evaluation of Endometrial Carcinoma: Results of an NCI Cooperative Study

Hricak H, Rubinstein LV, Gherman GM, Karstaedt N (Univ of California, San Francisco; Natl Cancer Inst, Bethesda, Md)

Radiology 179:829–832, 1991 9–12

Introduction.—The prognosis for patients with endometrial cancer depends on histologic tumor grade, tumor stage, depth of myometrial invasion, and presence of lymph node metastatis at the time of diagnosis. The role of MRI in the evaluation of tumor extent was evaluated in patients with endometrial carcinoma at 5 institutions.

Methods.—The 5 hospitals entered a total of 107 patients in the study, 88 of whom met the study's inclusion criteria. The mean patient age was 61.7 years. All 88 patients underwent hysterectomy. Of the 60 patients who had stage I disease, 43 had stage IA and 17 had stage IB disease. Eleven patients had stage II; 4, stage III; and 8, stage IV disease. There was no tumor invasion in 22 patients. Six different commercially available MR imagers, ranging in magnetic field strength from .15 tesla–1.5 tesla were used. The T1- and T2-weighted sequences in the transverse plane and the T2-weighted sequences in the sagital plane appropriate for each unit were used.

Results.—The overall image quality was rated poor in 18% of patients, adequate in 75%, and excellent in 7%. Imaging was judged adequate for pelvic lymph node evaluation in 92% of the patients but it was adequate for evaluation of the paraaortic nodes in only 8%. The abnormality within the endometrial cavity was identified correctly in 81% of the patients. The overall staging accuracy with MRI was 85%. When staging analysis included separate evaluation of each stage, the accuracy decreased to 65%. In the evaluation of the depth of myometrial invasion for stage I disease, the overall accuracy with MRI was 74%; the overall accuracy was 66% if all stages were analyzed. The sensitivity for detecting deep myometrial invasion with MRI was 54%, and the specificity was 89%.

Conclusion.—Magnetic resonance imaging is useful in the preoperative staging of endometrial carcinoma. As image quality improves and techniques advance, the accuracy is evaluating patients with endometrial carcinoma will probably improve even further.

▶ Although the staging of endometrial cancer is clinical, understaging can occur in as many as 22% of patients; overstaging, although less common, does occur. Important prognostic factors such as the depth of myometrial invasion and lymph node involvement cannot be easily assessed by clinical staging. Investigators have sought more effective ways of enhancing the accuracy of presurgical staging in this disease. In the 1991 YEAR BOOK, we reviewed an article on MRI and its potential use in documenting the extent of myometrial invasion and pelvic and periaortic lymphadenopathy. This study supported by the National Cancer Institute is a more extensive 5-institution evaluation of the accuracy of MRI staging. There is good news and bad news. Although the accuracy of MRI in assessing tumors with superficial myometrial invasion was 89%, it decreased to 54% in assessing deep myometrial invasion. The specificity for detecting pelvic nodal enlargement was 74%, but the authors had excluded all the patients whose MR images were inadequate for evaluation of the pelvic nodes. The overall staging accuracy of MRI in this multi-institutional study was 85%, which is superior to the clinical staging reported by the Gynecologic Oncology Group. Nevertheless, this accuracy decreases in precisely those areas of greatest importance—namely, depth of myometrial invasion and the presence of pelvic and aortic adenopathy. Standardized techniques and a greater experience with the procedure may enhance this accuracy, but it seems unlikely to replace operative staging if the therapeutic decisions depend on staging accuracy.—R.C. Young, M.D., F.A.C.P.

A New Treatment for Endometrial Cancer With Gonadotropin Releasing-Hormone Analogue

Gallagher CJ, Oliver RTD, Oram DH, Fowler CG, Blake PR, Mantell BS, Slevin ML, Hope-Stone HF (Royal London Hosp; Royal Marsden Hosp; St Bartholomew's Hosp, London)

Br J Obstet Gynaecol 98:1037–1041, 1991 9–13

Objective.—Endometrial cancer that recurs after surgery has a poor outlook. In a majority of patients, this disease is found outside the pelvis.

The antitumor efficacy of gonadotropin-releasing hormone (GnRH) analogues was examined in 17 patients with recurrent endometrial cancer, all of whom had symptomatic and progressive disease.

Management.—Progesterone therapy was ceased at least a month before the start of analogue treatment. The patients received monthly depot injections of 7.5 mg of leuprorelin or 3.6 mg of goserelin. Two early patients received tamoxifen as well.

Results.—Serum gonadotropin levels declined to normal luteal-phase values within a month, and they remained suppressed for the duration of treatment. Six patients (35%) had a response, and 1 of them responded completely. Five patients were still in remission after as long as 30 months; 1 was lost to follow-up. Two other patients had stable disease, whereas 8 died of progressive disease. The median follow-up was 14 months.

Conclusion.—Treatment with a GnRH analogue is an effective and safe approach to recurrent endometrial cancer.

▶ Endometrial cancer is generally thought to have an excellent prognosis. This results primarily from the frequency with which it is discovered early (i.e., stage I). Stage for stage, patients with endometrial cancer have a prognosis similar to that of patients with ovarian cancer. However, the disease is seldom diagnosed in the advanced stage. Although therapy for localized disease is excellent, treatment of advanced endometrial carcinoma has generally been only modestly successful. Primary therapy with progesterone achieves response rates in the 20% to 30% range. Responses are more likely in tumors with progesterone receptors. When patients have recurrence after progesterone therapy, Adriamycin has generally been the chemotherapy of choice; however, only a minority of patients respond. These investigators used gonadotropin-releasing hormone analogues (either leuprorelin or goserelin) in the treatment of 17 patients who had recurrence after hormone treatment. The overall response rate of 35% and the median duration of response of 20 months are interesting. There were essentially no significant side effects from this therapy; however, the receptor status of the patients was not analyzed, and it is conceivable that these patients were selected for treatment because of unusually good responses to previous hormone therapy. Although this may be a selected population of patients, it does suggest that further investigation of this new therapeutic approach is warranted.—R.C. Young, M.D., F.A.C.P.

Cervix

Case-Control Study of Risk Factors for Cervical Neoplasia in Denmark: I. Role of the "Male Factor" in Women With One Lifetime Sexual Partner

Kjaer SK, de Villiers E-M, Dahl C, Engholm G, Bock JE, Vestergaard BF, Lynge E, Jensen OM (Danish Cancer Society, Copenhagen; Deutsches Krebsforschungszentrum, Heidelberg, Germany; Slagelse Hosp, Slagelse, Denmark; Rigshospitalet, Statens Seruminstitut, Copenhagen)

Int J Cancer 48:39–44, 1991 9–14

Introduction.—Epidemiologic studies show that number of male partners and age at first intercourse are closely related to a woman's risk of cervical cancer and its precursor lesions. However, some female populations have high incidences of cervical cancer, despite a tradition of few sexual contacts. The role of the "male factor" in the rate of cervical cancer among monogamous women was studied to determine whether human papillomavirus infection and/or herpes simplex virus type 2 infection in the male partner are responsible for an increased cervical cancer risk.

Methods.—Possible risk factors were investigated in 645 women (age, 20–49 years) with histologically confirmed cervical cancer or carcinoma in situ; 614 controls were randomly selected from the female population in the same area. Monogamous women and their husbands were examined further; 41 (89%) case couples and 90 (92%) control couples were included.

Results.—A history of genital warts in the male partner and having ever used condoms were the most significant risk determinants. Other potentially important but not statistically significant factors included having ever visited prostitutes, circumcision, and a history of genital warts in the female partner. Having a husband who had multiple sexual partners was also associated with an increased crude risk, but this risk was not significant after adjustment for the husband ever having genital warts, use of condoms, and age. Human papillomavirus DNA was found in 1 control and 2 case husbands.

Conclusion.—Certain characteristics of male sexual behavior increase the risk of cervical neoplasia in women, thereby supporting the proposed existence of "high-risk males" in the development of cervical cancer. These findings also support the infectious nature of this disease.

▶ Although the conventional medical literature has long emphasized that sexual promiscuity in women is a risk factor for cervix cancer, there is increasing evidence that the risk factor is not the promiscuity of women, but the promiscuity of men. Earlier studies have defined a group of "high-risk males," and this study focused on the "male factor" in monogamous women. It indicates that a history of genital warts in the male and the nonuse of condoms are significantly associated with the risk of cervical cancer in women. Other potential factors, although not statistically significant, were lack of circumcision, prostitute exposure (ever), and a male's history of multiple sexual partners. Table 3 in the original article highlights some of these relative risks. This study clearly confirms that certain characteristics of male sexual behavior increase the risk of cervical cancer in women, and it also documents the existence of "high-risk males."—R.C. Young, M.D., F.A.C.P.

Herpes Simplex Virus Type 2: A Possible Interaction With Human Papillomavirus Types 16/18 in the Development of Invasive Cervical Cancer

Hildesheim A, Mann V, Brinton LA, Szklo M, Reeves WC, Rawls WE (Natl Cancer Inst, Bethesda, Md; McMaster Univ, Hamilton, Ont; Johns Hopkins School of Hygiene and Public Health, Baltimore; Ctrs for Disease Control, Atlanta)

Int J Cancer 49:335–340, 1991 9–15

Background.—Laboratory and epidemiologic studies have supported an etiologic role for herpes simplex virus type 2 (HSV-2) and human papillomaviruses (HPVs) in cervical cancer. To evaluate the etiologic role of HSV-2 and to determine its interaction with other risk factors for cervical cancer, a case-control study was conducted.

Patients.—Patients with newly diagnosed invasive cervical cancer were recruited from 4 countries in Latin America. The 766 patients with histologically confirmed invasive cervical cancer were matched with 1,532 hospital and community controls. A total of 98% of the subjects and 91% of controls had a personal interview and donated blood samples and cervical swabs for assessment of exposure to HSV-2 and HPVs.

Findings.—The women who tested positive for HSV-2 antibodies had a 60% increased risk of cervical cancer compared with seronegative women. The nonviral factors of age, number of pregnancies, oral contraceptive use, or cigarette smoking did not modify the effect. There was a significant interaction between HSV-2 and HPV-16/18. The women who tested positive for HSV-2 alone had a relative risk (RR) of 1.2, whereas those positive for HPV-16/18 DNA alone had an RR of 4.3, and those positive for both viruses had an RR of 8.8. Early initiation of sexual activity significantly increased the risk of cervical cancer independent of HSV-2 and HPV-16/18.

Conclusions.—The finding of a 60% increased risk of cervical cancer in women positive for both HSV-2 and HPV-16/18 supports a possible biological interaction between HSV-2 and HPV-16/18 in the development of cervical cancer. Although this study may be limited by possible misclassification of the assays used to measure the viruses, the suggested interaction between HSV-2 and HPVs should be studied further.

▶ The major question is whether HSV-2 is playing an active role in the development of cervical cancer or whether it is simply an innocent bystander that is transmitted in the same way that HPVs are transmitted and also appears in the same place. Certainly, there seems to be no requirement for additional factors other than HPV to produce cervical cancer.

The mechanisms by which viruses can promote carcinogenesis are varied and ingenious. For example, the hepatitis B virus appears to integrate into the host genome into a region on chromosome 17p that structurally alters the *p53* gene (1). Recent reports from Taiwan (2) and Japan (3) suggest that the hepatitis C virus also may be involved in some way in the development of hepatocellular carcinoma. With the hepatitis B virus altering 1 allele and exposure to aflatoxin mutating the second *p53* allele, the etiology of hepatocellular carcinoma is believed to be understood. Therefore, what role is there for hepatitis C virus?—D.L. Longo M.D., F.A.C.P.

References

1. Slagel BL, et al: *Cancer Res* 51:49, 1991.
2. Yu M-W, et al: *Cancer Res* 51:5621, 1991.
3. Nishioka K, et al: *Cancer* 67:429, 1991.

High Risk of Squamous Cell Carcinoma of the Cervix for Women With HLA-Dqw3

Wank R, Thomssen C (Univ of Munich, Technische Univ, Munich)

Nature 352:723–725, 1991 9–16

Background.—The genes of the major histocompatibility complex (MHC) control many immune responses. In humans these include the loci encoding the HLA-A, -B, -C, -DR, -DQ, and -DP antigens. Many diseases have been linked with these. However, no one has been able to identify human HLA genes that might explain why an immune response against malignant tumors should be ineffective, although there has ben a reported association between the HLA-DR1 antigen and a susceptibility to a rare thyroid gland carcinoma. Another strong connection between a common malignant tumor and an HLA antigen was identified.

Methods and Results.—Blood samples were obtained during a 3-year period from 94 patients. Sixty-six had squamous cell carcinoma and 28 had other gynecologic diseases. The prevalence of HLA-DQw3 antigens between these 2 groups was compared. Of the 66 patients with squamous cell carcinoma of the cervix, 88% had HLA-DQw3. Normally, it would be found in only 50% of individuals.

Conclusions.—There is a strong connection between HLA-DQw3 and squamous cell carcinoma of the cervix. This invasive cancer will develop in 1 of every 63 newborn girls. Because squamous cell carcinoma is probably induced virally, the discovery of its association with an HLA antigen is important to the understanding of the immunogenetic basis of susceptibility to it.

▶ Human papillomavirus types 16 and 18 are the prototypical transforming papillomaviruses whose ability to transform epithelial cells has been studied and characterized and is considered to be relevant to the generation of cervical cancer. Although some other serotypes may be associated with cervical cancer, types 16 and 18 account for most cases. Two viral proteins are required for transformation, E6 and E7. Convincing data suggest that E6 promotes the degradation of wild-type *p53,* and E 7 interferes with the function of the retinoblastoma gene product RB. The expression and function of these 2 gene products is necessary and sufficient for transformation. So what does immunogenetics have to do with this? No one knows. The association of an autoimmune disease with a particular HLA allele is understandable in light of what we know about the dominant expression of responsiveness in immune response gene-controlled responses to antigens. Thus, individuals in whom HLA-B27 is expressed respond to something they shouldn't, and they get arthritis. However, the association of a particular class II MHC allele with susceptibility to cancer implies a contributory role for an immune response in the carcinogenesis. Because immune response genes are functionally dominant, the failure of patients in whom DQw3 is expressed to respond to HPV-infected cells is an unlikely explanation for the phenomenon. Other DR, DQ, or DP alleles should be expressed and should act as restriction elements for an antiviral response. This is not the pattern of immune response gene-related nonresponsiveness, which would be a clinically important problem only in those patients who are homozygous for DQw3 (or any other low-response allelotype). An interesting hypothesis that we might propose from the data in this paper is that HPV-specific T cells are restricted to recognition on DQw3 alleles, and that a product of the immune response is acting as a co-factor in the induction of transformation. Recently, my colleague Joost Oppenheim and his workers demonstrated that tumor necrosis factor can act as a tumor promoter in vitro. It is possible that cervical carcinogenesis is mediated in part by inflammatory cytokines acting as tumor promoters.—D.L. Longo, M.D.

The State of the P53 and Retinoblastoma Genes in Human Cervical Carcinoma Cell Lines

Scheffner M, Münger K, Byrne JC, Howley PM (Natl Cancer Inst, Bethesda, Md)

Proc Natl Acad Sci USA 88:5523–5527, 1991 9–17

Background.—Both the retinoblastoma tumor-suppressor gene pRB and the *p53* protein, which also has tumor-suppressor properties, can bind with virus-encoded oncoprotein. The *pRB*- and *p53*-encoding genes in a series of human cervical carcinoma cell lines that were known to be either positive or negative for human papillomavirus (HPV) DNA were studied.

Methods.—The cell lines studied were C-33A, HT-3, ME-180, SiHa, C-4II, HeLA, and CaSki. The C-33A and HT-3 lines were HPV DNA-negative. In each cell line, evidence of *p53* and *pRB* gene mutation were sought by polymerase chain reaction.

Findings.—All the HPV-positive cell lines expressed normal levels of pRB and low levels of wild-type *p53* proteins. These were thought to be altered in function because of their association with HPV E7 and E6 oncoproteins, respectively. The C-33A and HT-3 cell lines showed mutated *p53* and *RB* genes. The *p53* gene mutation mapped to codon 273 of the C33-A line and codon 245 of the HT-3 line; these codons are located in highly conserved *p53* regions, in which many human cancers show mutations. The *RB* mutations occurred at splice junctions, resulting in in-frame deletions. Exon 13 was affected in the HT-3 cell line and exon 20 in the C-33A cell line, resulting in aberrant, nonphosphorylated proteins that could not bind with adenovirus E1A oncoprotein.

Conclusions.—The *p53* and *pRB* tumor suppressor proteins appear to be relevant in cervical carcinogenesis. Inactivation of their normal functions, whether by mutation or formation of complexes with the HPV E7 and E7 oncoproteins, may be an important step in tumor development.

▶ The unfolding story for the development of cervical cancer depicts an intricate interaction between viral protein and normal genes. Human papilloma viruses (HPV) encode oncoproteins (E6 and E7) that interact specifically with important cell-regulatory proteins (in this case, the tumor-suppressor protein *pRB,* which is a transcription factor that inhibits cell proliferation) to alter their normal function. The "high-risk" HPVs such as HPV-16 and HPV-18 bind *pRB* with markedly greater (tenfold) affinity than do the E7 proteins of the "low-risk" HPVs such as HPV-6 and HPV-11. This study also provides evidence that mutation of the *p53* suppressor gene may also be playing a role in cervical cancer carcinogenesis, particularly in those cervical carcinomas that are negative for HPV. Although many questions remain about the molecular events associated with HPV infection and cervical cancer, there seems to be little doubt that inactivation of the suppressor genes, either by complexes with viral protein or by mutation has an important role.—R.F. Ozols, M.D., Ph.D.

Laser Conization: Follow-Up in Patients With Cervical Intraepithelial Neoplasia in the Cone Margin

Andersen ES, Nielsen K, Larsen G (Aalborg Hosp, Aalborg, Denmark)
Gynecol Oncol 39:328–331, 1990 9–18

Background.—Cervical intraepithelial neoplasia (CIN) is managed effectively by laser conization. The combination of laser conization and vaporization has obvious advantages. The efficacy of laser conization was studied, and histologic and cytologic findings were compared in patients who had CIN in the cone margins.

Methods.—A total of 469 patients with CIN was treated by laser conization during a 3½-year period. Of these, 58 had CIN in the margins of the cone, for a rate of 12.4%. Fifty-one of these patients (mean age, 36.1 years) were readmitted approximately 3 months later for colposcopy, cytologic evaluation using the Ayre spatula and the Cytobrush, cervical biopsy, and endocervical curettage.

Results.—The histologic examination was positive in 6 patients. In 3 of the 6, cytoloci examination was positive as well. Five patients underwent hysterectomy, although only 1 of them had a significant lesion of the uterus. None of the 45 patients whose first postconization examination was negative had a positive follow-up examinating during mean follow-up of 44 months.

Conclusions.—In patients with CIN who undergo laser conization and have involvement of the cone margins, conservative, expectant management based on colposcopy and cytology is justified. The physician should bear in mind that many of these patients wish to maintain their fertility. Outpatient follow-up may be more economical than hospital follow-up.

▶ Less aggressive surgical management is increasingly being used to treat CIN. Laser conization has been used to accomplish a more precise excision while preserving a large part of the cervix. The excision allows the pathologist adequate material to exclude invasive disease, and the laser vaporization may eliminiate disease in the excisional margins. This study indicates that the vast majority of patients are well handled by this technique. However, it focuses on the 12.4% of women who have CIN in the margins of the cone after the procedure is complete. Although incomplete excision was found in this 12.4% of women, subsequent postconization evaluation showed persistent disease in only 1.3%. The authors conclude that it is appropriate to follow patients with Ayre spatula and Cytobrush cytology and with repeat colposcopy. Continued conservative management is acceptable, because the majority of women with positive margins ultimately do not require hysterectomy. Although this conservative approach clearly can reduce the frequency with which hysterectomy is required, it does require careful and diligent follow-up and a cooperative patient population.—R.C. Young, M.D., F.A.C.P.

Discrepancy of Cervical Cytology and Colposcopic Biopsy: Is Cervical Conization Necessary?

McCord ML, Stovall TG, Summitt RL Jr, Ling FW (Univ of Tennessee, Memphis)

Obstet Gynecol 77:715–719, 1991 9–19

Background.—Cervical conization traditionally is done when there is a discrepancy between the cytologic and histologic findings in women with cervical cytologic findings that are suggestive of cervical intraepithelial neoplasia (CIN). However, some studies have suggested that ablative therapy can be done in place of conization. The records of patients with a discrepancy between the Papanicolaou smear results and the colposcopically directed biopsy results were reviewed to determine whether diagnostic cervical conization was necessary.

Methods.—The records of 786 patients from a colposcopy clinic were reviewed to find cases with a discrepancy of at least 2 degrees, such as CIN III cytologic findings and CIN I or less on colposcopic biopdy, or CIN II cytologic findings with no dysplasia on biopsy. A total of 87 such patients were found, for an incidence of 11.1%. After elimination of 12 pregnant patients and 10 who did not return after their first colposcopic examination, 65 patients were left for analysis. Medical treatment was given in 30.8% of these cases, cryotherapy in 13.8%, and diagnostic cervical conization in 55.4%.

Results.—Microinvasive cervical carcinoma was found in 3 patients who underwent cervical conization. Of the 20 patients who had medical therapy, follow-up cytologic studies were negative in only 10% and they demonstrated CIN I in 10%. Additional therapy was given to 5 patients (25%), and 11 (55%) were lost to follow-up. Of these 11 patients, 7 failed to return for a follow-up Papanicolaou smear, and 4 failed to return after the follow-up smear showed persistent dysplasia. Six of 9 patients treated with cryotherapy had a negative Papanicolaou smear at their first follow-up.

Conclusions.—Cervical conization maximizes the chance of making the correct diagnosis in patients with a 2-stage or greater discrepancy between the findings of colposcopically directed biopsy and cervical cytologic study. The risk of missing a microinvasive or invasive carcinoma of the cervix far outweighs the risk of the conization procedure. Medical therapy may delay definitive treatment in a high-risk population with poor compliance with follow-up.

▶ What should you do when there is a significant discrepancy between the Papanicolaou smear and the results from colposcopically directed biopsies? This specific issue was addressed in this study analyzing 786 patients with CIN. Two-degree discrepancies were identified in 11% of patients; 30% were treated medically, 14% with cryotherapy, and 55% with a cervical cone. After medical therapy, 10% had a negative cytology. For those treated with cryotherapy, two thirds had a negative Papanicolaou smear. Those treated with cervical conization not only had definitive management of their disese, but 3 were found to have microinvasive carcinoma of the cervix. These data suggest that when substantial discrepancies exist between cervical cytology and colposcopically directed biopsies, the patient is appropriately managed with conization.— R.C. Young, M.D., F.A.C.P.

Carcinoma of the Cervix Treated With Radiation Therapy I: A Multi-Variate Analysis of Prognostic Variables in the Gynecologic Oncology Group

Stehman FB, Bundy BN, DiSaia PJ, Keys HM, Larson JE, Fowler WC (Indiana Univ, Indianapolis; Roswell Park Mem Inst, Buffalo, NY: Univ of California, Orange; Albany Med College, NY; Pennsylvania State Univ, Hershey, et al)

Cancer 67:2776–2785, 1991 9–20

Background.—Locally advanced cervical carcinoma is primarily treated by radiation therapy. Clinical trials suggest that para-aortic (PA) lymph node status, International Federation of Gynecology and Obstetrics (FIGO) stage, tumor grade, and pelvic node status are significantly related to progression-free interval. Data from 3 trials of locally advanced carcinoma of the cervix, International Federation of Gynecology and Obstetrics clinical stages I to IVA, were pooled to identify the factors related to an increased risk of failure or differing patterns of failure.

Methods.—The trials, conducted during an 8-year period included 626 patients with primary carcinoma of the uterine cervix. Each patient underwent surgical assessment of PA node status before entry into a protocol. Treatment was with standardized external radiation either to the pelvis alone or to the pelvis and the PA lymph nodes; it also included 1 or 2 brachytherapy applications. Radiation alone was given to 150 patients, radiation plus corynebacterium parvum to 136, radiation plus misonidazole to 156, and radiation plus hydroxyurea to 184. Metastases to the PA lymph nodes were documented in 14.6% of the patients, and pelvic node metastases were found in 35.9% of the patients who had pelvic node sampling.

Results.—In none of the 3 studies was a significant difference in progression-free interval or survival noted between treatment arms. Positive

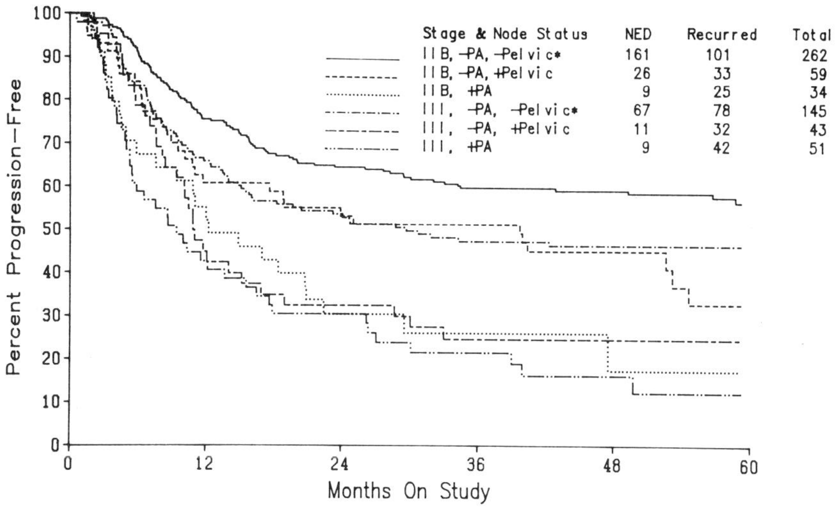

Fig 9–5.—Progression-free interval by stage and node status. *Asterisk* indicates unknown pelvic node status. (Courtesy of Stehman FB, Bundy BN, DiSaia PJ, et al: *Cancer* 67:2776–2785, 1991.)

PA and pelvic lymph nodes, tumor size, patient age, and performance status were significantly associated with progression-free interval on multivariate analysis. All of these, as well as clinical stage and bilateral extension, were significantly associated with survival. Cell type, histologic grade, hematocrit level, and peritoneal washings were not associated with progression-free interval or survival.

Conclusions.—In locally advanced carcinoma of the cervix, the positive PA lymph nodes are an important prognostic factor. This powerful risk factor, in combination with International Federation of Gynecology and Obstetrics stage, clearly separates (by stage) patients with negative nodes (Fig 9–5); the distinction made by stage decreases as the extent of node positivity increases. Clinical studies must stratify for this important risk factor.

▶ The Gynecologic Oncology Group analyzed a large experience with cervical cancer, further refining information on the prognostic factors influencing survival. This multivariant analysis of more than 600 patients indicated that patient age, performance status, tumor size, pelvic and aortic nodal status, clinical stage, and bilateral extension significantly influenced long-term survival. The patients were a part of a series of clinical trials using radiation alone and radiation plus either C-parvum, misonidazole, or hydroxyurea. Despite a variety of efforts to enhance the impact of surgery and radiation therapy, the long-term survival of patients with stage III disease and periaortic or pelvic adenopathy remains poor (see Fig 9–5). At four-year follow-up, only approximately 20% to 25% of the patients remained free of disease. These prognostic factors clearly define a population of patients requiring more effective therapy.—R.C. Young, M.D., F.A.C.P.

Radical Hysterectomy *Versus* Radiation Therapy for Stage IB Squamous Cell Cancer of the Cervix

Hopkins MP, Morely GW (Univ of Michigan, Ann Arbor)

Cancer 68:272–277, 1991 9–21

Background.—Treatment for early squamous cell cervical carcinoma consists of either radiation therapy or radical surgery. There have been few comparative studies of these forms of treatment. A total of 345 patients was studied to determine whether there was any survival difference between the 2 forms of treatment.

Patients.—The patients (mean age, 44.6 years) were given a diagnosis of stage IB squamous cell carcinoma of the cervix during a 16-year period. Radiation therapy consisted of 1,980 cGy to the pelvis, followed by 2 intracavitary applications totaling 7,000–8,000 mg of radiation/hr. Treatment was with radical hysterectomy in 213 patients radiation therapy in 111, and extrafascial hysterectomy plus radiation in 21. The overall 5-year survival rate was 89%.

Observations.—The 5-year survival for the surgical group was 92%. Fourteen patients in the radiation group underwent exploration for radical hysterectomy, which was not performed because of high-risk findings; their 5-year survival rate was 50%. Excluding this group, the survival for radiation-treated patients was 86%; the difference from the surgical group was nonsignificant. In patients with lesions measuring 3 cm or less, the survival rates were 94% for the surgical group and 88% for the radiation group. With lesions larger than 3 cm, the survival rates were 82% in the surgical group and 73% in the radiation group. Twenty-six of the surgically treated patients had lymph node metastases. Of the 19 patients with involvement of as many as 3 nodes, 16 survived; of the 7 patients with involvement of as many as 10 nodes, 3 survived. Four of the patients undergoing surgery and 1 of the patients undergoing radiation had fistulas. Six of the surgically treated patients and 7 of the patients given radiation needed a second operation for a complication.

Conclusions.—In patients with early squamous cell carcinoma of the cervix, radical surgery and radiation therapy give similarly high survivals and low complication rates. The overall survival is approximately 89%, with a worse prognosis for patients with lymph node metastases. The larger lesions do not appear to do any better with radiation than with surgical therapy.

▶ Stage IB squamous cell carcinoma of the cervix has commonly been managed with either radiation therapy or radical surgery. Although there are no prospective randomized trials comparing these interventions, the results from the 2 modalities appear to be similar. This retrospective analysis of a single-institution experience from the University of Michigan confirms results of earlier studies. Although 213 patients were managed with radical hysterectomy and only 111 were managed with radiation therapy, the long-term survivals for both groups were 91.3% vs. 87.3%, respectively—an insignificant difference. Unfortunately, nonrandomized retrospective analyses make such comparisons difficult.

Fourteen of 227 patients (6%) had their planned radical surgery aborted because of intraoperative findings. These patients would obviously be included in any radiation therapy series, and it has long been argued that these selection differences account for the small difference in the 2 therapeutic approaches. It certainly would be nice to see a large randomized trial resolving this issue; however, this appears to be unlikely. Nevertheless, we can take some solace from the fact that the long-term survival in stage IB cancer of the cervix managed by either approach is excellent.—R.C. Young, M.D., F.A.C.P.

Concurrent Chemoradiation in Advanced Cervical Cancer

Thomas G, Dembo A, Fyles A, Gadalla T, Beale F, Bean H, Pringle J, Rawlings G, Bush R, Black B (Univ of Toronto; Toronto Bayview Regional Cancer Centre; Princess Margaret Hosp, Toronto)

Gynecol Oncol 38:446–451, 1990 9–22

Introduction.—After radical radiotherapy (RT) for locally advanced cervical cancer, failure occurs most commonly in the pelvis. This problem cannot be addressed by increasing the radiation dose. A sequence of phase I and II studies was performed to develop an appropriate combination of concurrent RT and chemotherapy for testing in a phase III study.

Methods.—The studies included 200 patients with advanced cervical carcinoma. The cancer could be of any International Federation of Gynecology and Obstetrics stage or type as long as it measured more than 5 cm in diameter. Pelvic irradiation alone was used in 154 patients, with 46 patients receiving pelvic and para-aortic irradiation. The patients receved 5-fluorouracil (5-FU), 1 g/m^2/day by infusion, on the first and last 4 days of 5 weeks of continuous RT, or with both halves of split RT. In addition, 78 patients received mitomycin-C, 6 mg/m^2 by bolus, once or twice with the start of 5-FU infusion. The patients received a median external RT dose of 46 Gy; 90% of the patients also had a single intracavitary 40-Gy dose using a linear source of cesium-137. The patients were followed for a median of 2.5 years.

Results.—Significant acute toxicities developed in 23 patients—transient oral mucositis in 13, enteritis necessitating interruption of RT in 7, febrile neutropenia in 3, and thrombocytopenic tumor bleeding in 1. Three patients died of serious late toxicities; 6 patients had late toxic effects in the bladder, and 25 had such effects in the bowel, including 8 patients with recurrent tumors. Toxicity to the bowel was associated with specific therapies, and it decreased with successive protocols. Treatment with mitomycin-C was the only variable with a significant effect on complications. Only 4 of the 105 patients who received RT and 5-FU only had complications (fewer than are seen with RT alone). In patients with stage Ib/II disease, the 3-year pelvic control rate was 85% and the survival rate was 71%. In those with stage III/IV disease, the pelvic control rate was 50% and the survival rate was 42%.

Conclusions.—Preliminary study suggests that concurrent RT and chemotherapy can improve survival and reduce toxicity in advanced cervical cancer. A phase III trial to determine whether concurrent 5-FU and continuous partially hyperfractionated pelvic RT can improve local control and survival has begun.

▶ Although surgery and radiation therapy form the backbone of treatment for cancer of the cervix, the management of advanced disease continues to be suboptimal. Based on encouraging results of the use of concurrent chemoradiation therapy in anal and esophageal cancer, these investigators embarked on a series of phase I–II studies testing several chemotherapeutic agents in conjunction with radiation therapy for advanced cervical carcinoma. Their initial studies with 5-FU and mitomycin-C were encouraging, but the addition of mitomycin-C was associated with increased hematologic toxicity. Because of both the limited evidence of a radiation-sensitizing effect of mitomycin-C and the increased toxicity, the authors no longer believe that that combination is preferred. They have concluded that 5-FU infusions with partially hyperfractionated pelvic radiation therapy improve local control, and that they may have an impact on long-term survival. Although this may be true, the authors point out that a phase-III randomized trial will be required to establish the radiation-enhancing effect of infusional 5-Fu in this clinical setting.—R.C. Young, M.D., F.A.C.P.

Other

Results With the EMA/CO (Etoposide, Methotrexate, Actinomycin D, Cyclophosphamide, Vincristine) Regimen in High Risk Gestational Trophoblastic Tumours, 1979 to 1989

Newlands ES, Bagshawe KD, Begent RHJ, Rustin GJS, Holden L (Charing Cross Hosp, London)

Br J Obstet Gynaecol 98:550–557, 1991 9–23

Objective.—The efficacy and safety of EMA/CO chemotherapy were examined in an open study of 148 patients with high-risk gestational trophoblastic tumor (GTT) who were consecutively referred in a 10-year period. Of the 148, 76 had not previously received chemotherapy.

Patients.—Twenty-seven patients were seen after a nonmolar miscarriage, 53 after term delivery, and 68 after a hydatidiform mole. The risk status was based on age (younger or older than 39 years), the chorionic gonadotropin level, the size of the largest tumor mass, and the number and site of metastases.

Outcome.—The remission rates were 82% for previously untreated patients and 89% for those previously given chemotherapy. Overall survival was 85% (table). Ten previously untreated patients died of extensive disease within 3 weeks of starting chemotherapy. Adding cisplatin salvaged 9 of the 11 patients who became drug resistant. Salvage surgery alone yielded complete remission in 7 of 8 cases. Six of 8 patients with relapse after EMA/CO therapy achieved a further sustained remission after further chemotherapy and/or surgery. Complications were acceptable, although acute myeloid leukemia developed in 1 patient. Menses usually

Overall Survival of High-Risk Patients Entering EMA/CO Series (November 1989)

	No. prior chemotherapy (%)	Prior chemotherapy (%)	Total series (%)
Total	76	72	148
Alive	62 (82)	64 (89)	126 (85)
Dead	14 (18)	8 (11)	22 (15)
Relapsed	2 (2·6)*	6 (8·3)†	8 (5·4)

*Both alive and well after further treatment.
†Four patients are alive and well.
(Courtesy of Newlands ES, Bagshawe KD, Begent RHJ, et al: *Br J Obstet Gynaecol* 98:550–557, 1991.

returned within a few months of treatment. No fetal anomalies have occurred to date.

Recommendations.—The currently preferred treatment for patients with high-risk GTT is EMA/CO therapy. Salvage surgery is helpful in those who become drug resistant.

▶ A gestational trophoblastic tumor is one of the most highly curable forms of disseminated malignancy. Although relatively simple therapy is capable of curing almost every patient with trophoblastic disease with good prognosis, attention has focused increasingly on the group of patients with poor prognostic features. Patients with human chorionic gonadotropin levels $>10^5$ IU/L, 8 or more metastases, brain metastasis, failure of previous combination therapy, and those whose disease develops for longer than 1 year after antecedent pregnancy are included in this group. Patients with characteristics of poor pronosis have a 50% to 60% long-term survival with standard-combination chemotherapy.

These investigators now report substantial experience with a regimen called EMA/CO, which includes etoposide, methotrexate, actinomycin D, cyclophosphamide, and vincristine. A group of 148 consecutive patients was treated, and an 85% overall survival was achieved for the entire group. The acute myelotoxicity was consistent with intensive standard combination therapy, but late complications were rare. The regimen was not sterilizing, and no fetal abnormalities were noted in subsequent pregnancies. Of note is that acute myelogenous leukemia developed in a single patient, and that this development may relate in part to the presence of etoposide in the regimen. On the basis of this extensive experience, EMA/CO should be considered the treatment of choice for patients with high-risk gestational trophoblastic disease.—R.C. Young, M.D., F.A.C.P.

Changing Concepts in the Management of Vulvar Cancer

Thomas GM, Dembo AJ Bryson SCP, Osborne R, DePetrillo AD (Toronto Bayview Regional Cancer Centre, Toronto; Univ of Toronto)

Gynecol Oncol 42:9–21, 1991 9–24

Introduction.—Vulvar epidermoid carcinoma is an uncommon tumor that generally has been treated by radical vulvectomy and inguinal lymphadenectomy. However, several factors have been recognized to lead to improved treatment results, including earlier detection, understanding of tumor features predicting nodal involvement, and the use of radiation therapy. New directions in the management of vulvar carcinoma were examined.

Surgery.—Conventional surgical therapy can achieve an overall uncorrected 5-year survival rate of approximately 65% in an elderly population. The operability rates are now approximately 95%, with substantial mortality and morbidity. There are varying opinions on the role of pelvic node dissection; however, if it does have a survival benefit, it is very small—even when done selectively. The definition of radical surgery has been extended, with trends toward less extensive vulvar surgery, separate groin incisions, and less radical inguinal node therapy. Very good results have recently been seen with radical wide excision and selective groin node dissections.

Radiation.—Despite vulvar necrosis and other concerns, physicians use radiation therapy either radically or preoperatively, sometimes in patients who are unfit for radical surgery and sometimes in earlier disease. That vulvar cancer is probably as sensitive to radiation as other epidermoid cancers is supported by several studies. There is also some evidence that radiation can eliminate microscopic disease without surgery in clinically negative groins.

Future Directions.—The advantages of surgery and radiation now need to be integrated to tailor new treatment strategies to the extent of disease. For patients with well-lateralized disease and no evidence of multifocal disease, wide local excision is recommended. Radical vulvectomy and bilateral groin node dissection remain the standard for early, centrally located disease, but alternative therapies should be explored. Those patients with clinically positive nodes should have superficial bilateral groin node dissections. Those with extensive primary lesions may be treated with preoperative chemoradiotherapy followed by surgery. For primary lesions in an unfavorable location, preoperative chemoradiotherapy should be followed by bilateral groin node dissection.

Discussion.—These new approaches to treatment will be difficult to test in randomized studies; also, treatment may need to be individualized. Integration of different treatment modalities should improve anatomical and functional preservation in early disease and improve locoreginal control in advanced disease.

▶ Vulvar carcinoma is a relatively uncommon tumor that is generally diagnosed in elderly patients. It typically has been managed with radical vulvectomy and inguinal lymphadenectomy; however, the morbidity is high and the 5-year survival rate is less than ideal (65%). Recently, considerable effort has been made to reduce the use of extensive surgery in an effort to minimize morbidity in this elderly population. These investigators suggest that locoregionally advanced disease with high-risk features predict for local failure and define a patient population that should receive combined-modality chemotherapy/radiation and surgery. They advocate postoperative adjuvant inguinal and deep nodal irradiation for patients with 2 or more inguinal nodes; they also advocate the use of concurrent radiation and 5FU as a radiation sensitizer. The rarity of this tumor makes definitive randomized trials difficult; however, the overall thrust of these approaches and those of other investigators is to reduce the extensiveness of surgery and use combined-modality approaches to reduce morbidity.—R.C. Young, M.D., F.A.C.P.

10 Gastrointestinal Cancer

Esophageal

Rising Incidence of Adenocarcinoma of the Esophagus and Gastric Cardia
Blot WJ, Devesa SS, Kneller RW, Fraumeni JF Jr (Natl Cancer Inst, Bethesda, Md)
JAMA 265:1287–1289, 1991 10–1

Objective.—Recent clinical and epidemiologic data suggest that adenocarcinomas of the esophagus and gastric cardia may be increasing in frequency. The incidence data from 9 areas of the United States during 1976–1987 were analyzed.

Findings.—Increases of 4% to 10% per year were seen in men during the review period, exceeding those for any other type of cancer. In contrast, squamous cell cancers of the esophagus occurred at a relatively stable rate, and the number of cases of adenocarcinoma of more distal regions of the stomach decreased slightly. Adenocarcinomas of the esophagus and gastric cardia tended to occur in white men and were rare in women. In white men, adenocarcinomas accounted for one third of all esophageal cancers by the mid-1980s, and cardia cancers represented approximately half of all stomach cancers for which the subsites were specified.

Implications.—It is not clear whether the use of endoscopy contributes to the observed racial disparity in rates of esophageal and gastric cardia adenocarcinomas. The higher rates seen in whites suggest that alcohol intake and cigarette smoking are less important in gastric cardia cancer than they are in squamous cell carcinoma of the esophagus.

▶ More evidence accumulates as to the real increase in the incidence of adenocarcinomas of the distal esophagus and gastric cardia. Whether these tumors have the same natural history as other gastric cancers is unknown, but the outcome after either single-modality or multimodality therapy is known to be considerably worse (almost half the expected 2-year and 5-year stage-for-stage survival rates of patients with distal gastric adenocarcinomas) (1). A second important question is whether squamous cell carcinomas of the upper and middle third of the esophagus and distal esophageal adenocarcinomas can or should be studied together when various multimodality treatment plans are being investigated. By and large, they are lumped together in many clinical studies. A third important question is the relationship between gastroesophageal reflux, Barrett's esophagus, and the development of adenocarcinomas of the distal third of the esophagus and gastric cardia. A subset of this last question is whether effective reflux prevention changes either the natural course of Barrett's esophagus or the incidence of subsequent epithelial transformation. Finally, when esophagitis is defined after endoscopy in a patient with symptomatic reflux—particularly in a patient with documented Barrett's esophagus—there is still no quantitatable predictor of transformation or impending transformation.

In the case of a patient with known ulcerative colitis, 1 of our major research goals should be to develop molecular biological definitions that can be applied to tissue samples obtained at endoscopy or, even better, to blood samples, thereby allowing for a more reasonable screening procedure in patients with known but unpredictable predisposition to transformation. Such investigations are underway, and they should produce clinically valuable information soon (2–4).—G.D. Steele, Jr., M.D.

References

1. Gastrointestinal Tumor Study Group: *Cancer* 49:1116, 1982.
2. Andrews CW, et al: *Human Pathol,* in press.
3. Wiltz O, et al: *Gastroenterology* 100:1266, 1991.
4. Wiltz O, et al: *Surgery* 108:269, 1990.

Barrett's Esophagus: Prevalence and Incidence of Adenocarcinoma

Williamson WA, Ellis FH Jr, Gibb SP, Shahian DM, Aretz HT, Heatley GJ, Watkins E Jr (Lahey Clinic Med Ctr, Burlington, Mass; New England Deaconess Hosp, Boston)

Arch Intern Med 151:2212–2216, 1991 10–2

Background.—The reported incidences of adenocarcinoma in patients with Barrett's esophagus vary greatly. Some physicians have found a frequent association between severe dysplasia and the development of ade-

TABLE 1.—Comparison of Risk Factors in Patients With Barrett's Esophagus

Risk Factor	No. (%) No Carcinoma	No. (%) Carcinoma Present	P	Difference % (95% Confidence Interval of Difference %)
Median age, y (range)	56.0 (19-85)	61.0 (40-83)	.013†	. . .
Family history of esophageal carcinoma	2/168 (1.2)	4/62 (6.5)	.053‡	5.3 (−1.8 to +14.6)
Sex				
Male	111/171 (64.9)	60/65 (92.3)	<.0001‡	. . .
Female	60/171 (35.1)	5/65 (7.7)	<.0001‡	. . .
Smoking	49/164 (30.0)	26/61 (42.6)	.08‡NS	12.7 (−6.4 to +32.1)
Alcohol consumption	83/164 (50.6)	30/61 (49.2)	.85‡NS	. . .
Heavy alcohol consumption	20/164 (12.2)	8/61 (13.1)	.84‡NS	. . .

**Abbreviation: NS,* not significant.
†Wilcoxon rank sum test.
‡Miettinen's modification of the Fisher Exact Test.
(Courtesy of Williamson WA, Ellis FH Jr, Gibb SP, et al: *Arch Intern Med* 151:2212–2216, 1991.)

TABLE 2.—Incidence of Carcinoma in Barrett's Esophagus as Determined by Endoscopic Screening

Source, y	No. of Patients	No. of Carcinomas	Patient-Years of Follow-up Study	Patient-Year Incidence
Hameeteman et al, 1989	50	5	260	1/52
Robertson et al, 1988	56	4	224	1/56
Spechler et al, 1984	105	2	350	1/175
Skinner, 1989	45	3	145	1/48
Ovaska et al, 1989	32	3	166	1/55
Sampliner et al, 1985	25	1	92	1/92
Present study	176	5	497	1/99
Total	**489**	**23**	**1734**	1/75

(Courtesy of Williamson WA, Ellis FH Jr, Gibb SP, et al: *Arch Intern Med* 151:2212–2216, 1991.)

nocarcinoma in these patients. The prevalence and incidence of adenocarcinoma were established in 1 patient series.

Patients and Findings.—From 1973 to 1989, 241 patients with Barrett's esophagus were treated at the Lahey Clinic Medical Center in Burlington, Massachusetts. Sixty-five of these patients initially had adenocarcinoma in Barrett's esophagus, for a prevalence rate of 27%. A total of 176 patients was followed for a total of 497 patient-years. Adenocarcinoma developed in 5 patients, for an incidence of 1 per 99 patient-years. All 5 of these patients had severe dysplasia before the development of adenocarcinoma. Heartburn and regurgitation were more common in patients with benign Barrett's esophagus. There were significant differences in age, sex, and family history of esophageal carcinoma between those with benign conditions and those with malignant conditions (Table 1). Of the patients in whom adenocarcinoma occurred, 92% were men. These patients were also older (median age, 60 years), and they had a higher incidence of a family history of esophageal carcinoma.

Conclusions.—Long-term endoscopic and histologic surveillance of patients with Barrett's esophagus is important. An annual endoscopic follow-up examination is recommended for all patients. When mild dysplastic changes are found, case surveillance should be more frequent. Those patients who have severe dysplasia and are acceptable surgical candidates should be advised to have esophageal resection (Table 2).

▶ Carcinoma of the esophagus remains an enormous therapeutic challenge. It occurs in an increased frequency in those patients who have Barrett's esophagus. Such patients certainly need close surveillance as a minimum. This report from the Lahey Clinic shows adenocarcinoma occurring in 27% of the patients with Barrett's esophagus. In addition, in a large number of patients who were followed up, an incidence of 1 per 99 patient-years was seen. The presence of known Barrett's esophagus should send a signal to the physician to look carefully for carcinoma, not only when the diagnosis of Barrett's esophagus is made, but also in the follow-up of such patients.—E. Glatstein, M.D.

Esophageal Ultrasound and the Preoperative Staging of Carcinoma of the Esophagus

Rice TW, Boyce GA, Sivak MV, Loop FD (Cleveland Clinic Found)

J Thorac Cardiovasc Surg 101:536–544, 1991 10–3

Introduction.—The International Union Against Cancer (UICC) and the American Joint Committee on Cancer (AJCC) recently issued new guidelines for the staging of esophageal cancer. The new guidelines are still based on the tumor/node/metastasis staging classification, but evaluation of the primary tumor now involves assessing the depth of wall invasion rather than evaluating anatomical location, tumor length, or the percentage of wall circumference involved. Because the traditionally used methods for clinical staging are not useful in determining tumor invasion depth, the usefulness of esophageal ultrasonography (EUS) in preoperative staging was evaluated.

Esophageal Wall.—The normal esophageal wall consists of 5 distinct layers. Previous studies have shown that these 5 layers, as well as the regional lymph nodes, can be visualized with EUS. Periesophageal tissue is also well visualized by EUS. Lymph node shape, margin, and internal structure can also be assessed.

Methods.—Preoperative staging by EUS was attempted in 6 women and 22 men (age, 46–83 years) less than 2 weeks before operation. All patients had carcinomas involving the thoracic esophagus by AJCC definition. The EUS probe could not be passed through the malignant stricture in 6 patients (21%). The studies in the remaining 22 patients were evaluable. All studies were performed with a flexible endoscope and were videotaped. The depth of tumor invasion was confirmed by pathologic review.

Results.—Depth of tumor invasion was correctly identified in 13 of the 22 patients, yielding a 59% accuracy. Tumor depth was overstaged in 4 patients (18%) and understaged in 5 (23%). Lymph node staging at operation was adequate to allow comparison with the EUS findings in 20 patients. The disease was correctly identified by EUS as node negative in 7 patients and as node positive in 7 patients, yielding a 70% accuracy. There were 3 false positive and 3 false negative assessments.

Conclusion.—Esophageal ultrasonography provides a useful alternative method for clinical staging of esophageal cancer. It is anticipated that refinements of technique and increasing experience will improve the diagnostic accuracy of EUS.

▶ A generic problem in the application of any so-called neoadjuvant (i.e., preoperative) combination chemotherapy approach or any cancer treatment technique that attempts to tailor therapy and decrease morbidity of surgery by preoperatively defining disease stage is our continued dependency on the pathologic evaluation of the removed tissue specimen to obtain accurate prognostic information. The recent development of EUS will lead to numerous trials that hopefully will refine at least the "T" part of tumor/node/metastasis staging, with potential applicability to better preoperative prognostic data gathering.

This report from the Cleveland Clinic is such a preliminary attempt. Obviously, the deficits in study specificity are apparent. After the appropriate series of correlative studies have been done, using pathologic staging as the reference, this technique should have application to the entire gastrointestinal tract, and it should open up more rational approaches to neoadjuvant and more tailored cancer therapy techniques.—G.D. Steele, Jr., M.D.

A Randomized Trial Comparing Radiation Therapy *Versus* Concomitant Radiation Therapy and Chemotherapy in Carcinoma of the Thoracic Esophagus

Araújo CMM, Souhami L, Gil RA, Carvalho R, Garcia JA, Froimtchuk MJ, Pinto LHJ, Canary PCV (Instituto Nacional de Câncer, Rio de Janeiro)

Cancer 67:2258–2261, 1991 10–4

Background.—Studies of 5-fluorouracil (5-FU), mitomycin C, and radiation therapy (RT) have given promising results in patients with esophageal carcinoma. The chemotherapy (CT) acts as a radiation sensitizer to enhance the effects of RT. In a prospective randomized trial, the use of RT alone was compared with the use of RT plus CT.

Methods.—The subjects were 59 previously untreated patients with stage II squamous cell carcinoma of the thoracic esophagus. Fifty-two of the patients were men (age range, 30–69 years). The patients were randomized to receive either RT alone, 5,000 cGy given in 200-cGy daily fractions 5 days per week, or RT plus CT. The CT regimen consisted of 5-FU, 1,000 mg/m^2/day, given intravenously as a continuous infusion for 72 hours; mitomycin C, 10 mg/m^2, given as a bolus injection on day 1; and bleomycin, 15 units/week, given intramuscularly for 5 weeks starting on week 1.

Results.—A complete local response was attained by 58% of the RT group and 75% of the RT plus CT group. The response lasted a median of 8 months in both groups. After 5 years, the overall survival was 6% for the RT group and 16% for the RT plus CT group. All the patients had mild-to-moderate esophagitis, but it was more pronounced in the RT plus CT group. However, this did not affect treatment.

Conclusions.—Combined RT and CT in patients with esophageal carcinoma appears to offer no improvement in outcome compared with RT alone. However, because of the small size of this sample, these results should be interpreted cautiously. Larger clinical trials, whose full results are forthcoming, suggest that combined treatment has some advantages.

▶ The key question concerning RT, CT, and surgical treatment of squamous cell carcinoma of the thoracic esophagus is whether surgery will be necessary for anything but purely palliative purposes in the future. This small trial by Araujo et al. exemplifies the difficulties of clinical studies that have sample sizes too small for any appropriate conclusions. The study does, however, give one an excuse for referring to numerous larger studies that are presently asking a series of compromised questions concerning the treatment of squamous cell carcinoma of the esophagus. The most often asked questions are a function of the inability of multi-institutional groups to accrue patients if surgery is not a part of each alternative treatment method. The questions are also compromised because chemotherapy is not as effective as one would hope, and because staging is still dependent on the definitive pathologic evaluation of a resected specimen. Thus, surgery is rationalized as a part of neoadjuvant or combination CT/RT approaches for either palliative intent.

If patients fail, they most often fail locally, and their symptoms of dysphagia, bleeding, and pain ultimately may not be as easily ameliorated if resection of the esophagus is delayed. Surgery is justified to obtain histologic confirmation of what may be a complete or major partial clinical response after preoperative therapy. To date, however, there is little evidence that patients who have microscopic residual disease documented in the resected specimen after combination CT will be cured. With the development of more effective CT or the concomitant application of RT and CT drugs that are not only cytotoxic but radiosensitizing, we will probably begin to move closer to answering the important question of whether surgery can be used as 1 of the initial treatments in most of these unfortunate patients.—G.D. Steele, Jr., M.D.

Stomach

Resectable Gastric Carcinoma: An Evaluation of Preoperative and Postoperative Chemotherapy

Ajani JA, Ota DM, Jessup JM, Ames FC, McBride C, Boddie A, Levin B, Jackson DE, Roh M, Hohn D (Univ of Texas, Houston)
Cancer 68:1501–1506, 1991 10–5

Background.—In locoregional gastric carcinoma, the rate of curative resection is low, and distant metastases—especially to the peritoneum and liver are common. Thus, survival is low. The use of adjuvant systemic chemotherapy has been emphasized, but there is no standard approach. The feasibility of preoperative and postoperative chemotherapy was studied in 25 patients with potentially resectable locoregional gastric carcinoma.

Methods.—The subjects included 17 men and 8 women (median age, 62 years), 19 of whom had proximal carcinomas. All the patients received 2 preoperative courses of etoposide, 5-fluorouracil, and cisplatin (EFP). Three more courses were given 4–6 weeks postoperatively if there was any objective response to the first course. Postoperative radiation was given to patients who had microscopic or gross residual carcinoma. A total of 98 courses was given (median, 5 per patient). The median follow-up time was 25 months.

Results.—Therapy with EFP caused a major response in 6 patients. Resection was curative in 18 patients, and microscopic tumor only was found in 3 specimens. Only 1 patient had radiation therapy. The median survival was 15 months, and the most common indicator of failure was peritoneal carcinomatosis. One patient who responded to EFP died postoperatively, but there were no deaths from chemotherapy. The toxic effects were moderate and appeared to be worse during postoperative EFP.

Conclusions.—The use of EFP chemotherapy before and after surgery appears to be feasible for patients with locoregional gastric carcinoma. Before randomized trials are done, regimens that result in a 5% to 10% rate of complete pathologic response should be developed.

▶ The search for an adjuvant therapy that is effective in gastric cancer continues. Truly appropriately designed studies have given positive results only intermittently. Thus, the Gastrointestinal Tumor Study Group's adjuvant trial showing the effectiveness of 1 particular combination of chemicals after complete surgical resection of gastric adenocarcinoma (1) has not been substantiated by other concurrent or subsequent well-designed multi-institutional studies. The interesting results obtained by Preusser et al. (2) have not been substantiated in terms of toxicity (3) or outcome (4) in the United States. Thus, new trials will be based either on extrapolation of the conceptual or real benefits of the treatment modality used in other parts of the gastrointestinal tract (as in the present Intergroup multimodality study of gastric adjuvant chemoradiation therapy post-surgical resection), or on the application of such preliminary data on the potential effectiveness of EFP (as presented in this pilot study by the M.D. Anderson group). Ideally, in all of these studies, the meticulous detailing of surgical and surgical/pathologic staging will be upgraded from past studies, thereby eliminating the possibility that stage shifting will complicate the interpretation of minor differences in outcome between the control and experimental arms.—G.D. Steele, Jr., M.D.

References

1. Gastrointestinal Tumor Study Group: *Cancer* 49:1116, 1982.
2. Preusser P, et al: *J Clin Oncol* 7:1310, 1989.
3. Lerner A, et al: *Proc Am Soc Clin Oncol* 9:103, 1990.
4. Ajani JA, et al: *J Clin Oncol* 8:1231, 1990.

Hepatic

Hepatitis C Antibody in Patients With Chronic Liver Disease and Hepatocellular Carcinoma

Colombo M, Rumi MG, Donato MF, Tommasini MA, Del Ninno E, Ronchi G, Kuo G, Houghton M (Univ of Milan, Italy; Chiron Corp, Emeryville, Calif)
Dig Dis Sci 36:1130–1133, 1991 10–6

Introduction.—Hepatocellular carcinoma (HCC) is increasingly being recognized as a major health problem in European countries of the Mediterranean basin (where it is associated with cirrhosis). There is evidence that, in addition to hepatitis B virus and alcohol excess, chronic non-A, non-B hepatitis may be an important factor in the development of HCC.

Methods.—Sera from 132 patients with HCC and 139 with non-A, non-B chronic liver disease were tested for antibody to hepatitis C virus

(HCV). Eleven patients with mild hemophilia with no liver disease, 15 housestaff members living in a community for drug users, and 11 patients with miscellaneous liver diseases also were studied.

Findings.—Anti-HCV was found in 65% of the patients with HCC. It was comparably frequent in patients who were either positive or negative for serum hepatitis B surface antigen. Anti-HCV also was present in 74% of the patients with non-A, non-B chronic liver disease. Only 18% of the patients with miscellaneous diseases and 8% of all controls were positive for anti-HCV. The prevalence of anti-HCV was relatively low (28%) in HBsAg-positive patients with cirrhosis.

Implications.—These findings suggest that HCV is an important factor associated with HCC. It is possible that patients may be infected by both HCV and the hepatitis B virus.

Hepatitis B and C Viruses and Their Interaction in the Origin of Hepatocellular Carcinoma

Kaklamani E, Trichopoulos D, Tzonou A, Zavitsanos X, Koumantaki Y, Hatzakis A, Hsieh CC, Hatziyannis S (Harvard School of Public Health, Boston; Univ of Athens Med School, Greece)

JAMA 265:1974–1976, 1991 10–7

Objective.—Hepatocellular carcinoma (HCC) is 1 of the most frequently occurring cancers worldwide. The interactive roles of hepatitis B virus (HBV) and hepatitis C virus (HCV) in the origin of HCC were determined by obtaining sera from patients in a large case-control study in Athens. An enzyme immunoassay was used to estimate the amount of anti-HCV antibody in sera obtained from 185 patients with HCC, 35 patients with metastatic liver cancer, and 432 hospital controls.

Findings.—Strongly positive anti-HCV titers were significantly related to HCC, with a relative risk of 6.3. Weakly positive sera were associated more closely with metastatic liver cancer than with HCC. The association between HCV antibody and HCC was strongest in those patients with serum hepatitis B surface antigen. It appears that HBV and HCV interact to produce HCC.

Hepatitis C and Hepatitis B in the Etiology of Hepatocellular Carcinoma in the Japanese Population

Tanaka K, Hirohata T, Koga S, Sugimachi K, Kanematsu T, Ohryohji F, Nawata H, Ishibashi H, Maeda Y, Kiyokawa H, Tokunaga K, Irita Y, Takeshita S, Arase Y, Nishino N (Kyushu Univ School of Medicine, Fukuoka; Iizuka Hosp, Iizuka-shi; Bureau of Public Health of Fukuoka City; Fukuoka Red Cross Blood Ctr; Tokai Univ Fukuoka Junior College, Munakata-shi, Japan; et al)

Cancer Res 51:2842–2847, 1991 10–8

Introduction—Past studies have suggested that chronic hepatitis B virus infection is the predominant risk factor for hepatocellular carcinoma

(HCC). Ninety-one patients with HCC, 75 patients with hepatic cirrhosis who had no evidence of HCC, and 410 controls from the general Japanese population were enrolled in a case-control study.

Methods.—The serum titers of antibody to hepatitis C virus (HCV) were estimated by both enzyme-linked immunosorbent assay and recombinant immunoblot assay. Serum hepatitis B surface antigen (HBsAg) also was determined.

Findings.—Approximately half the patients with HCC or cirrhosis and only 3% of the controls had serum HCV antibody. Serum HBsAg was found in 21% of the patients with HCC, 11% of those with cirrhosis, and 2% of the control subjects. The relative risk of anti-HCV being present was estimated as 52 for HCC and 64 for cirrhosis. Among men with either disease, blood recipients and heavy drinkers had especially high rates of anti-HCV, as did those without identifiable risk factors. Anti-HCV was much less frequent in HBsAg-positive patients with HCC or cirrhosis than in those who tested negative for HBsAg.

Conclusion.—In Japan, HCV may be more important than chronic hepatitis B virus infection in the development of HCC and cirrhosis.

▶ The studies by Colombo et al., Kaklamani et al., and Tanaka et al. (Abstracts 10–6, 10–7, and 10–8) are studies of Mediterranean, Greek, and Japanese patient populations, respectively, in which serotyping (with appropriate case controls) was used to address questions concerning the possible synergy between HCV and HBV damage to the liver and HCC. Although the results in these different studies vary, a shared theme is that there is undoubtedly synergy between HBV and HCV, either in hepatocellular carcinoma development or in promoting the underlying conditions that cause liver damage as a precedent to HCC. The implications for diagnosis, prevention, and treatment by more conventional means are innumerable because, in terms of frequency, HCC remains the most important solid tumor worldwide.—G.D. Steele, Jr., M.D.

Hepatitis B Virus Integration in Hepatitis B Virus-Related Hepatocellular Carcinoma in Childhood

Chang M-H, Chen P-J, Chen J-Y, Lai M-Y, Hsu H-C, Lian D-C, Liu Y-G, Chen D-S (Natl Taiwan Univ, Taipei)

Hepatology 13:316–320, 1991 10–9

Introduction.—Hepatocellular carcinoma (HCC), a leading malignancy in Taiwan, is much less prevalent in children than in adults. Nevertheless, it is an important malignancy in children aged 5–14 years. The close relationship between HCC and hepatitis B virus (HBV) infection is well documented, and HBV infection in hyperendemic areas usually begins in infancy and early childhood.

Methods.—The status of HBV DNA was determined in HCC tissue and uninvolved liver tissue obtained from 8 children (mean age, 10.5 years) with hepatitis B serum antigen whose mothers also had HBsAg. An

HBV genome probe was prepared from a dimer of HBV DNA cloned in the *Eco*RI site of *pBR* 322.

Results.—Of the 8 samples of HCC, 5 showed integration of HBV DNA. In most patients, a single distinct band was observed, suggesting single-site integration of HBV DNA into liver-cell DNA. Of 4 samples of nontumorous liver tissue, 1 showed multiple integration bands of HBV DNA. Studies using subgenomic fragments of the HBV genome as probes showed the X gene fragment and the surface antigen gene fragment to be the most conserved sequences.

Conclusion.—The single-site integration pattern seen in childhood HCC in Taiwan provides a useful model with which to study the carcinogenicity of HBV. An integrative process affecting the critical region of the gene may lead to insertional mutagenesis and the early development of HCC.

▶ Not only can HBV make you sick, it can also substantially increase the risk of subsequent development of HCC. The HBV vaccine is available and effective. Although the connection is indirect, this is a case in which a vaccine can prevent the subsequent development of cancer.—J.V. Simone, M.D.

Depot-Medroxyprogesterone Acetate (DMPA) and Risk of Liver Cancer

Thomas DB, for the WHO Collaborative Study of Neoplasia and Steroid Contraceptives (Fred Hutchinson Cancer Research Ctr, Seattle)

Int J Cancer 49:182–185, 1991 10–10

Background.—Depot-medroxyprogesterone acetate (DMPA), which has been available as a long-acting progestational contraceptive for as long as 25 years in some countries, may have carcinogenic effects in the human liver. Oral contraceptives do not appear to potentiate the carcinogenic effects of hepatitis B virus, but this conclusion is not necessarily applicable to DMPA. A hospital-based case-control study was done to assess the relationship between DMPA and liver cancer in developing countries in which hepatitis B virus is endemic.

Methods.—The analysis included findings from 3 centers in Thailand and 1 in Kenya. Breast, uterine cervix and corpus, ovarian, and hepatobiliary cancers were identified in women who were at risk of exposure to steroid contraceptives during their reproductive years. The 71 patients identified were matched to 530 controls. The mean patient age was 41.7 years. Of the Kenyan and Thai women, 18.2% and 8.2%, respectively, had been exposed to DMPA. Each subject completed a standard questionnaire that included information about previous DMPA use and potential confounders.

Results.—The relative risks of liver cancer in DMPA users were 1.64 in Kenya and .33 in Thailand; neither association was significant. Risk was not affected in any significant way by the duration of DMPA use, time since last use. or time since first use. There were no significant associations between the use of DMPA and the risk of hepatocellular carcinoma or cholangiocarcinoma.

Conclusions.—The use of DMPA does not appear to significantly affect the risk of liver cancer in areas where hepatitis B virus is endemic.

▶ With the increased use of DMPA as a long-acting contraceptive, particularly in countries in which hepatocellular carcinomas are indigenous, the question of whether DMPA is a potentiator of the carcinogenic effects of hepatitis B virus is an important one. It has previously been established that oral contraceptives do not appear to potentiate hepatitis B virus and the development of hepatocellular carcinomas. This World Health Organization Collaborative Study provides the first evidence that hepatitis B is endemic, and that the relative risk of liver cancer in DMPA users is not greater than that found in individuals who do not use DMPA.—G.D. Steele, Jr., M.D.

Hepatocellular Carcinoma in Italian Patients With Cirrhosis

Colombo M, de Franchis R, Del Ninno E, Sangiovanni A, De Fazio C, Tommasini M, Donato MF, Piva A, Di Carlo V, Dioguardi N (Policlinico Hosp, Milan, Italy; Univ of Milan)

N Engl J Med 325:675–680, 1991 10–11

Introduction.—Hepatocellular carcinoma has an extremely poor prognosis. Several studies have identified cirrhosis of the liver as a risk factor for hepatocellular carcinoma. Studies among Asian patients have demonstrated that early detection increases the number of lesions that are resectable, but this has not yet been confirmed in the West. The prevalence, incidence, and natural history of hepatocellular carcinoma were determined in Italian patients with cirrhosis.

Methods.—Real-time ultrasonography (US) and serum α-fetoprotein assays were performed at baseline and every 3–12 months thereafter in 447 patients with well-compensated cirrhosis. The 308 men and 139 women were 36–76 years of age, and all were of Italian descent. The average follow-up period was 33 months.

Results.—Hepatocellular carcinoma was detected at baseline in 30 patients (7%) and during follow-up in 29 of the 417 patients (7%) who were free of tumor at baseline. The cumulative hazard of hepatocellular carcinoma among patients without tumors at enrollment was higher among those with persistently elevated serum α-fetoprotein levels than it was among those with fluctuating or consistently normal levels. Thirteen of the 30 tumors (43%) detected at baseline (but only 4 of the 29 tumors [14%] detected during follow-up) were potentially resectable. Five patients refused operation. The postoperative survival in the 12 patients who underwent tumor resection ranged from 25 days to 36 months. Survival at 1 year was 67%, and the tumor recurrence rate was 60%. The outcome with tumor resection did not differ appreciably from that in the 5 patients who refused resection.

Conclusion.—In the West, patients with liver cirrhosis also are at substantial risk for hepatocellular carcinoma. Screening did not appreciably increase the detection rate of potentially curable tumors.

▶ This small study by Colombo et al. challenges many of the assumptions that have been made but have never been proven in the Japanese literature. It also extrapolates a set of important questions concerning hepatocellular carcinoma to a Western population. Specifically, the predisposition of patients with liver cirrhosis to subsequent risk for hepatocellular carcinoma is shown. The ineffectiveness of screening to define disease at an early stage that might be more amenable to cure is also shown. The only arguable aspect of the article is the implication that the Japanese have shown both the benefit of surveillance in high-risk populations and the increased curative potential of early application of treatment for smaller hepatocellular carcinomas. In fact, the Japanese have never shown any plateaus in their survival curves after treatment of hepatocellular carcinoma, which will remain the "proof in the pudding" for any claim of early diagnosis equating to increased chance for cure (whether by surgical resection or by other means). The real emphasis on hepatocellular carcinoma, regardless of whether it is based on cirrhosis or not, should be its prevention. This should become ever more approachable in the next several years, at least in populations located in areas where the hepatitis B virus is endemic.—G.D. Steele, Jr., M.D.

A 5-Year Study of Cryosurgery in the Treatment of Liver Tumors

Ravikumar TS, Kane R, Cady B, Jenkins R, Clouse M, Steele G Jr (Yale Univ School of Medicine, New Haven, Conn; Harvard Med School, Boston)

Arch Surg 126:1520–1524, 1991 10–12

Introduction.—Cryosurgery has been shown to be effective in controlling liver tumors, especially when combined with intraoperative ultrasonographic monitoring. Thirty-two patients were treated in this way in 1985–1990. Twenty-four of these patients had colorectal cancer, 3 had hepatoma, and 2 had neuroendocrine tumors.

Results.—Nine patients were free of disease after a median follow-up of 2 years. Eleven others were living with disease, whereas 12 patients had died. More than half the patients who died had disease in both the liver and extrahepatic sites, whereas one third had liver disease only. The latter group included 3 patients with recurrent disease at the site of treatment. Three fourths of the patients with colorectal cancer were free of disease after cryosurgery. Two of 3 patients with hepatoma and both patients with neuroendocrine tumor metastases exhibited long-term control of disease.

Conclusion.—Both the ability of cryosurgery to conserve normal liver tissue and the availability of retreatment make this approach an effective means of treating both primary liver tumors and hepatic metastases.

▶ These investigators initially attempted to apply cryosurgical ablation together with intraoperative ultrasonography monitoring freeze margins to extend the application of regional therapy to 2 groups of patients: (1) those who had metastatic colon and rectum adenocarcinoma of the liver and too many liver lesions to justify a resection (more than 3); and (2) those patients whose isolated liver lesions were at particular locations that would prohibit adequate resection (contiguous to the vena cava or at the junction of the vena cava and a major hepatic vein). Unfortunately, they have disproven both initial hypotheses in terms of application of the cryosurgical ablation technique. However, they have shown that when freeze margins can be adequately monitored in real time by the intraoperative ultrasonography, and when these margins are comparable to good surgical resection margins (i.e., 1–2 cm around the tumor), then the results are similar to those of conventional resection. This means that, in some groups of patients (particularly those with small lesions in the depths of the right and left liver lobe), removal of more than 1–2 cm of the normal liver tissue that surrounds the tumor is not necessary to ensure the best possible chance of regional or distant freedom from recurrence. Obviously, this decreased destruction of normal tissue is reflected in the decreased morbidity and absent mortality associated with this technique. Even though the application is limited to a subset of a relatively small group of patients with isolated, potentially resectable liver recurrence from rectum and colon cancer, the cryosurgical technique should be available in institutions when patients are frequently seen as candidates for potential liver metastasis resection.—G.D. Steele, Jr., M.D.

Pancreas

Ras Gene Mutations in Intraductal Papillary Neoplasms of the Pancreas: Analysis in Five Cases

Tada M, Omata M, Ohto M (Chiba Univ, Chiba, Japan)
Cancer 67:634–637, 1991 10–13

Introduction.—Intraductal papillary neoplasm of the pancreas is a rare neoplasm that grows papillary in the pancreatic duct; it is considered a low-grade malignancy because of its good prognosis. It may be hard to determine whether this tumor is a carcinoma or an adenoma on the basis of clinical and pathologic findings. The presence of *ras* gene mutations was sought in 5 patients with intraductal papillary neoplasms of the pancreas.

Methods.—Surgical specimens were obtained from 3 men and 2 women (age, 44–70 years) with intraductal papillary neoplasm. None of the patients had metastatic disease at the time of operation. The *ras* gene mutations were sought by polymerase chain reaction and direct sequencing.

Results.—There was a *ras* gene mutation in codon 12 of the K-*ras* gene in 3 patients. Compared with the 93% incidence reported for ordinary pancreatic adenocarcinoma, this incidence was considered to be low. There was no correlation between the presence of mutations and the severity of cellular atypia; however, the 3 tumors with mutations were larger than those without mutations.

Conclusion.—The *ras* gene mutation does not appear to be the first genetic alteration of tumor progression in intraductal papillary neoplasm of the pancreas; rather, it appears to occur during the development of pancreatic neoplasms. The *ras* gene mutations are less common in these tumors than in other pancreatic tumors.

▶ The K-*ras* gene is an oncogene with mutational activation that is associated with the malignant transformation of the colon and rectum as well as of the pancreas. The activation of K-*ras* through mutation is considered to be an early event in the induction of adenocarcinomas of the colon or rectum. It also may be an early event in the induction of adenocarcinoma of the pancreas, because between 93% and 95% of pancreatic adenocarcinomas have K-*ras* gene mutations (1,2). The series reported by Tada et al. is important because, although the number of patients studied is small, intraductal papillary neoplasms of the pancreas have a good prognosis and may represent a subset of carcinoma that is not nearly as aggressive as the more common pancreatic adenocarcinomas. Thus, when Tada et al. demonstrate that these less aggressive intraductal papillary neoplasms of the pancreas have a lower incidence of K-*ras* mutation, the mutation of K-*ras* may not be an early inductive event but, rather, an event associated with aggressive cancer. Furthermore, because this is a small series, it is difficult to really draw any conclusions about the frequency of K-*ras* mutations. Nonetheless, this is an important paper, because it points out the necessity of considering the clinical entity as well as the oncogene or tumor suppressor gene that is altered genetically. It is hoped that, as more aggressive screening for pancreatic cancer occurs, K-*ras* gene mutations will be analyzed so that the true frequency of mutation and the association with malignant characteristics can be determined.—J.M. Jessup, M.D.

Pancreatic Cancer in Illinois: A Report by 88 Hospitals on 2,401 Patients Diagnosed 1978–84

Sener SF, Fremgen A, Imperato JP, Sylvester J, Chmiel JS (American Cancer Society, Chicago)

Am Surg 57:490–495, 1991 10–14

Introduction.—The survival results for pancreatic cancer were analyzed in a series of 2,401 patients whose cancer was diagnosed at Illinois hospitals in 1978–1984. More than two thirds of the patients had cancer in the head of the pancreas. Laparotomy was carried out in 68% of the group, and 12% of the patients underwent resection. Approximately one fourth of the patients who underwent resection received radiotherapy and/or chemotherapy afterwards.

Outcome.—Survival after 3 years was enhanced by radiotherapy/chemotherapy in patients undergoing laparotomy/bypass surgery (Fig 10–1). The median survival for patients with stage I disease was 12.5 months after resection and 6.8 months after laparotomy/bypass. Resection appeared to be advantageous in patients without metastatic disease. When resection was not carried out, patients lacking gross metastasis

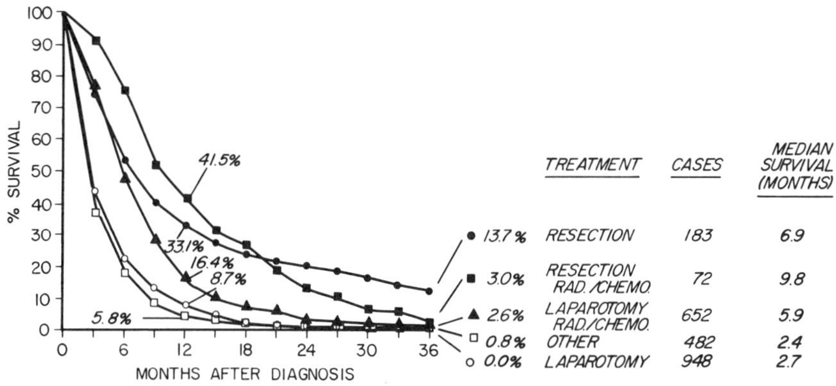

Fig 10–1.—Observed survival for patients with adenocarcinoma (according to treatment). (Courtesy of Sener SF, Fremgen A, Imperato JP, et al: *Am Surg* 57:490–495, 1991.)

lived longerthan those who were found at laparotomy to have metastatic disease.

Conclusion.—Postoperative treatment warrants further evaluation in patients with unresectable pancreatic cancer and in those undergoing resection. Both the value of hyperthermia added to full-dose irradiation and the use of multidrug chemotherapy are currently being studied.

▶ This is a large population-based retrospective study of 2,401 patients in whom pancreatic cancer was diagnosed at 88 hospitals in Illinois. The strength of this study is that a large number of patients was accrued during a 6-year interval, allowing little chance for change in the natural history of the disease. The report suggested that, in a heterogeneous community with surgeons, medical oncologists, and radiotherapists of varied abilities, resection of the pancreatic cancer is associated with an improvement in 3-year survival compared with unresectable lesions. However, the important finding is that the addition of radiation and chemotherapy to surgical resection tends to improve median survival. Analysis of the patients who had stage I lesions at initial presentation further supports an aggressive approach to the management of this grim cancer. The median survival after resection alone was 12.5 months vs. survival of 6.8 months after laparotomy and 3.8 months after other nonoperative treatment. Thus, aggressive surgical treatment of pancreatic cancer, especially in lesions confined to the pancreas, may improve the survival of patients.—J.M. Jessup, M.D.

Factors Influencing Survival After Pancreaticoduodenectomy for Pancreatic Cancer

Cameron JL, Crist DW, Sitzmann JV, Hruban RH, Boitnott JK, Seidler AJ, Coleman J (Johns Hopkins Med Insts, Baltimore)

Am J Surg 161:120–125, 1991 10–15

Multivariant Analysis Using Cox Proportional Hazards Model

Variable	Coefficient	p Value	Relative Risk
Lymph node involvement	1.197	0.0065	3.31
Blood vessel invasion	0.785	0.025	2.19
Blood transfusion	0.757	0.015	2.13

(Courtesy of Cameron JL, Crist DW, Sitzmann JV, et al: *Am J Surg* 161:120–125, 1991.)

Background.—A significant decline in hospital morbidity and mortality was recently reported after pancreaticoduodenectomy for periampullary carcinoma. Patients treated between 1969 and 1990 were studied to determine the factors influencing long-term survival.

Methods.—A group of 89 patients underwent pancreaticoduodenectomy for head of the pancreas carcinoma in this period. The 81 hospital survivors were analyzed.

Findings.—Overall, the actuarial 5-year survival was 19%. The median survival was 11.9 months. Long-term survival was more likely in patients with negative lymph nodes and no blood vessel invasion. Negative lymph node status was the strongest predictor of long-term survival (median survival, 55.8 months), compared with 11 months among patients with lymph node involvement. Blood transfusions also predicted long-term survival. Those patients receiving 2 or fewer units had a median survival of 24.7 months, whereas those receiving 3 or more had a median survival of 10.2 months.

Conclusions.—The biology of the tumor, including lymph node status and blood vessel invasion, appears to be the most important determinant of long-term survival after pancreaticoduodenectomy (table). However, whether resection was done also seems to influence survival in such cases.

▶ This is the latest review of pancreaticoduodenectomies from the Johns Hopkins Hospital. Dr. Cameron and his associates have compiled an excellent series and, in this article, they analyze the impact of various prognostic factors on outcome. Unfortunately, the actuarial 5-year survival rate is only 19%, with a median survival of only 11.9 months. The univariant prognostic factors that had a significant impact on prognosis were tumor size less than or equal to 2 cm, the absence of blood vessel or lymphatic invasion, the absence of metastases to regional lymph nodes, and a less than 3-unit blood transfusion. When the multivariant analysis was performed, the most important variables were lymph node involvement, blood vessel invasion, and blood transfusion. Those patients who lacked lymph node involvement and had tumors less than 2 cm in diameter had a median survival of approximately 56 months. This data serves as a benchmark for comparison with future series. It also suggests the need for further therapy and implies that the addition of chemoradiotherapy may improve outcome.—J.M. Jessup, M.D.

Risk Factors for Septicemia Following Endoscopic Biliary Stenting

Motte S, Deviere J, Dumonceau J-M, Serruys E, Thys J-P, Cremer M (Université Libre de Bruxelles, Brussels

Gastroenterology 101:1374–1381, 1991 10–16

Background.—Endoscopic biliary drainage is the palliative treatment of choice for bile duct tumors. However, septicemia is a major complication of this technique. The risk factors for septicemia after endoscopic biliary drainage were investigated.

Method.—Using discriminant regression analysis, the clinical, biological, and radiologic data on 34 patients who had septicemia within 3 days of endoscopic biliary stenting were reviewed retrospectively and compared with data on 71 patients who did not have septicemia.

Results.—When only data available before the procedure were used, both prior cholangitis and leukocytosis were identified by discriminant analysis as risk factors. However, even in linear combination, only 50% of the cases of septicemia could be predicted on the basis of these 2 risk factors. When information on the quality of drainage after the procedure was added to the analysis, 91% of the cases could be identified. Those patients from centers where duodenoscopes may have been poorly disinfected were at higher risk for *Pseudomonas aeruginosa* septicemia.

Conclusion.—The quality of drainage plays a critical role in risk of the septicemia. Diagnostic endoscopic retrograde cholangiopancreatography should be avoided unless drainage can be performed as part of the same procedure. Drainage should be as complete as possible. Antibiotics should be administered before every procedure and should cover *P. aeruginosa* if a problem with disinfection of the endoscope is suspected. The quality of the drainage should be the important factor in determining the duration of antibiotics.

▶ Bile duct and pancreatic cancers frequently require endoscopic biliary drainage for palliative management. These authors attempt to identify the factors in the procedure that predisposed to septicemia. In analyzing 347 patients who underwent biliary stenting, they documented 34 episodes of septicemia. This was most frequently seen either in patients undergoing diagnostic procedures without drainage or in situations in which *P. aeruginosa* bacteriemia was closely associated with contaminated endoscopes. The authors emphasize the importance of periodic surveillance culture of the endoscopic equipment, strict disinfection of the duodenoscopes, the use of prophylactic antibiotics active against *Pseudomonas,* and the importance of establishing adequate biliary decompression and satisfactory drainage.—R.C. Young, M.D., F.A.C.P.

Colorectal

Cancer Incidence Among Parents of Patients With Colorectal Cancer

Søndergaard JO, Bülow S, Lynge E (Danish Cancer Society, Copenhagen; Hvidovre Hosp, Hvidovre, Denmark)

Int J Cancer 47:202–206, 1991 10–17

Introduction.—A recent study of the spouses of patients with colorectal cancer found no increased risk of colorectal cancer, even among those who had been married for more than 30 years. Thus, the probable dietary component in the etiology of colorectal cancer was not detectable among these genetically unrelated individuals. To determine the genetic component in the etiology of colorectal cancer, the incidence of disease was studied among parents of patients with colorectal cancer.

Methods.—According to the Danish Cancer Registry, from 1982 to 1984, 1,524 patients younger than 60 years of age received a diagnosis of colorectal cancer. The parents of these patients were identified from public population registers. The index patients had a total of 1,478 eligible mothers, of whom 1,411 (96%) were traced, and a total of 1,414 eligible fathers, of whom 1,364 (96%) were traced. The Cancer Register was then searched for colorectal cancer diagnosed in parents from 1943 through 1986.

Results.—There were 83 cases of colorectal cancer among the mothers of index patients; 51.08 had been expected based on the incidence rates for the Danish population. There were 103 cases of colorectal cancer among the fathers; 55.17 cases had been expected. The mothers had a 1.62-fold increased risk compared with all Danish women, and the fathers had a 1.87-fold increased risk compared with all Danish men. Statistically, the incidence of colorectal cancer was increased significantly among mothers and fathers. The excess risk among parents was slightly higher if the index patient was a son rather than a daughter. The excess risk among parents was not related to the index patient's age at diagnosis. The excess risk was particularly strong if colorectal cancer had been diagnosed in both the parent and the index patient before the age of 50. There appears to be a possible genetic factor in the etiology of colorectal cancer.

▶ This study adds to a study published in the *New England Journal of Medicine* several years ago (1), in which the intuitive belief in the genetic predisposition to "sporadic" colorectal cancer (nonulcerative colitic; non-Lynch syndrome; or nonfamilial, polyposis coli-related) was supported by a variety of scientific approaches. In this study, the investigators looked at the mothers and fathers of index cases and found not only an increase from the expected incidence among the parents, but also a synergistic increase if the index case was 50 years or younger at the time of colorectal cancer diagnosis. The practical consequences of such data may relate to screening recommendations, and they probably support the implications of the earlier study's recommendation that first-degree relatives undergo endoscopic screening of their large bowel mucosa at some reasonable age (probably between 40 and 50 years), even if they are asymptomatic and have signs of colorectal pathology at the time of routine physical examination. If the index case occurs at an earlier age, then screening should probably be started at an earlier age. Obviously, the most rational approach to screening will await molecular biological definitions of precise genetic predisposition. However, at present, epidemiologic studies have provided most of the clinically relevant data that are available.—G.D. Steele, Jr., M.D.

Reference

1. Leppert M, et al: *N Engl J Med* 322:904, 1990.

Aspirin Use and Reduced Risk of Fatal Colon Cancer

Thun MJ, Namboodiri MM, Heath CW Jr (American Cancer Society, Atlanta)

N Engl J Med 325:1593–1596, 1991 10–18

Background.—There is growing evidence from animal and human epidemiologic studies that nonsteroidal anti-inflammatory drugs (e.g., aspirin) may have a protective effect against colon cancer. Data from an ongoing prospective cancer mortality study were used to test this hypothesis.

Methods.—The analysis included data on 662,424 adults enrolled since 1982 in the American Cancer Society's Cancer Prevention Study II. The average patient age at enrollment was 57 years. The study sample included all white subjects who specified their frequency and duration of aspirin use at entry into the study. The mortality data were completed through 1988. Multivariate analysis was done on 598 patients and 3,058 matched controls to address the potential effects of other risk factors for colon cancer.

Results.—The deaths from colon cancer decreased with more frequent aspirin use among both men and women. For patients who took aspirin at least 16 times per month for at least 1 year, the relative risks were .60 for men and .58 for women. These risks were unchanged after exclusion of factors that might affect aspirin use and motility, including arthritis, cancer, heart disease, and stroke at entry. The results were not significantly affected by adjustment for diet, obesity, physical activity, or family history. Acetaminophen use had no significant effect on risk.

Conclusions.—Frequent use of low doses of aspirin might reduce the risk of fatal colon cancer. No conclusions can be drawn as to the mechanism of this effect, whether direct, (e.g., by inhibition of prostaglandin synthesis), or indirect (e.g., by inducing bleeding in subjects with polyps or early cancer leading to early diagnosis). Controlled trials in high-risk patients may be useful.

▶ In the absence of any exact knowledge of the cause of such a major scourge as colorectal cancer, and in the absence of any easy way of defining the incidence of asymptomatic early disease, the simple appeal of a true panacea is almost overwhelming. Two modern-day candidates for "true pancreas" are tamoxifen for women and aspirin for almost everybody. This intriguing epidemiologic, statistical approach by Thun et al. is minimally based upon scientific data. Nevertheless, it is extraordinarily appealing because so many individuals are currently taking 1 aspirin every day or every other day to prophylax against numerous dietary, genetic, and environmental indiscretions (either controllable or uncontrollable). If this article and its conclusions are valid, then we may be benefitting our gastrointestinal tracts as well as our cardiovascular systems. The fact that such benefits is based on largely empiric or retrospectively derived epidemiologic evidence will, of course, be irrelevant until we have more exact knowledge of the causes of premalignant and malignant bowel disease.—G.D. Steele, Jr., M.D.

Colonoscopic Surveillance After Polypectomy: Considerations of Cost Effectiveness

Ransohoff DF, Lang CA, Kuo HS (Yale Univ, New Haven, Conn; Univ of Colorado, Denver)

Ann Intern Med 114:177–182, 1991 10–19

Introduction.—Regular colonoscopic examinations are recommended for individuals who have had an adenomatous colon polyp removed. However, small adenomatous polyps are quite common, and they may not have a high malignant potential. The cost-effectiveness of periodic follow-up colonoscopy was determined for the millions of Americans who have had adenomatous colon polyps.

Method.—Using data from the medical literature, a simulation model was constructed to estimate both the costs and the risk of perforation associated with colonoscopic surveillance of a 50-year-old man followed for 30 years. For the baseline analysis, the surveillance was considered to be 100% effective, thus providing a minimum estimate of cost-effectiveness or of cost per cancer-associated death prevented. The calculations were then repeated, assuming efficacies of 75% and 50%.

Results.—With colonoscopy done every 3 years, a 50-year-old patient can expect to have an average of 7 examinations. In 1 example, the 30-year cumulative risk for mortality from colon cancer after the removal of an index polyp was assumed to be 2.5%. To prevent a single death from colon cancer, 283 examinations would have to be performed, with a direct physician cost of $82,825. There would be .6 perforations and .4 perforation-related deaths. With a lower 30-year cumulative risk for mortality, there would be more examination, greater costs, and more perforation-related deaths before a single death from colon cancer would be prevented.

Implications.—Because the risk of death from colon cancer appears to be low in patients who have had a single small adenoma removed, the costs and effort involved in regular and indefinite surveillance are deemed excessive. With frequent examinations, the cumulative risk of colonic perforation may even exceed the risk of death from colon cancer.

▶ Questions concerning both the screening of asymptomatic patients for the development of polyps or colorectal cancer and the use of colonoscopic surveillance after polypectomy are hard to answer with clinical trials. Until very recently, there was a general consensus that no database existed to recommend asymptomatic screening, nor was it easy to be dogmatic about interval surveillance after initial polypectomy. However, Ransohoff's article and more recent articles by the Kaiser Permanente group and the St. Mark's Group (1, 2) have added to the arguments of those who would suggest that (1) some limited endoscopic screening is probably warranted in asymptomatic individuals aged 40–50 years; (2) interval screening in the absence of any sentinel polyp or cancer is probably unnecessary for a longer interval than we had previously suspected (perhaps every 10 years); and (3) in patients who are found to have polyps, the subsets that can be defined are probably not at any greater risk for the subsequent development of colorectal premalignancies or malignancies than is the general population. All of these recent approaches were formulated either by statistical modeling or by case-control methods, instead of by a prospective randomized trial that would have been extraordinarily costly and equally difficult to interpret.

There is a "pot of gold" at the end of the conceptual rainbow: if a reasonable (i.e., small) subset of the population could be considered at risk for the development of colon or rectal cancers, then most such tumors could be prevented by regular surveillance and endoscopic polypectomy. Interestingly, in a recent editorial accompanying the Kaiser group study and the St. Mark's paper, Bernard Levin (3) approached what had been suggested by a few of us earlier: (1) the cost side of the cost/effectiveness equation must be challenged; and (2) we must begin to move toward training technicians to provide endoscopic surveillance to our patients, much in the same manner that we have tried to define lower cost mammographic techniques for screening patients who are at risk for breast cancer. Hopefully, this will gain momentum in the near future, and issues concerning litigation can be neutralized by assuring that quality assessment of colonoscopy will continue to be done by adequately trained supervising physicians.—G.D. Steele, Jr., M.D.

References

1. Selby JV, et al: *N Engl J Med* 10:653, 1992.
2. Atkin WW, et al: *N Engl J Med* 10:658, 1992.
3. Levin B: *N Engl J Med* 10:700, 1992.

Mucin Production by Human Colonic Carcinoma Cells Correlates With Their Metastatic Potential in Animal Models of Colon Cancer Metastasis

Bresalier RS, Niv Y, Byrd JC, Duh Q-Y, Toribara NW, Rockwell RW, Dahiya R, Kim YS (VA Med Ctr, San Francisco; Univ of California, San Franciso)

J Clin Invest 87:1037–1045, 1991 10–20

Background.—Patients with mucinous adenocarcinoma of the colon frequently are seen initially with advanced disease and reportedly have a poor prognosis. Inconsistent correlations between survival and the presence of mucinous cancer may reflect a lack of adequate quantitation of mucin production by cancer cells in most histochemical studies.

Study Design.—The production and secretion of metabolically labeled mucin were compared in LS LiM 6, a colon carcinoma cell line with a high ability to metastasize to liver in nude mice, and in LS174T, a poorly metastatic parental cell line. The variants of LS174T selected for high and low mucin synthesizing ability were evaluated.

Observations.—Cells of LS LiM 6 produced twofold more intracellular mucin and secreted fourfold to fivefold more mucin into the culture medium than did the LS174T cells. Blot hybridization with a human intestinal mucin complementary DNA probe showed an increase in poly(A)$^+$ RNA in LS LiM 6. Increased mucin core carbohydrate antigens were evident immunohistochemically. The variants of LS174T produced metastases and colonized the liver in proportion to their ability to produce mucin. Liver colonization was reduced markedly when an arylglycoside was used to inhibit mucin glycosylation.

Conclusions.—Mucin production by human colon cancer cells appears to correlate with the metastatic potential of the cells and their ability to colonize the liver.

Mucinous Carcinomas of the Colon and Rectum: An Analysis of 62 Stage B and C Lesions

Connelly JH, Robey-Cafferty SS, Cleary KR (Univ of Texas, Houston)

Arch Pathol Lab Med 115:1022–1025, 1991 10–21

Background.—The importance of the finding of a large extracellular mucinous component in colorectal adenocarcinomas continues to be debated. To resolve some of the associated conflicts, 62 stage B and C lesions were analyzed.

Methods.—Stage B or C mucinous carcinoma was defined by the presence of a mucinous component of 60% or more. The patients were 35 women and 27 men (mean age, 62.6 years). The clinical records of each patient were reviewed. Each of 60 patients was matched for sex, stage, site, and age with 2 patients with nonmucinous carcinoma.

Results.—Survival was significantly better in patients with mucinous carcinoma and residual adenoma than in those without residual adenoma. The 5-year survival rate was 64% for patients with both mucinous and nonmucinous adenocarcinoma. Patients with stage B mucinous carcinoma had significantly worse survival and more local sites of treatment failure than did those with stage B nonmucinous carcinoma.

Conclusions.—There is no overall difference in survival between patients with mucinous and nonmucinous adenocarcinomas; however, when stages are considered separately, those with stage B mucinous carcinoma do much worse. This may result from the presence of extracellular mucin, which can make complete surgical extirpation more difficult.

▶ The production of mucin by human colorectal carcinomas is probably associated with some significant effect on tumor function and prognosis. The difficulty in defining the exact effect on prognosis is demonstrated in the article by Connelly et al. (Abstract 10–21), in which a limited number of patients with stage II or III lesions were examined with crude morphologic definitions of mucin production (which are all that pathologists have at present); as expected, the prognostic information was equivocal at best. An interesting contrast is the application of molecular biological techniques, such as those discussed in the article by Bresalier et al (Abstract 10–20); one can begin to see more precise genetic and phenotypic quantitation of mucin production. This will help clinical pathologists establish more precisely the capability of human colorectal carcinoma cells to produce 1 or another of a variety of mucins that are associated with gastrointestinal cancers. It will also help to quantitate expression in primary or metastatic tumors. Until such cell biological and molecular biological definitions catalyze a switch from the 19th century clinical morphologic descriptions to more modern concepts, will we be unable to define subsets of patients by a correlation between mucin production and tumor course.

The most important question is why mucin production should be associated with poor outcome. The answer is certainly not as simple or straightforward as is suggested by the M.D. Anderson Cancer Center article (Abstract 10–21), which states that it is simply harder for the surgeon to fully resect large bowel tumors if there is mucin production. Undoubtedly, the mucin either creates a functional advantage for the tumor cells or it is a fellow traveler with other characteristics that give the highly mucin-producing transformed gastrointestinal epithelium an advantage in invasion, spread, or site-specific seeding.—G.D. Steele, Jr., M.D.

A Prospective Evaluation of the Effect of Tumor Cell DNA Content on Recurrence in Colorectal Cancer

Armitage NCM, Ballantyne KC, Sheffield JP, Clarke P, Evans DF, Hardcastle JD (Univ Hosp, Nottingham, England; St Mark's Hosp, London)

Cancer 67:2599–2604, 1991 10–22

Background.—Although it is accepted that patients with either localized colorectal cancer or distant disease will have either a good or poor prognosis, the ability to estimate tumor aggressiveness using cellular factors such as DNA ploidy may help clarify the likelihood of survival in patients in an intermediate group. The influence of tumor-cell DNA content on recurrence and survival after resection of colorectal cancer was investigated.

Methods.—Tumor-cell DNA content was measured in both fresh and paraffin-embedded tissues obtained from 320 patients who were followed for 2 years or longer after surgery.

Findings.—Recurrences developed in 32% of the 236 patients who underwent potentially curative surgery. They were significantly more frequent in patients with aneuploid tumors than in those with diploid tumors (37% vs. 24%). Ploidy was a prominent factor in patients with stage B tumors, those with mobile tumors, and those older than 65 years of age. Local recurrences were twice as frequent in patients with aneuploid tumors, and distant disease occurred threefold more often.

Implications.—Estimates of DNA ploidy can identify patients with colorectal cancer who have a relatively high risk of recurrent disease. Therefore, this study may prove helpful in planning adjuvant treatment, as well as in analyzing the results of clinical trials.

▶ Exactly who is at risk for recurrence after primary therapy for bowel cancer remains an important question. An offshoot of this question has clinical significance: What proportion of patients with stage II colon cancer has high enough risk to justify adjuvant treatment? Those patients with stage II disease (i.e., penetration of the entire bowel wall and no positive regional lymph nodes) with obstructing or perforating carcinomas are currently considered to have high enough risk to justify adjuvant systemic therapy after cancer surgery. An additional group has been hinted at, but it continues to allude unequivocal confirmation. This group includes patients whose primary tumors are aneuploid, although they are pathologically staged as Dukes B lesions (stage II by tumor/node/metastasis staging criteria). Analysis of the most recent colon cancer study of the North Central Cancer Treatment Group has indicated a possible benefit of DNA ploidy studies: definition of the biological subsets of patients with stage II colon lesions who are at high enough risk for recurrence to justify postoperative adjuvant treatment as standard therapy. This institutional study by the group at University Hospital in Nottingham provides additional data implying that ploidy will soon become an important stratifier—if not a conventionally accepted prognostic criterion independent of tumor/node/metastasis or Dukes staging.—G.D. Steele, Jr., M.D.

Colorectal Carcinoma: Preoperative TNM Classification With Endosonography

Tio TL, Coene PPLO, van Delden OM, Tytgat GNJ (Academic Med Ctr, Amsterdam)

Radiology 179:165–170, 1991 10–23

Background.—In patients with colorectal carcinoma, the prognosis and risk of local recurrence after surgery are often related to the depth of carcinomatous infiltration and the presence of lymph node involvement. However, it is difficult to apply Dukes classification for staging colorectal carcinomas clinically before surgery. Transcolorectal endosonography (TES) might enable preoperative staging of colorectal carcinoma according to the 1987 tumor/nodes/metastasis (TNM) classification system.

Methods.—Transcolorectal endosonography was performed in 61 patients with rectal carcinoma and in 30 patients with colonic carcinoma proved at endoscopic biopsy. Both flexible and inflexible nonoptic instruments and an echocolonoscope were used. The results of the examinations were correlated with the findings at histologic examination of resected specimens. Findings from both procedures were used to stage carcinomas according to the 1987 TNM classification.

Results.—In most cases, TES correlated well with histologic analysis. The overall accuracy of TNM staging of rectal carcinomas was 81%; the accuracy of staging colonic carcinomas was 93% with TES. Of the cases, 13% were overstaged and 2% were understaged. The TES procedure could not accurately stage T2 tumors, possibly because these tumors were often accompanied by peritumoral inflammation or abscess. The accuracy of staging regional lymph nodes with TES was 70%; sensitivity was 94% and specificity was 55%. The correlation between TES findings and Dukes classification for rectal carcinomas was 48% for class A, 50% for class B, and 96% for class C. For colonic carcinomas, the correlation was 67% for class A, 46% for class B, and 91% for class C, for an overall accuracy of 67%.

Conclusions.—Transcolorectal endosonography can become an important imaging technique for clinical TNM staging of colorectal carcinomas. Abdominal CT or ultrasound should be added to the evaluation of distant metastases to reduce the risk of false positive diagnoses of lymph node metastases.

▶ As in other parts of the gastrointestinal tract, current staging criteria for colorectal carcinoma can be definitively determined only by pathologic examination of the surgically resected specimen. Obviously, this limits any rational initiation of preoperative or so-called neoadjuvant therapy approaches. It also limits the "tailoring" of any operative approach, because there is an inability to define accurately before surgery the T stage, node positivity or negativity, and presence or absence of metastases. The resolution capacity for defining pre- and intraoperative node and metastasis stage remains suboptimal (without major improvement on the horizon, except perhaps for intraoperative radioscintigraphy using a variety of labeled anticarcinoembryonic antigen antibodies); however, there is hope for accurate preoperative T staging through the careful stepwise application of endoscopic ultrasonography. Initial approaches at either end of the gastrointestinal tract, with ultrasonic esophagography and with intrarectal ultrasonography, will soon be expanded by the availability of ultrasonic equipment on the ends of colonoscopes and gastroscopes. As exemplified by this relatively small study, routine application with histopathologic correlation shows the beginnings of what will hopefully be a valuable addition to T staging that will lead to a much more rational design of therapy, one that can be precisely tailored to the particular stage of the patient being treated.—G.D. Steele, Jr., M.D.

Carcinoembryonic Antigen Expression of Resurgent Human Colon Carcinoma After Treatment with Therapeutic Doses of ^{90}Y-α-Carcinoembryonic Antigen Monoclonal Antibody

Esteban JM, Kuhn JA, Felder B, Wong JYC, Battifora H, Beatty JD, Wanek PM, Shively JE (City of Hope Natl Med Ctr, Duarte, Calif; Hybritech, Inc, San Diego)
Cancer Res 51:3802–3806, 1991 10–24

Background.—Human colon carcinoma xenografts from athymic mice that have undergone radioimmunotherapy with ^{90}Y-labeled anticarcinoembryonic antigen (CEA) monoclonal antibody (MAb) ZCE025 do not express significant amounts of CEA in comparison with untreated tumors. Whether the resulting tumor immunophenotype results from CEA-specific therapy and whether it is permanent were investigated.

Methods.—Human colon carcinomas (cell line LS174T) were implanted into athymic mice. The animals received 120 μCi of either ^{90}Y-labeled ZCE025 or ^{90}Y-labeled 96.5, a nonspecific MAb. Another group of mice received no treatment. The treated tumors grew to a diameter of approximately 1.5 cm 6 weeks after therapy. At that time, they were resected and aliquoted for transplantation into other mice, plating in tissue culture, fixation in formalin, and homogenization for CEA quantitation. The procedure was done a total of 3 times, 4 months after treatment. At 2 weeks, 6 weeks, and the time of transplantation, the CEA content was evaluated. To evaluate other possible therapy-induced changes in immunophenotype, the resurgent tumors were studied by immunohistochemistry, using MAbs detecting various epitopes of CEA, keratin, TAG-72, and epithelial membrane antigen.

Results.—The resurgent tumors treated with ^{90}Y-ZCE025 had a fourfold decrease in CEA at 6 weeks, which was 2 times greater than the decrease in tumors treated with nonspecific MAb. This result suggested that CEA-expressing cells were being killed specifically and in substantial numbers. On each new pass of the tumor in mice, the CEA content increased somewhat; at the end of the study, the values were almost half those found in controls. Immunohistochemical studies showed that only TAG-72 expression increased immediately after therapy, and that it returned to baseline levels by the end of the study.

Conclusions.—Cells that express higher levels of CEA can be selectively killed by radioimmunotherapy with ^{90}Y-ZCE-25; however, in the surviving part of the tumor, the immunophenotype appears to revert slowly to its original form. A similar effect may be noted in other tumor markers that are unrelated to CEA. These findings should be considered in the design of clinical trials using anti-CEA MAbs.

▶ One of the major limitations in defining mechanisms for tumor escape or tumor resistance to chemo- or immunotherapy is the lack of ability to define with resolution or specificity the genotypic or phenotypic markers of the multiple subsets of cell populations that comprise heterogeneous solid tumor primaries. Thus, in patients with adenocarcinomas of the bowel, primary tumors that have been removed and subsequently followed by either regional or distant failure are usually found to be of the same morphologic type. Therefore, we are left with the dogma that these tumors do not change when they fail, either under natural host evolutionary pressure or under "environmental" influences such as chemotherapy or radiation chemotherapy after surgery. However, as we become more adept at following precise markers such as the various CEA epitopes seen in the athymic nude mouse model of Esteban et al., we will probably begin to see either a selection for or a natural drift in cellular subsets as the tumors progress from primary tumors to metastatic or recurrent secondary tumors. Accentuation of subset selection may be seen as we more precisely target our therapy (as in the case with the radiolabeled anti-CEA MAb approach used in this experimental radioimmunotherapy model). The kinetics of suppression of the CEA epitope-containing subsets will be quite important, both in the design of "remission induction" as well as in maintenance therapy. They will have to be described carefully in elegant experimental models (such as this interesting study) before clinical utility can be expected.—G.D. Steele, Jr., M.D.

A Prospective Randomized Comparison of Protracted Infusional 5-Fluorouracil With or Without Weekly Bolus Cisplatin in Metastatic Colorectal Carcinoma: A Mid-Atlantic Oncology Program Study

Lokich JJ, Ahlgren JD, Cantrell J, Heim WJ, Wampler GL, Gullo JJ, Fryer JG, Alt DE (Cancer Ctr, Boston; George Washington Univ, Washington, DC: Birmingham Hematology-Oncology, Birmingham, Ala; Hematology and Oncology Associates of Northeastern PA, Scranton, Pa; Med College of Virginia, Richmond, et al)

Cancer 67:14–19, 1991 10–25

Introduction.—A bolus infusion of 5-fluorouracil (5-FU) has been used in the treatment of patients with advanced metastatic colorectal cancer. A previous trial found that therapy with protracted 5-FU infusion (PIF) increased the response rate when compared with therapy via bolus infusion, but it did not increase survival time.

Methods.—To determine whether the addition of weekly cisplatin infusion would improve the efficacy of PIF, 184 patients (median age, 63 years) with metastatic colorectal carcinoma (who had not previously been treated with chemotherapy) received a continuous 24-hour infusion of 5-FU through a battery-operated pump for 10 of every 12 weeks. An additional weekly bolus of cisplatin was administered to 92 randomly selected patients. The patients were evaluated for response at weeks 6 and 12, and at 12-week intervals thereafter. Complete survival and toxicity data were available for 179 patients, and tumor response data were available for 168 patients.

Results.—Of the 83 patients treated with PIF alone, 29 (35%) responded to therapy, 2 of whom had a complete response. Of the 85 patients treated with PIF plus weekly cisplatin, 28 (33%) responded to therapy, 2 of whom had a complete response. The median survival time was 11.8 months for the cisplatin-added group and 11.2 months for the

PIF-only group. Approximately 75% of the patients had died by the time of this analysis. Based on these figures, the projected 2-year survival was 14% for PIF alone and 17% for PIF plus cisplatin. None of the differences was statistically significant.

Conclusion.—The addition of weekly cisplatin to PIF in the treatment of metastatic colorectal cancer does not increase the effectiveness of PIF.

▶ Unless interesting new biological modulation approaches make the transition from laboratory models to human studies, most of the conventional treatment approaches that have shown effectiveness in advanced colorectal cancer and are available for possible inclusion in earlier disease or adjuvant settings will soon be exhausted. Attempts to increase the efficacy of known treatment by adding new single agents to standard chemotherapy combinations are exemplified in this study by the old Mid-Atlantic Oncology program. In patients with metastatic colon and rectum adenocarcinoma who had not been exposed to any previous chemotherapy, the addition of cisplatin to a protracted FIP protocol did not significantly increase the response rate. Thus, the justification for any pursuit of this combination in an earlier disease setting is not rational.

Questions about the implied benefit of FIP compared with intermittent or bolus administration in the adjuvant setting, particularly with regard to combination chemoradiotherapy for patients whose surgery leaves them at high risk for recurrence of rectal cancer, should soon be answered by several national studies. Continued questions concerning leucovorin, either added to levamisole or in place of levamisole, α-interferon-2a, and PALA modulators of 5-FU, may soon be answered as well. Combinations containing cisplatin will not be included in future treatments.—G.D. Steele, Jr., M.D.

Intraoperative Electron Beam Radiation Therapy for Recurrent Locally Advanced Rectal or Rectosigmoid Carcinoma

Willett CG, Shellito PC, Tepper JE, Eliseo R, Convery K, Wood WC (Harvard Med School, Boston; Univ of North Carolina, Chapel Hill)

Cancer 67:1504–1508, 1991 10–26

Introduction.—Surgery and radiation therapy are, by themselves, inadequate to provide palliation for patients with recurrent rectal or rectosigmoid carcinoma. Data were reviewed on 30 patients who were treated with a multimodality approach of moderate- to high-dose preoperative irradiation, surgical resection, and intraoperative electron beam radiation therapy (IORT) during an 11-year period.

Methods.—A total preoperative radiation dose of 50.4 Gy in 28 fractions was administered during a 5–6 week period. Those patients treated most recently also were administered 5-fluorouracil, 500 mg/m^2/day intravenously, for 3 days in the first and last weeks of radiation treatment. Surgical exploration was performed 4–6 weeks after external beam radiation was completed. The IORT was given at doses of 10–16 Gy for microscopic and 15–20 Gy for macroscopic residual tumor, after which the operation was completed. The mean follow-up was 30 months.

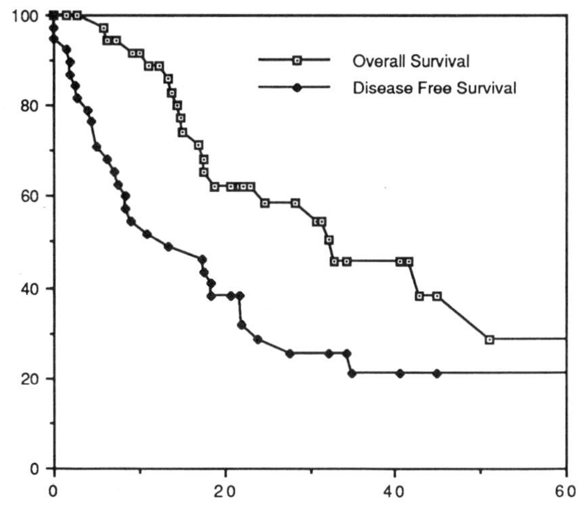

Fig 10–2.—The 5-year actuarial overall survival and disease-free survival for patients with recurrent rectal or rectosigmoid carcinoma. (Courtesy of Willett CG, Shellito PC, Tepper JE, et al: *Cancer* 67:1504–1508, 1991.)

Results.—The 5-year actuarial survival rate was 29%, and the disease-free survival rate was 21% (Fig 10–2). The 5-year actuarial local control rate was 26%, and the disease-free survival rate was 19%. Complete resection, with negative pathologic margins, was the most important factor in a favorable outcome. For 13 patients who had complete resection, determinate local control was 62% and disease-free survival was 54%, compared with 18% and 6%, respectively, for patients who had partial resection (table). The original surgical resection did not appear to affect local control or survival, but patients who had a previous low anterior resection had a greater chance of obtaining a complete resection than those who had a previous abdominoperineal resection. Soft-tissue or sacral injury and pelvic neuropathy were the most significant toxicities.

Determinate Local Control and Disease-Free Survival

	No. of patients	Local control	Disease-free survival
All patients	39	36% (14/39)	23% (9/39)
Unresectable at laparotomy	2	0% (0/2)	0% (0/2)
Liver metastases at laparotomy	1	100% (1/1)	0% (0/1)
Resection with IORT	30	37% (11/30)	27% (8/30)
Complete resection	13	62% (8/13)	54% (7/13)
Partial resection	17	18% (3/17)	6% (1/17)
Resection without IORT	6	33% (2/6)	33% (2/6)

(Courtesy of Willett CG, Shellito PC, Tepper JE, et al: *Cancer* 67:1504–1508, 1991.)

Conclusion.—The local failure rate is high in patients with rectal or rectosigmoid carcioma, despite this aggressive treatment. Additional postoperative radiation therapy and chemotherapy are being used concurrently to modify the radiation dose during IORT.

▶ This is a very provocative and interesting study of a subset of patients that has traditionally done particularly poorly. It seems clear from the paper that, if the surgeon can remove the recurrent mass with negative margins, then there is a finite chance of achieving a cure. The exact contribution of IORT remains unclear. These patients represent a continuing challenge to the physician, and this study would suggest that IORT deserves an objective assessment, probably manifested as a controlled clinical trial with a randomized control population.—E. Glatstein, M.D.

High Dose Preoperative Irradiation for Cancer of the Rectum, 1976–1988
Mohiuddin M, Marks G (Thomas Jefferson Univ, Philadelphia)
Int J Radiat Oncol Biol Phys 20:37–43, 1991 10–27

Introduction.—Rectal cancer has been treated primarily by surgery alone. Integrated programs using high, effective doses of radiation to minimize postoperative recurrence have been developed in the past 10–15 years. Data on 220 patients treated with adjunctive high-dose preoperative radiation and sphincter preservation during a 12-year period were reviewed.

Methods.—All patients were followed for 1–12 years (median, 32 months). The cancers were classified according to their mobility (stage I, mobile to stage IV, unresectable). There were 74 mobile, 49 partially fixed, 85 totally fixed, and 12 unresectable tumors. The patients received

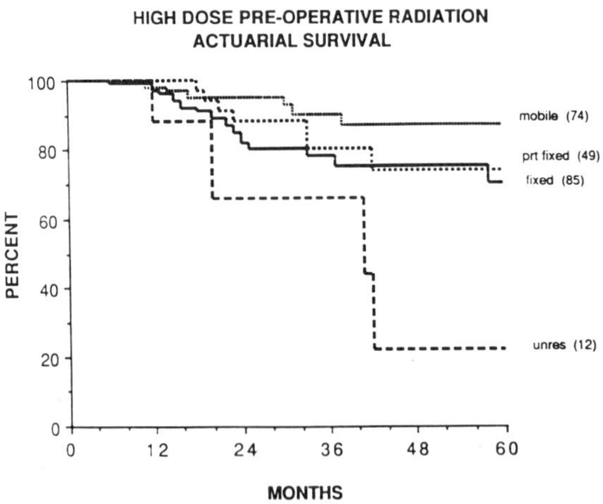

Fig 10–3.—Actuarial (Kaplan-Meier) survival by clinical stage of disease. (Courtesy of Mohiuddin M, Marks G: *Int J Radiat Oncol Biol Phys* 20:37–43, 1991.)

Patterns of Failure by Clinical Stage

Clinical stages	No. of pts.	Local only	Local and distant	Distant
I (mobile)	74	3 (4%)	5 (7%)	8 (11%)
II (partially fixed)	49	2 (4%)	3 (6%)	7 (14%)
III (fixed)	85	6 (7%)	8 (9%)	12 (13%)
IV (unresectable)	12	2 (17%)	3 (25%)	3 (25%)
Total	220	13 (6%)	19 (9%)	30 (14%)

(Courtesy of Mohiuddin M, Marks G: *Int J Radiat Oncol Biol Phys* 20:37–43, 1991.)

high-energy photons using a 4-field box technique. The total radiation dose ranged from 4,000 to 6,000 cGy, and surgery was performed a mean of 5.2 weeks after radiation, longer for patients with higher radiation doses.

Results.—Most patients had significant tumor shrinkage. There was local recurrence in 15% of the patients. The highest incidence was 20% in patients with fixed and unresectable tumors, and the lowest was 10% in those with mobile and partially fixed tumors. The overall failure rate was 14% (table). There was local recurrence in 6% of the patients with 0, A, and B1 stages of disease, compared with 20% of those with stage B2 and C disease. The 5-year survival rate was 67% for the overall group, 87% for patients with mobile tumors, 74% for those with partially fixed tumors, 70% for those with fixed tumors, and 22% for those with unresectable tumors (Fig 10–3). At 5 years, 90% of the patients with stage 0, A, and B1 disease were alive, compared with 71% of those with stage B2, 75% of those with stage C1, and 47% of those with stage C2 disease.

Conclusion.—Rectal carcinoma is best treated by careful patient selection based on prognostic factors and an integrated approach to radiation and surgical resection. Judicious high-dose preoperative radiation can allow sphincter preservation and improve survival, as well as reduce the rate of local recurrence. Further improvements can be expected as new techniques of combined chemotherapy and radiation and intraoperative radiation are incorporated.

▶ This is an important study dealing with a common, but unfortunate problem that generally does not have a good prognosis. The large majority of patients in this series had partial or total tumor fixation, and they would not be included in many analyses. Nonetheless, preoperative irradiation for this particular group of patients resulted in a 5-year survival figure of 67%. Of the small subset of patients who had a frozen pelvis, 22% survived 5 years. These results are excellent, and one wonders why this form of treatment has not been more popular. In many ways, one suspects that the major obstacle is the reluctance of the surgeon to delay the surgical procedure, despite data like these.—E. Glatstein, M.D.

Effective Surgical Adjuvant Therapy for High-Risk Rectal Carcinoma

Krook JE, Moertel CG, Gunderson LL, Wieand HS, Collins RT, Baert RW, Kubista TP, Poon MA, Meyers WC, Mailliard JA, Twito DI, Morton RF, Veeder MH, Witzig T, Cha S, Vidyarthi S (Duluth Community Clinical Oncology Program, Duluth, Minn; Mayo Clinic and Found, Rochester, Minn; Mayo Clinic, Scottsdale, Ariz; Saskatchewan Cancer Found, Regina, Sask, Canada; Duke Univ, Durham, NC; et al)

N Engl J Med 324:709–715, 1991 10–28

Introduction.—As an adjunct to surgery, radiation therapy reduces local recurrence, but it does not improve survival in patients with rectal cancer. One study has suggested that combined radiation and chemotherapy improve survival compared with surgery alone—but not compared with adjuvant radiation, which is often regarded as standard therapy. A combination regimen was designed to optimize the effects of chemotherapy, decrease recurrence, and improve survival compared with adjuvant radiation alone.

Methods.—The study included 204 patients with rectal carcinoma that was either deeply invasive or metastatic to regional lymph nodes. All patients had undergone a potentially curative resection. The patients were randomly assigned to receive postoperative radiation alone or sequential postoperative chemotherapy and radiation therapy. Postoperative radiation consisted of 4,500–5,040 cGy delivered during a 5-week period. The combined-therapy group received radiation plus fluorouracil, which was both preceded and followed by a cycle of systemic therapy with fluorouracil plus semustine (methyl-CCNU). The median follow-up period was more than 7 years.

Results.—The combined therapy reduced rectal cancer recurrence by 34%, initial local recurrence by 46%, and distant metastasis by 37%. The combined-therapy group had a 36% reduction in the rate of cancer-related deaths and a 29% reduction in the overall death rate. Nausea, vomiting, diarrhea, leukopenia, and thrombocytopenia were acute toxic effects of the combined regimen, but they were seldom severe. Of all patients receiving radiation, 6.7% had severe, delayed treatment-related reactions, usually small bowel obstruction requiring surgery. The 2 treatment groups had comparable frequencies of these complications.

Conclusion.—In patients with rectal carcinoma with a poor prognosis, combined postoperative local therapy with radiation plus fluorouracil and systemic therapy with a fluorouracil-based regimen improves results compared with postoperative radiation alone. Improvements are seen in both recurrence and survival rates. The addition of fluorouracil appears to be crucial in reducing rate of local recurrence.

▶ This article by Krook et al. summarizes the North Central Cancer Treatment Group's study of adjuvant therapy in patients who are at high risk after rectal cancer resection. It substantiated the core of earlier studies of rectal adjuvant treatment by the Gastrointestinal Tumor Study Group, and it provided a foundation for the recent National Institutes of Health Consensus Conference, which proposed routine postoperative treatment of patients with stage II and III rectal cancers, using a combination of 5-FU and external beam irradiation. The potential for saving lives was outlined in an accompanying editorial (1), and current questions on the topic concern the application of existing data to different ways of administering 5-FU (infusion vs. intermittent bolus), the decrease in the time patients have to be treated (without sacrifice of benefit), and the possible preoperative application to patients who might be at highest risk for recurrence. Several of these questions are being addressed by 1 or another of the national, multimodality, rectal cancer adjuvant treatment follow-up studies. The area is remarkably fast moving, and clinical benefit is beginning to be translated to the approximately 45,000 patients with rectal cancer.

That multimodality treatment may allow a decrease in the number of patients who need permanent colostomy—that is, those patients with the most distal adenocarcinomas of the rectum—is almost as exciting. Even if there was no increase in survival in this group of patients, the diminution in the psychological as well as functional aspects attendant to sphincter removal would be of huge benefit not only to the 4,000–5,000 patients who are at risk for abdominoperineal resection each year, but also to many other patients with more proximal lesions who ignore changes in their bowel habits because they fear that when they finally do go to their doctors, they will need a colostomy.—G.D. Steele, Jr., M.D.

Reference

1. Steele G Jr: *N Engl J Med* 324:764, 1992.

Anus

Chemotherapy and Radiation Therapy for Anal Carcinoma: Survival and Late Morbidity

Tanum G, Tveit K, Karlsen KO, Hauer-Jensen M (Norwegian Radium Hosp, Oslo)

Cancer 67:2462–2466, 1991 10–29

Background.—The usual treatment for anal squamous cell carcinoma is either combined chemotherapy and radiation therapy or radiation therapy alone, with abdominoperineal resection (APR) being reserved for resistant neoplasms. There have been no randomized, comparative studies of various chemotherapy/radiation therapy regimens. Long-term survival and late morbidity were evaluated for a standardized, widely used regimen of combination therapy.

Methods.—A total of 106 patients was treated during a 6-year period. Of these, 79% were women (mean age, 64.3 years) and 21% were men (mean age, 67.8). There were 94 primary tumors and 23 local recurrences after primary surgery. Radiation therapy consisted of 5,000 cGy given by 2 anteroposterior-posteroanterior opposed fields, and chemotherapy included mitomycin C and 5-fluorouracil. A split course of 2–3 weeks was used in 48 patients.

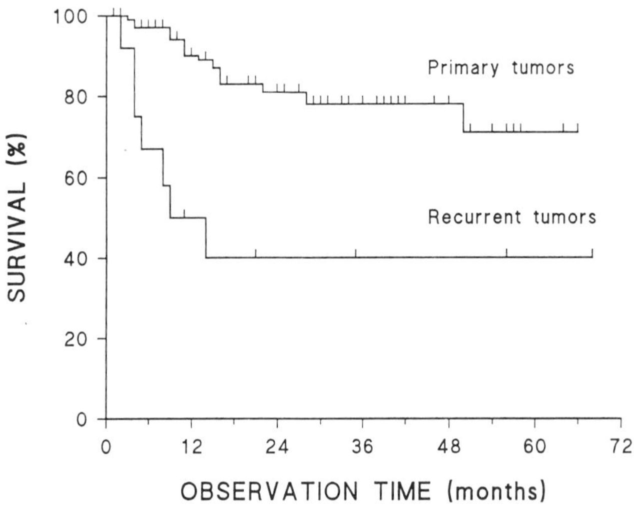

Fig 10–4.—The survival time of patients receiving combined chemotherapy and radiation therapy for anal carcinoma. "Recurrent tumors" are local recurrences after APR. (Courtesy of Tanum G, Tveit K, Karlsen KO, et al: *Cancer* 67:2462–2466, 1991.)

Results.—Of the patients with primary tumors, 84% had a complete response, the remainder later undergoing APR. Eleven patients (48%) with local recurrence had a complete response. The 5-year survival rates were 72% for those with primary tumors and 40% for those with recurrence (Fig 10–4). In the primary tumor group, tumor stage and survival were not significantly correlated (Fig 10–5). Metastases occurred after

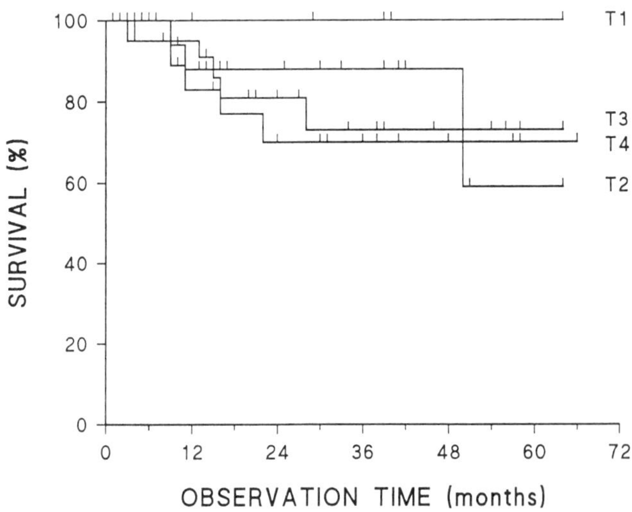

Fig 10–5.—The survival time of patients receiving combined chemotherapy and radiation therapy for anal carcinoma relative to tumor stage. (Courtesy of Tanum G, Tveit K, Karlsen KO, et al: *Cancer* 67:2462–2466, 1991.)

treatment in 18 patients, most commonly in the liver. Late treatment-related symptoms, including anal incontinence, intestinal obstruction, and chronic pelvic pain, occurred in 15% of the patients.

Conclusions.—The described combination chemotherapy and radiation therapy regimen for anal carcinoma, although effective, is associated with a high risk of complications. Patients with small tumors should probably have less extensive locoregional treatment than those with advanced tumors. They would probably have fewer late side effects and no decrease in survival.

▶ This large series of patients with anal carcinoma demonstrated an excellent outcome with combined-modality treatment. The morbidity figures are somewhat higher than those in other reports, but not strikingly so. To some degree, they may be explained by the inclusion of recurrent patients in this series. Nonetheless, the overall outcome for these patients appears to be remarkably good, and one wonders why more gastrointestinal problems have not been approached with combined-modality efforts.—E. Glatstein, M.D.

11 Sarcomas

Soft Tissue

Twenty Years Experience of Interstitial Iridium Brachytherapy in the Management of Soft Tissue Sarcomas

Habrand JL, Gerbaulet A, Pejovic MH, Contesso G, Durand S, Haie C, Genin J, Schwaab G, Flamant F, Albano M, Sarrazin D, Spielmann M, Chassagne D (Institut Gustave Roussy, Villejuif, France)

Int J Radiat Oncol Biol Phys 20:405–411, 1991 11–1

Background.—Adult patients with soft tissue sarcoma (STS) are commonly treated with limited surgery and radiation therapy. Few reported series have used brachytherapy (CT) alone or with external radiotherapy. A series of 48 patients treated with wide excision and BT was studied.

Patients.—The patients, all older than 10 years of age, were treated during a 20-year period. Of 41 sarcomas for which a pathologic grade was established, 20 were grade 3; 15, grade 2; and only 6, grade 1. The lesions were mainly of small or medium size, 36 being smaller than 5 cm and 12 being larger than 5 cm. The tumor was in the limbs in 32 patients, in the trunk in 9, and in the head and neck in 7. Four patients had metastases at the time of treatment. Twenty-two patients had BT as a part of their initial therapy. Twenty-six had BT as part of a salvage procedure after previous excision, either alone or in combination with other

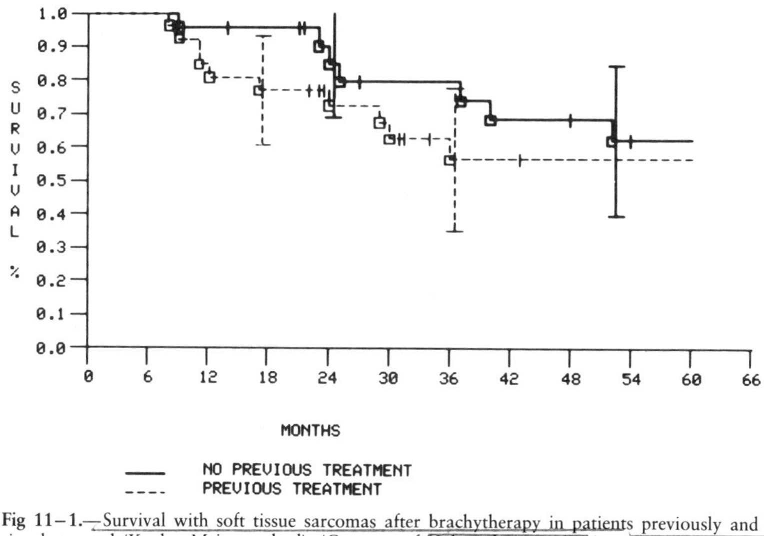

Fig 11–1.—Survival with soft tissue sarcomas after brachytherapy in patients previously and not previously treated (Kaplan-Meier method). (Courtesy of Habrand JL, Gerbaulet A, Pejovic MH, et al: *Int J Radiat Oncol Biol Phys* 20:405–411, 1991.)

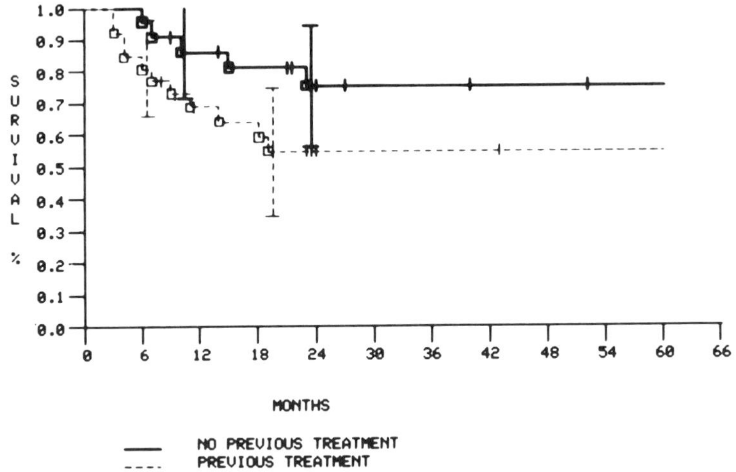

Fig 11–2.—Survival without local relapse of soft tissue sarcomas after brachytherapy in patients previously and not previously treated (Kaplan-Meier method). (Courtesy of Habrand JL, Gerbaulet A, Pejovic MH, et al: *Int J Radiat Oncol Biol Phys* 20:405–411, 1991.)

treatment. The standard technique of BT was done with iridium 192 wires afterloaded in plastic tubing. The median dose was 60 Gy, both in the patients who received BT alone and in the 4 patients who also had external radiation. Adjuvant chemotherapy was used in 16 patients.

Outcome.—The median follow-up was 82 months, and 58.4% of the patients were alive at 5 years. Survival rates were 62% in patients who had no previous treatment and 56.5% in those who had previous treatment; the difference was not significant (Figs 11–1 to 11–3). Only 4%

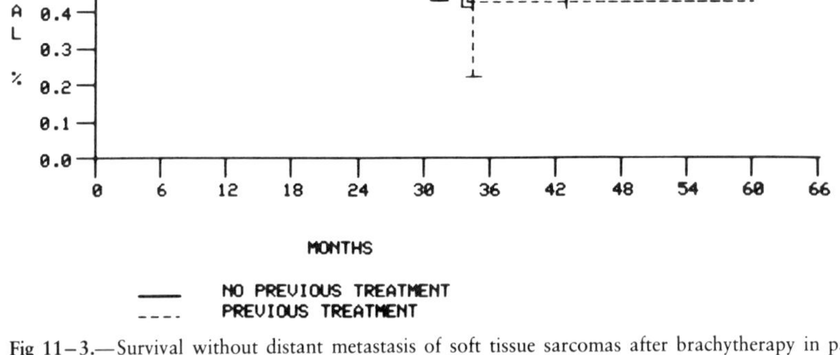

Fig 11–3.—Survival without distant metastasis of soft tissue sarcomas after brachytherapy in patients previously and not previously treated (Kaplan-Meier method). (Courtesy of Habrand JL, Gerbaulet A, Pejovic MH, et al: *Int J Radiat Oncol Biol Phys* 20:405–411, 1991.)

of the patients had failure in the irradiated volume, but there was a surprisingly high rate of marginal failures (14 of 31). A second, similar procedure achieved salvage in 43% of the failures. Tumor location in the chest was the only factor predictive of local failure, and it was strongly associated with metastatic outcome. A total of 35% of the patients had necrosis, the course of which was usually benign.

Conclusions.—Combined treatment with high-dose BT and conservative surgery appears to be effective in patients with small and medium-sized STS of the extremities and the head and neck. The procedure is fast and the rate of complications is reasonable. For patients with STS of the trunk and recurrent STS, large-field external radiation and possibly polychemotherapy appear necessary.

▶ This is a good-sized series (with excellent follow-up) from a major radiotherapy center in Europe. The management that they have used for STS includes wide excision and intraoperative interstitial BT using iridium. The results that they reported are excellent. A similar paper was published several years ago by the Memorial Surgical Radiotherapy team, which was headed by Dr. Shiu (1).

In addition, a small series with similar outcome was reported by the University of Kansas (2). These series of BT papers, along with the preoperative data of MGH and the postoperative data from the M.D. Anderson Cancer Center, University of California (San Francisco), and the National Cancer Institute all show excellent local control, especially in the extremities. That the local control is as excellent as it appears to be suggests that this neoplasm is not "radioresistant," as has been traditionally taught. Obviously, the cells are being destroyed, because the local recurrence rate with wide excision alone is expected to be anywhere from 35% to 70%, depending on which series one wishes to quote. The point is that a combination of surgery and radiation therapy can achieve excellent local control (regardless of how the 2 have been put together), as long as high doses of radiation are used. It is interesting to note that the only area in which there is a suggestion of the efficacy of adjuvant chemotherapy is in the extremity, where local control is so excellently achieved; in the head and neck, in the torso, and in the retroperitoneum, where local control is less likely, the putative benefit of adjuvant chemotherapy has not yet been reported. The precise benefit of adjuvant chemotherapy is still awaiting a definitive study of sufficient size.—E. Glatstein, M.D.

References

1. Shiu MH, et al: *Cancer* 53:1385, 1984.
2. Gemer LS, et al: *Int J Radiat Oncol Biol Phys* 20:587, 1991.

A Prospective Randomized Trial of Adjuvant Chemotherapy With Bolus *Versus* Continuous Infusion of Doxorubicin in Patients With High-Grade Extremity Soft Tissue Sarcoma and an Analysis of Prognostic Factors

Casper ES, Gaynor JJ, Hajdu SI, Magill GB, Tan C, Friedrich C, Brennan MF
(Meml Sloan-Kettering Cancer Ctr, New York; Cornell Univ, New York)
Cancer 68:1221–1229, 1991 11–2

Background.—Extremity-sparing surgery for soft tissue sarcoma (STS) of the extremity has generally replaced amputation as the standard surgical treatment for most patients with localized disease. Radiation therapy and chemotherapy have been used as adjuvants to wide surgical excision to reduce the frequency of local recurrence and distant metastases. Doxorubicin-containing regimens have been found effective, but they are associated with cardiac toxicity. The cardiotoxic and therapeutic effects of doxorubicin given by bolus or 72-hour continuous infusion were studied in eligible patients after resection of high-grade STS of the extremity or superficial trunk.

Methods.—Eighty-two patients were enrolled in the prospective randomized trial. Doxorubicin was given in a dose of 60 mg/m^2 every 3–4 weeks. Cardiac toxicity was defined as a decrease of 10% or more in left ventricular (LV) ejection fraction, as assessed by radionuclide cineangiography. It was evaluated in 69 patients.

Results. Cardiac toxicity occurred in 61% of those treated by the bolus method, with a median total dose of 420 mg of doxorubicin per m^2. Of those who received doxorubicin by continuous infusion, 42% had cardiac toxicity, with a median dose of 540 mg of doxorubicin per m^2. The cardiac toxicity rate as a function of the cumulative dose of doxorubicin was significantly greater in the bolus treatment arm. Two patients in each group had clinical congestive heart failure. One patient in each group died of cardiac causes. Those patients in the bolus group had a trend toward a lower rate of metastasis and a significantly lower rate of death from disease. According to Cox model analysis, there were 3 unfavorable characteristics for the rate of developing a distant metastasis: blood transfusion within 24 hours of surgery, tumor deep to the fascia and 5 cm or more in size, and a histologic subtype other than liposarcoma.

Conclusions. Adjuvant chemotherapy for patients with STS who undergo extremity-sparing surgery is still being investigated. The effect of perioperative blood transfusion in such cases needs further study.

▶ This is an important study from the Memorial Sloan-Kettering Cancer Center, which has had extensive experience in the management of STS. In this study, the authors randomized patients to receive 60 mg of adriamycin per m^2, given either by bolus or infusion during a 72-hour period. Those patients who received the bolus therapy had a higher incidence of cardiac toxicity. However, the patients also had a significantly better survival than did the controls who received prolonged infusion. This interesting finding is somewhat negated by the fact that there was a significant imbalance in the distribution of liposarcomas between the 2 arms, because liposarcomas comprised 47% of the patients on the bolus therapy arm and only 16% of the patients on the prolonged infusion arm. Because the patients with liposarcoma had a better overall outcome than patients with other subtypes of STS, the outcome in the bolus therapy arm may be caused by the distribution to the subtypes of STS rather than the method of administration of the drug. This is an important point, because it illustrates the importance of stratification in the performance of randomized trials. The authors have also observed that perioperative transfusion had a significantly bad effect on outcome. Interestingly, although the size and depth of penetration of the tumor were poor prognostic factors, a negative surgical margin was not a significant factor in multivariant analysis. This is hard to believe, because most other studies have shown such an effect. This may result from the use of radiotherapy to control local disease.—J.M. Jessup, M.D.

Intraoperative Electron Beam Radiation Therapy for Retroperitoneal Soft Tissue Sarcoma

Willett CG, Suit HD, Tepper JE, Mankin HJ, Convery K, Rosenberg AL, Wood WC (Harvard Med School, Boston; Univ of North Carolina, Chapel Hill)
Cancer 68:278–283, 1991 11–3

Background.—Although significant advances in the management of soft tissue sarcomas of the extremities have occurred, management of ret-

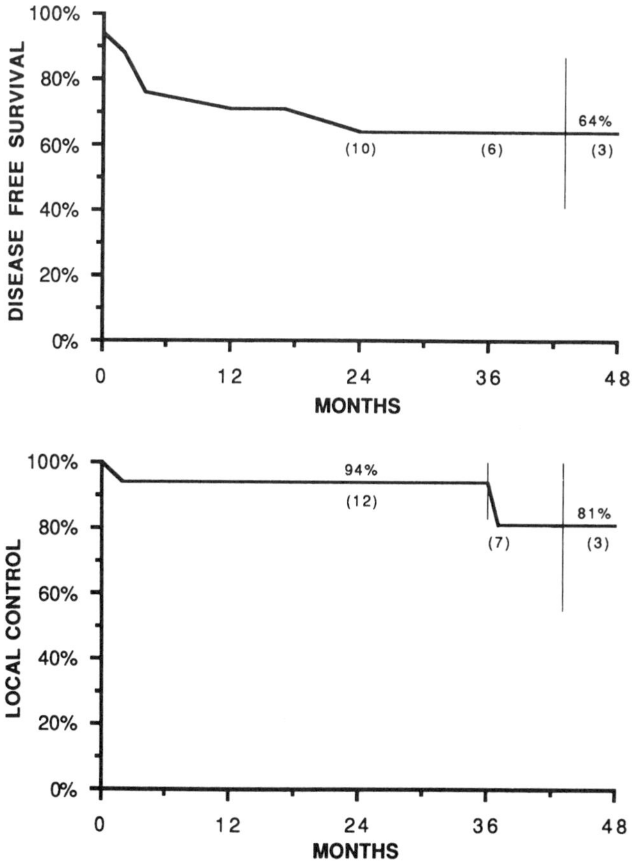

Fig 11–4.—Actuarial disease-free survival and local control of 17 patients undergoing resection with and without IORT. (Courtesy of Willett CG, Suit HD, Tepper JE, et al: *Cancer 68:278–283, 1991.)*

roperitoneal sarcomas has been less successful. Intraoperative radiation therapy (IORT) and external beam radiation therapy (EBRT) were combined in an attempt to improve local control and survival in patients with retroperitoneal sarcoma.

Methods.—Twenty patients with retroperitoneal sarcoma were treated during an 8-year period. There were 14 primary and 6 recurrent tumors. The patients were 11 women and 9 men (median age, 41 years). Treatment included EBRT, 4,000–5,000 cGy, followed by surgical resection and IORT 4–6 weeks later. Seventeen patients underwent resection, 14 complete and 3 partial; metastases had occurred by the time of surgery in 3 patients. Doses of IORT ranged from 1,000 to 2,000 cGy. Intraoperative radiation was used for microscopic disease in 10 patients and for gross residual sarcoma in 2.

Results.—For the 17 patients who had resection, the 4-year actuarial local control rate was 81%, and the 4-year disease-free survival rate was 64% (Fig 11–4). Three patients who received IORT for microscopic residual tumor died, 1 of local failure and peritoneal sarcomatosis and 2 of distant metastases only. The other 7 patients were disease free. One patient treated for gross residual sarcoma died of local failure, but the other was alive 7 years after salvage chemotherapy for local failure. The extensive size of the tumor bed precluded IORT for 5 patients. At last follow-up, 3 were disease free, 1 was alive with lung metastases, and 1 had died of hepatic metastases.

Conclusions. Combined treatment with preoperative EBRT, aggressive resection, and IORT appears to yield satisfactory resectability and local control rates. The treatment is acceptably tolerated. The high-dose preoperative regimen may minimize the risk of tumor implantation in the peritoneal cavity; the partial regression of EBRT may allow complete gross resection; and normal tissue radiation may be reduced.

▶ This study reviewed a small series of patients with retroperitoneal sarcomas who were treated with radiation therapy preoperatively, followed by surgery and IORT. The results of this series from Massachusetts General Hospital are excellent; they appear to be superior to those from the National Cancer Institute's study (1). In that study, the benefit of IORT appeared to be a reduction in the likelihood of enteritis; there was no suggestion of improvement in survival.

The issue of local control is complex. If one talks about local control and means only the retroperitoneum, in which the radiation was used, then the local control figures can be made to appear quite good. On the other hand, when one tries to resect these retroperitoneal sarcomas, it is almost impossible to excise the lesion without cutting across the tumor at some point. This predisposes the patient to subsequent sarcomatosis and peritoneal seeding. Thus, local control needs careful definition, because, at least in the National Cancer Institute's experience, a large proportion of these patients did ultimately seed the peritoneal cavity. In any event, this kind of approach to the retropertineal sarcomas may ultimately prove to be valuable. If so, it will likely have to be combined with some means of preventing peritoneal seeding. The lesions tend to be large, and as noted above, it is extremely difficult to obtain negative margins for most of these lesions.—E. Glatstein, M.D.

Reference

1. Kinsella TJ, et al: *J Clin Oncol* 6:18, 1988.

Phase III Comparison of Doxorubicin and Decarbazine Given by Bolus Versus Infusion in Patients With Soft-Tissue Sarcomas: A Southwest Oncology Group Study

Zalupski M, for the Southwest Oncology Group (Wayne State Univ, Detroit)
J Natl Cancer Inst 83:926–932, 1991 11–4

Objective.—The influence of the dosing regimen was examined in patients with disseminated soft tissue sarcoma who received both doxorubicin and dacarbazine. Those patients with Ewing's sarcoma, Kaposi's sarcoma, mesothelioma, and bone sarcoma were excluded.

Treatment.—A group of 118 patients received bolus treatment with 60 mg of doxorubicin per m^2 and 750 mg of dacarbazine per m^2, given intravenously on day 1. Another 122 patients received the same doses by continuous infusion for 4 days. Chemotherapy was planned at 3-week intervals. Residual disease was resected both in patients who responded partially and in those with stable disease after chemotherapy.

Results.—Survival did not differ between the patients given bolus treatment and those given infusion therapy. The median survival was 10–11 months in both treatment groups. Survival times also were similar. Of the 12 patients who responded completely, 7 had lung involvement only. Both hematologic and cardiac side effects were most frequent after bolus treatment, and the same was true for moderate or severe nausea/vomiting.

Conclusion.—Infusion of doxorubicin and decarbazine is as effective as bolus dosing and is better tolerated by patients with soft tissue sarcoma.

▶ This report contrasts with the report from the Memorial Sloan-Kettering Cancer Center group (Abstract 11–2), because it shows that there is no difference in survival between patients given bolus treatment with an Adriamycin regimen and those given prolonged infusion therapy. The setting is different, because this study (Abstract 11–4) treated patients with advanced disease (the Memorial series had a post-surgical adjuvant setting); nevertheless, the use of bolus dosing produced the same response rate and overall survival as did continuous infusion. This is important, because bolus is easier to administer. Further trials are encouraged to confirm the usefulness of bolus vs. continuous infusion.— J.M. Jessup, M.D.

Reoperative Pulmonary Resection in Patients With Metastatic Soft Tissue Sarcoma

Pogrebniak HW, Roth JA, Steinberg SM, Rosenberg SA, Pass HI (Natl Cancer Inst, Bethesda, Md)
Ann Thorac Surg 52:197–203, 1991 11–5

Introduction.—As many as 30% of patients with pulmonary metastases of soft tissue sarcoma have lived for 3 years after the resection of these metastases; however, the role of multiple resections of recurrent lung metastases is uncertain.

Series.—Outcome was reviewed in 43 patients who, since 1976, had had 2 or more thoracic explorations for metastasis of adult soft tissue sarcoma. The most frequent tumor types were synovial sarcoma, malignant fibrous histiocytoma, and leiomyosarcoma.

Outcome.—There were no operative deaths in a total of 89 reoperations. Thirty-one patients (72%) were free of disease after the second thoracotomy. Those patients with resectable disease lived for a median of 25 months after the second operation, and those with unresectable disease lived for 10 months. The outlook was best when the disease-free interval between the first and second operations exceeded 18 months. Younger patients did better than those who were older.

Recommendations.—Patients who had as many as 6 or 7 lesions on CT were reviewed. An attempt to remove all disease is warranted if this can be done without compromising pulmonary reserve.

▶ This series is from a group that had 1 of the largest experiences with the resection of pulmonary metastases from soft tissue sarcoma. The focus of this paper is on those patients who failed the original resection and required a second or third resection for removal of all metastases. It is not clearly stated in this study whether the patients who had multiple thoracotomies did so as part of a planned procedure, or because of recurrence after being rendered disease free. Some patients will have staged thoracotomies because there are too many nodules to resect at one operation. Nonetheless, those patients who were rendered disease free after the second thoracotomy had a better outcome than those patients who were not rendered disease free. In addition, a prolonged interval between the first and second thoracotomy is also associated with a better outcome. This suggests that if patients can be made disease free with 1 operation and the tumor has a long doubling time, then the outcome may be more favorable. This is certainly in concert with the early results of Morton (1). This interesting approach should be vigorously pursued, because these patients are otherwise destined to die.—J.M. Jessup, M.D.

Reference

1. Morton DL, et al: *Ann Surg* 178:360, 1973.

Sarcomas of Soft Tissue and Bone

Mazanet R, Antman KH (Harvard Med School, Boston)

Cancer 68:463–473, 1991 11–6

Introduction.—Considering that 75% of the average body weight represents somatic soft tissue and the skeleton, it is surprising that sarcomas constitute only 1% of adult malignancies and 15% of those found in children. Sarcomas originate in mesenchymal tissues. Approximately 5%

of the diagnoses of new sarcoma are associated with a history of radiotherapy. Certain sarcomas occur more often in the setting of familial retinoblastoma or neurofibromatosis.

Soft Tissue Sarcomas.—These lesions usually are pseudoencapsulated tumors that grow along histologic planes, and they require wide excision for control in the absence of radiotherapy. Malignant fibrous histiocytoma and liposarcoma are the most common types in adults. Optimally, the surgical margins exceed 3 cm. Recently, radiotherapy has been administered before conservative surgery. At present, the risks of adjuvant chemotherapy are not warranted in patients with low-grade lesions. One or several lung metastases can be removed in selected patients with soft tissue sarcoma.

Bone Sarcomas.—Osteosarcoma is the most common form of bone sarcoma. As is the case for soft tissue sarcomas, survival correlates with grade of tumor. Primary lesions must be removed with several centimeters of microscopically clear margin. Preoperative combination chemotherapy is being studied as a possible means of avoiding amputations. Radiotherapy controls many cases of Ewing's sarcoma with good functional results. Chondrosarcomas are relatively resistant to radiotherapy and must be adequately resected at the outset.

▶ This is an excellent overview of the management of soft tissue and skeletal sarcomas. The authors have reviewed the literature concerning the preoperative, adjuvant, and standard therapy for sarcomas of soft tissue and bone. The conclusion that adjuvant herapy is of benefit for osteosarcomas has not yet been established. As the authors indicate, 1 of the 3 prospective randomized trials does not confirm either a disease-free or overall survival advantage for adjuvant therapy. Furthermore, the Mayo Clinic has noticed an improvement in outcome for patients who have just undergone surgical resection. Two prospectively randomized trials do suggest that adjuvant therapy may improve the outcome of patients with osteosarcoma, although these trials are relatively small. It is hoped that, in the future, larger trials will be performed to establish the role of adjuvant therapy in osteosarcoma.—J.M. Jessup, M.D.

Bone

Changing Pattern of Pulmonary Metastases With Adjuvant Chemotherapy in Patients With Osteosarcoma: Results From the Multiinstitutional Osteosarcoma Study

Goorin AM, Shuster JJ, Baker A, Horowitz ME, Meyer WH, Link MP (Children's Hosp, Boston; Pediatric Oncology Group Statistical Office, Gainesville, Fla; National Cancer Inst, Bethesda; St Jude Children's Research Hosp, Memphis, Tenn; Stanford Univ School of Medicine)

J Clin Oncol 9:600–605, 1991 11–7

Introduction.—The Multi-Institutional Osteosarcoma Study (MIOS) of adjuvant therapy enrolled 113 patients in 1982–1984. Seventy-seven patients received adjuvant chemotherapy, whereas 36 formed a concur-

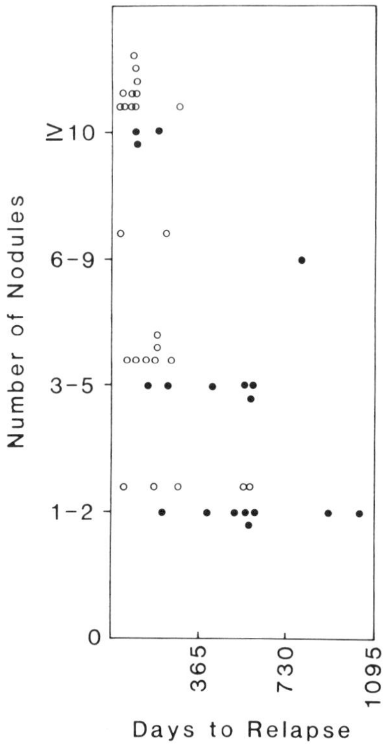

Fig 11–5.—For patients with pulmonary relapse, the distribution of nodule groups was analyzed as a function of days to relapse. *Filled circles* indicate the adjuvant group; *open circles*, the observation group. (Courtesy of Goorin AM, Shuster JJ, Baker A, et al: *J Clin Oncol* 9:600–605, 1991).

rent control group. Chemotherapy began 2–4 weeks after operation on the primary tumor.

Findings.—Those patients who relapsed after surgery alone tended to relapse earlier than those given adjuvant chemotherapy; they also had more pulmonary nodules and experienced bilateral lung involvement more frequently (Fig 11–5). The lungs were the initial site of relapse in more than 80% of the patients who relapsed. In contrast, the interval to further progression of disease was longer in patients who relapsed after surgery alone, and their final survival was better than that for patients who received chemotherapy. The only factor predicting survival after relapse was whether the patient could be made surgically free of disease after initial relapse.

Conclusions.—The use of adjuvant chemotherapy after surgery on primary osteosarcoma can delay or prevent relapse in many instances, and it is recommended for all patients with high-grade tumors. Ultimately, the cure rate can be improved only by preventing relapses.

▶ The efficacy of adjuvant chemotherapy is determined not only by the prolongation of disease-free or overall survival, but also by the pattern of tumor progression. In the study by Goorin et al., adjuvant therapy used in patients with osteosarcoma changed the pattern and kinetics of recurrence. Those patients who received adjuvant therapy had fewer recurrences that took longer to appear than the recurrences in patients who were treated with surgery only. However, once the patients failed, those who initially had surgery only had a significantly better outcome than did the patients who failed adjuvant chemotherapy. This suggests that chemotherapy retards the growth of a subset of these tumors. Furthermore, adjuvant therapy reduces or forestalls the recurrence of osteosarcoma. If recurrence can be forestalled, then the outcome may be improved. When failures are analyzed in the 2 groups, the adjuvant chemotherapy group has a better outcome, because 81% of the patients were free of disease at the end of the study, compared with 61% of the controls who had surgery alone ($P < .05$). This study reinforces the concept that prevention of recurrent disease is better than treatment of regional or distant failure.—J.M. Jessup, M.D.

Pulmonary Metastases and Bone Sarcomas: Surgical Removal of Lesions Appearing After Adjuvant Chemotherapy

Burk CD, Belasco JB, O'Neill JA Jr, Lange B (Univ of Pennsylvania School of Medicine, Philadelphia)

Clin Orthop 262:88–92, 1991 11–8

Background.—Pulmonary metastasis is the outstanding cause of death in pediatric patients with malignant bone tumors. Multiple thoracotomies are done to remove individual lesions at some centers, and many series have reported long-term survival rates of 40% to 60% or even better.

Series.—The outcome of 43 thoracotomies performed in 24 children with pulmonary metastases from primary bone tumors was evaluated. Twenty patients had osteosarcoma, 3 had Ewing's sarcoma, and 1 had a synovial-cell sarcoma of bone. At the time of thoracotomy, the lungs were the only site of metastatic disease.

Outcome.—Four patients (17%) were well without disease after a mean follow-up of 29 months. There were no significant intraoperative or postoperative complications. Those patients in whom metastases developed more than 1 year after diagnosis lived longer than those with metastasis less than a year after diagnosis. Approximately half the latter patients had bilateral pulmonary lesions.

Conclusions.—Removal of isolated lung metastases, combined with chemotherapy, can prolong survival in children with osteogenic and synovial-cell sarcomas. Ewing's sarcoma can often be managed in other ways. Thoracotomy is safe, and it is especially effective in patients in whom metastatic disease develops more than 1 year after diagnosis. The best procedure is complete wedge resection.

▶ This single institutional series describes the overall dismal prognosis of pulmonary metastases in pediatric patients with primary bone tumors treated between 1970 and 1987. The degree of adjuvant therapy and the type of adjuvant therapy that were given to these patients before surgical resection are not described. It is unlikely that adjuvant therapy would have been used for the patients accrued early in this series. Thus, the authors' discussion of the effects of adjuvant therapy decreasing the biological aggressiveness of the metastases seems unwarranted. Nonetheless, this series demonstrates and confirms the conclusion of other series: patients who have a longer disease-free interval between primary tumor resection and recurrence have a better outcome than patients who have less than a 12-month disease-free interval. The overall outlook for these patients is quite bleak, because the actuarial survival curves indicate that, essentially, all patients will recur. However, recurrences may occur more than 5 years after thoracotomy. It is hoped that adjuvant chemotherapy will have a favorable impact on survival in the future.—J.M. Jessup, M.D.

Others

Ewing's Sarcoma: Prognostic Factors, Disease Control, and the Reemerging Role of Surgical Treatment

O'Connor MI, Pritchard DJ (Mayo Graduate School of Medicine and Mayo Clinic and Foundation, Rochester, Minn)
Clin Orthop 262:78–87, 1991 11–9

Prognosis.—Ewing's sarcoma consists of a spectrum of tumors ranging from the classic lesion to primitive sarcoma of bone. The histologic response to chemotherapy holds significant prognostic value in patients who undergo surgery for local disease. Age and leukocyte count also are prognostic factors in patients with localized Ewing's tumor; younger patients tend to have a better prognosis.

Management.—Modern multidrug chemotherapy can prevent disseminated disease in many patients with localized Ewing's sarcoma of bone. Radiation-induced malignancies have become an increasing problem. Surgical excision of the primary tumor is considered whenever feasible. Intensive chemotherapy is often given as a preliminary measure. Surgery may be required to correct complications of nonoperative treatment. The role of surgery probably will widen as more patients are at risk of radiation-induced sarcoma.

▶ This is an excellent review of the management of Ewing's sarcoma, which has long been thought to be the responsibility of the medical oncologist in radiotherapy. Recent data suggest a role for surgical control of the primary tumor. The authors provide an excellent review of this aspect—and other facets—of the management of Ewing's sarcoma. Ewing's sarcoma is an uncommon tumor, and this review is recommended for all oncologists who may treat this tumor.—J.M. Jessup, M.D.

Radiation Therapy for Aggressive Fibromatosis: The Experience at the University of Florida

McCollough WM, Parsons JT, Van Der Griend R, Enneking WF, Heare T (Univ of Florida, Gainesville)
J Bone Joint Surg 73-A:717–725, 1991 11–10

Background.—It has been suggested that radiation therapy can control unresectable aggressive fibromatosis and decrease the risk of local recurrence when the resection margin is close to the tumor. An 11-year experience with radiation therapy for aggressive fibromatosis was analyzed.

Patients.—Thirty sites in 29 patients with histologically confirmed aggressive fibromatosis were treated with radiation. Twenty-one patients were female and 24 were white; the mean patient age was 32 years. All patients were followed for at least 2 years, and 76% were followed for more than 5 years. At least 5,000 cGy were administered to 27 sites, and 12 lesions received twice-a-day treatments. Postoperative radiation was given for 14 sites with known or presumed microscopic residual aggressive fibromatosis; local control was achieved in 11 of these. Postoperative treatment was given for 16 sites with grossly apparent residual disease; local control was achieved in 14 of these.

Outcome.—Control of disease was achieved in 83% of sites, and the 6-year actuarial rate of local control was 79% (Fig 11–6). There were 5 local recurrences at 4, 11, 34, 61, and 68 months after the start of therapy, 2 of them occurring in the high-dose radiation field in patients treated for grossly apparent disease. Some regression was noted in all 9 patients with grossly apparent disease in whom a response was quantified (Table 1). Three recurrences occurred at the margin of the irradiated field in patients treated for microscopic residual disease. The rate of local control appeared to be no different between patients treated for primary aggressive fibromatosis and those treated for recurrences.

Conclusions.—Local control of aggressive fibromatosis appears to improve substantially with postoperative radiation therapy when the operative margins are less than wide. This was also found in 6 interpretable

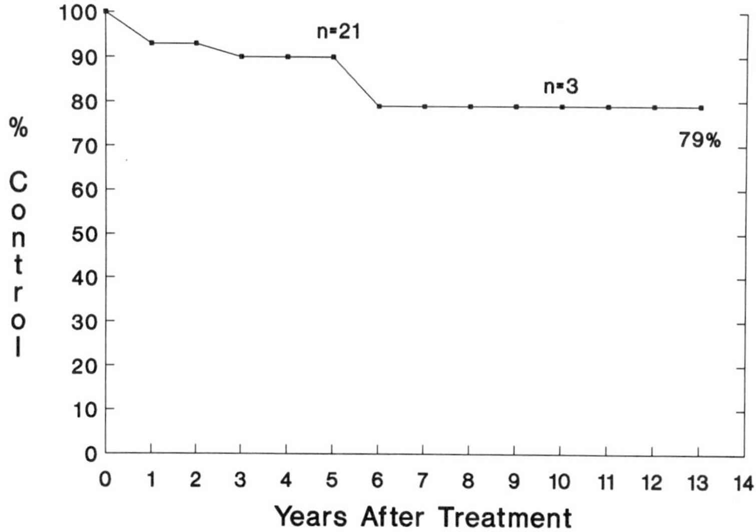

Fig 11–6.—Local control graphed by the life-table method. Thirty sites were treated. (Courtesy of McCollough WM, Parsons JT, Van Der Griend R, et al: *J Bone Joint Surg* 73-A:717–725, 1991.)

TABLE 1.—Clinical Response of Grossly Apparent Disease to Radiation Therapy

Site	Known Dimensions *(cm)*	Maximum Response†	Length of Time Free of Disease After Radiat. Therapy *(Mos.)*
Dorsum of foot	6 × 4	100% at 3 mos.	24
Left lower quadrant	14 × 12	100% at 12 mos.	126
Axilla	15 × 8	100% at 14 mos.	64
Paraspinous	18 × 10	100% at 19 mos.	25
Groin	10 × 8	100% at 30 mos.	90
Subscapular	25 × 20	90% at 10 mos., no regrowth	64
Achilles tendon	5 × 4	50% at 7 mos., no regrowth	62
Right upper quadrant	20 × 20	30% at 2 mos., no regrowth	88
Forearm	8 × 5	50% at 5 mos., local failure at 11 mos.	Amputation

Does not include 7 patients in whom grossly apparent disease was too small in volume or was in a location that prevented assessment of clinical response or both.

†Estimated reduction in volume of the tumor.

(Courtesy of McCollough WM, Parsons JT, Van Der Griend R, et al: *J Bone Joint Surg* 73-A:717–725, 1991.)

TABLE 2.—Aggressive Fibromatosis Treated With Radiation Therapy

Institution	Range of Follow-up *(Mos.)*	Local Control* Microscopic Evidence of Disease	Local Control* Gross Evidence of Disease	Proportion of Failures in Areas Treated with 5000 Centigrays or More†
Joint Center for Radiation Therapy[14]	24-96	1/1	7/8	0/1
Univ. of California, San Francisco[22]	24-132	4/6	9/13	1/6
Massachusetts General Hospital[20]	9-94	3/3	8/10	1/2
Netherlands Cancer Institute[18]	29-106	15/17	4/4	1/2
Westminster Hospital[34]	60-303	22/29	6/9	3/10
Institut Curie[1]	12-240	3/3	9/12	0/3
Present series	24-151	11/14	14/16	2/5
Total		59/73 (81%)	57/72 (79%)	8/29 (28%)

*Does not include patients treated with preoperative radiation therapy or those who had an operation soon after radiation therapy, without definitive evidence of progressive disease. When the authors failed to state clearly whether or not gross evidence of disease was present at the initiation of postoperative radiation therapy, patients were included in the group that had assumed microscopic quantities of residual disease.

†Other failures occurred at the margin of or outside the irradiated field, or in an area that received less than 5,000 cGy.

(Courtesy of McCollough WM, Parsons JT, Van Der Griend R, et al: *J Bone Joint Surg* 73-A:717–725, 1991.)

reports from the literature (Table 2). Radiation therapy appears to be an effective alternative to radical surgery.

▶ Aggressive fibromatosis (sometimes known as "desmoid" tumor) is a benign but locally aggressive neoplasm. Because it has no potential at all for metastasis, it is different from a low-grade sarcoma. Even so, its local behavior can be even more aggressive than that of a sarcoma, and the need for wide excision is important. Sometimes, however, wide excision cannot be achieved, and radiation alone may be successful. These results from an outstanding center of radiation therapy show excellent control, even when gross disease is being treated. High doses are required, and considerable time frequently is required before regression can be assessed. Ideally, radiation should occur after a wide excision.

As Figure 11–6 shows, these results are excellent, even when there is microscopic residual disease or gross residual disease. Local control is excellent, assuming that high doses of radiation therapy have been used. A common mistake in managing this problem is to fail to consider radiation therapy—or to use it in an inadequate dose.—E. Glatstein, M.D.

Intentions and Outcomes in the Radiotherapeutic Management of Epidemic Kaposi's Sarcoma

Cooper JS, Steinfeld AD, Lerch I (New York Univ)

Int J Radiat Oncol Biol Phys 20:419–422, 1991 11–11

Background.—Radiotherapeutic management of epidemic Kaposi's sarcoma in patients with AIDS has become more widespread. Epidemic Kaposi's sarcoma is radioresponsive, and doses of the level used for classic Kaposi's sarcoma induce regression of the disease. As the approach to treatment became more selective, the lesions were irradiated for palliation of pain or to improve cosmetic appearance only.

Methods.—There were 226 lesions irradiated in 129 patients with AIDS-related Kaposi's sarcoma. The rationales for radiotherapy included pain, cosmetic improvement, palliation of incapacitating edema or impaired function, healing of ulcerated lesions, local control of a mass, or staunching of a bleeding lesion.

Results.—The likelihood of obtaining complete regression of the tumor masses was 68%. Residual purple pigmentation remained in 20%, and local recurrence developed in 9%. Treatment intention, anatomical site, and Karnovsky score are important predictors of the short-term and long-term tumor response. The intention of treatment was closely linked to the anatomical site, and the 2 combined directly influenced outcome. The host's Karnovsky score independently predicted the tumor's long-term response, although it had less impact on outcome than on treatment site and intention.

Conclusion.—Epidemic Kaposi's sarcoma is a radiosensitive tumor, and moderate doses of radiotherapy can produce palliation. The response of Kaposi's sarcoma is influenced by both tumor and host factors of treatment intention, anatomical site, and Karnofsky score. Case selection can alter the observed response rate of epidemic Kaposi's sarcoma to radiotherapy.

▶ More and more, the radiotherapist is called upon to be involved in the management of Kaposi's sarcoma in patients with AIDS. This study indicates some of the determinants of outcome as far as the Kaposi's sarcoma itself is concerned. Obviously, the overall outcome is determined by the immunodeficiency itself, with its predisposition to many infectious complications. Nonetheless, the performance status, the site of involvement, and the intention of treatment are important predictors of tumor response, as is nicely demonstrated in this paper.—E. Glatstein, M.D.

12 Skin Cancer

Melanoma

A Community Study of Delay in Presenting With Signs of Melanoma to Medical Practitioners

Hennrikus D, Girgis A, Redman S, Sanson-Fisher RW (Univ of Newcastle, New South Wales, Australia)

Arch Dermatol 127:356–361, 1991 12–1

Introduction.—Australia has the highest rate of melanoma in the world, and the incidence is increasing. Melanoma is the leading cause of death from diseases of the skin in Australia, and it causes approximately 800 deaths per year. The prevalence of signs of melanoma, the length of delay in seeking medical advice, the reasons for the delay, and the actions of general practitioners when first confronted with these signs were investigated in a community sample.

Methods.—A questionnaire completed by 1,344 randomly selected individuals from 1,075 households included questions on the presence of signs of melanoma, the perceived susceptibility to melanoma, and attitudes toward early detection and treatment. Information regarding the actions by the family physician included questions on investigations performed at the first consultation, specialist referrals, and final diagnosis. All respondents were also interviewed in person.

Results.—Of the 1,344 respondents, 156 (11.9%) reported having observed signs of melanoma during the previous 12 months. Of the 115 respondents who reported signs of melanoma that first appeared in the previous 5 years, only 66 (57%) consulted a physician regarding their symptoms. The most common reason for delay or failure to see a physician for signs of melanoma was the belief that the sign was not serious or would clear. The most common reason for seeking medical advice was worry that the sign might be an indication of something serious. Of the 71 patients who provided information on the actions of their physicians, only 21 (30%) recalled being asked about a family history of melanoma; 23 (32%) were referred to a specialist; 13 (18%) had the mole removed for pathologic investigation; and 7 (10%) had their mole removed by burning or freezing. Melanoma was diagnosed in 5 (7%) individuals.

Conclusion. In Australia, the general public is insufficiently familiar with the signs of melanoma, the severity of the disease, and the potential risks associated with delay.

▶ Despite the fact that Australia has the highest incidence of melanoma in the world (a lifelong risk per individual of less than 1 in 50, which is twice the risk in the United States), this incidence is increasing at a relatively rapid rate. The cure rates are good if detected early and very poor if detected late. Despite the fact that Australia has extensive public education programs on melanoma, these authors have demonstrated, quite convincingly, that the average Australian is poorly informed about the clinical appearance of melanoma and is unaware of the dangers of a delay in diagnosis. In the United States, it is probably safe to say that, despite valiant efforts by the American Cancer Society and other educational organizations, further melanoma education is necessary in an effort to promote earlier diagnosis of melanoma.—J.S. Dover, M.D.

Dysplastic Nevi as Risk Markers of Sporadic (Nonfamilial) Melanoma: A Case-Control Study

Halpern AC, Guerry DP IV, Elder DE, Clark WH Jr, Synnestvedt M, Norman S, Ayerle R (Univ of Pennsylvania, Philadelphia)

Arch Dermatol 127:995–999, 1991 12–2

Introduction.—Familial melanoma can appear as dysplastic nevi that serve as phenotype markers for an increased risk of melanoma. The nevi are large, macular, variegated in color and have ill-defined borders. Data on 105 patients with newly diagnosed (without histories of familial melanoma) were compared with data on 181 controls to determine the risk of nonfamilial melanoma related to the presence of dysplastic nevi.

Methods.—All patients with 1 or more macular, color-varigated nevus greater than 4 mm were considered to be dysplastic nevus positive. All nevi greater than 2 mm were recorded on a body map. Biopsies were performed on patients with abnormal-appearing nevi. Both patients and controls participated in 20-minute interviews regarding personal and family melanoma history and sun exposure.

Results.—The mean total nevus counts differed significantly, with 31.1 for patients and 9.4 for controls. The mean dysplastic nevus number was 8.6 for patients and 1.7 for the controls. Those with dysplastic nevi were significantly younger than those who did not have dysplastic moles. Biopsy specimens confirmed 35 of the 38 patients with 1 or more dysplastic nevi. The sensitivity of the clinical diagnosis of the dysplastic nevi was 100%. The odds ratio for dysplastic nevi by multiple logistic regression analysis correcting for age, sex, eye, and hair color, actinic damages, freckles, and total number of dysplastic nevi was 6.8.

Conclusion.—Clinically diagnosed dysplastic nevi are associated with an increased risk of nonfamilial melanoma. Histologic dysplasia may serve as a more specific marker of the risk of melanoma than other atypical factors.

▶ The findings of this study help to confirm a belief held by many: dysplastic nevi are significant markers for melanoma, both in the familial and the *nonfamilial* settings.—J.S. Dover M.D.

Sunlight and Dysplastic Nevus Risk: Results of a Clinic-Based Case-Control Study

Weinstock MA, Stryker WS, Stampfer MJ, Lew RA, Willett WC, Sober AJ (Brown Univ, Providence, RI; Harvard Univ, Boston; Univ of Massachusetts, Worcester)

Cancer 67:1701–1706, 1991 12–3

Introduction.—The dysplastic nevus (DN) is the most important risk factor and precursor for malignant melanoma. The prevalence of DN in white individuals has been estimated to range from 2% to 9%.

Methods.—The risk factors for DN were examined in a case-control study of 557 white patients referred to a pigmented lesion clinic, of whom 132 had 1 or more DN, 186 had histologically confirmed cutaneous melanoma, and 239 had other diagnoses. Immediately before examination, all patients completed a self-administered questionnaire that included items regarding sun sensitivity, sun exposure, demographics, personal and family history of melanoma, smoking, and oral contraceptive use. The latitude of birthplace and location of summer residence during the preceding 5 years were also evaluated.

Results.—Patients with DN were younger than the controls and were of a higher social class (as determined by more years of formal education). After controlling for age and education, gender was not significantly related to DN risk, nor was it related to melanoma risk. A family history of melanoma was more common in controls than in patients with melanoma. Sun sensitivity, which was determined by reports of poor tanning after repeated sun exposures as a teenager, was significantly associated with DN risk. However, this association was nonlinear; the relative risks were 2.3 for average tanners, 2.8 for light tanners, and 1.6 for those who reported almost no tan after sun exposure. Thus, those who were least able to tan after sun exposure did not have the highest risk for DN. After controlling for age and education, exposure measures were not associated with DN risk.

Conclusion.—There was a clear association between sun sensitivity and the risk of DN, but the association was nonlinear. No association between lifetime sun exposure measures and DN risk could be found. These findings suggest a role for either sunlight or a trait linked with sun sensitivity in the development of dysplastic nevi.

▶ The risk factors for melanoma are fairly well established. Having fair skin, blue eyes, blonde hair, sun sensitivity, and severe blistering sunburns in childhood are all individual risk factors for melanoma. However, the risk factors for dysplastic nevi are not nearly as well established. In this case-control study of the effect of sunlight on the prevalence of melanoma, risk was determined by an individual's ability to tan. The lack of a linear relationship between ability to tan and risk of DN is not entirely surprising, considering the complexity of the relationship between melanoma and the sun.—J.S. Dover, M.D.

Correlation of Clinical and Histopathologic Features in Clinically Atypical Melanocytic Nevi

Barnhill RL, Rousch GC (Massachusetts Hosp, Boston; Harvard Med School, Boston; Cancer Prevention Research Inst, New York)

Cancer 67:3157–3164, 1991 12–4

Objective.—A quantitative study that correlated individual clinical features with histologic features of clinically atypical nevi was conducted to define better the evolving entity of dysplastic melanocytic nevus (DMN).

Methods.—The most clinically atypical nevus was identified in 153 patients with newly diagnosed melanoma. This nevus was examined clinically and independently by 2–4 physicians, and it was studied histopathologically by a single dermatopathologist. Each of the 12 gross morphologic features studied, including size (mm), presence of a macular component, irregular border, ill-defined border, haphazard coloration, distortion of skin cleavage lines on tangential lighting, asymmetry, and individual colors present (tan, brown, black, or pink) were correlated with 19 histopathologic features, including architectural, nuclear, and cytoplasmic parameters ascribed to dysplastic nevi.

Findings.—A total of 17% of the nevi had a histologic diagnosis of DMN. Nevus size (mm), irregular border, ill-defined border, macular component, and pink color correlated significantly with a histologic diagnosis of DMN. Of these clinical features, nevus size and irregular borders correlated with the greatest number of individual histologic features. There were significant differences between the examiners in their clinicopathologic correlations. These differences could be related both to different thresholds among examiners for recognizing clinical features and to the fact that certain clinical parameters were deemed more important than others by individual examiners.

Conclusion.—There are significant correlations between individual clinical features and individual histologic parameters of clinically atypical melanocytic nevi, with the nevus size being most closely linked to histologic dysplasia. These observations may be relevant to the development of clinical criteria for dysplastic nevi.

▶ Finally, an attempt at systematic correlation of the clinical and pathologic features of dysplastic nevi! Of the 12 clinical features assessed, nevus size and irregular borders correlated best with the pathologic features of dysplastic nevi. These results have great potential for helping to develop clinical criteria for the diagnosis of dysplastic nevi. Further large studies will be required before the significance of each of the individual clinical parameters is known; however, a good starting point for determining whether a nevus is dysplastic would appear to be size greater than 6 mm in diameter, with associated notching or irregularity of the border.—J.S. Dover, M.D.

Narrow Excision (1-cm Margin): A Safe Procedure for Thin Cutaneous Melanoma

Veronesi U, Cascinelli N (Natl Tumor Inst, Milan)

Arch Surg 126:438–441, 1991 12–5

Background.—In 1988, the World Health Organization Melanoma Programme published study results that showed that, at 55-month follow-up, the disease-free and overall survival rates were similar in patients with cutaneous melanomas no thicker than 2 mm, whether they received narrow or wide excision. The results of the randomized, multicenter, international study were updated to reflect 90 months of follow-up.

Methods.—Data were analyzed from 612 patients; 189 were male. All patients had clinical stage I melanomas. The mean thickness of the primary melanoma was 1.009 mm. A group of 305 patients was randomly assigned to receive excisions with 1-cm margins; 307 received excisions with wide margins of at least 3 cm. The patients were examined every 2 months for 2 years, then every 3 months from the third to the fifth year. After this, the patients were followed up at 6-month intervals.

Results.—At 8 years, the actuarial survival rate of the entire group was 89%. Those patients who underwent narrow excision had an actuarial survival rate of 89.6%; the rate for those who received wide excision was 90.3%. The 8-year disease-free survival rate was 81.6% in the narrow-excision group and 84.4% in the wide-excision group. Neither of these differences was statistically significant. The patients with primary melanomas no thicker than 1 mm had better prognoses than those with thicker tumors, but there was no impact of the width of the margins on either disease-free or overall survival. Four patients had local recurrence, and all had melanomas greater than 1 mm in thickness that were excised with narrow margins. Two patients died of melanoma; 1 had local recurrence at 18 months and the other had a local recurrence at 7 years. Both died of distant metastases.

Conclusions.—Narrow excision is a safe procedure for primary melanomas no thicker than 1 mm. Conclusions regarding its use for melanomas ranging between 1.1 mm and 2 mm cannot be made based on this early information. For the procedure, the skin must be cut 1 cm from the visible margins of the primary melanoma. The excision should be 1 or 2 cm wider in the subcutaneous fat extending to the muscular fascia. The benefits of narrow excision are that primary closure is always possible, the cosmetic effects are good, and the procedure can be done on an outpatient basis under local anesthesia.

▶ In a follow-up to the 1988 World Health Organization narrow margin study, these well-known Italian investigators completed 90 months of follow-up. Narrow margin excision (1 cm margin of skin with 2–3 cm margins of subcutaneous fat to fascia) of melanomas that are 1 mm or less in Breslow thickness appears to be safe and effective, reducing the morbidity of melanoma surgery while maintaining high cure rates. Unfortunately, because of local recurrences that occurred in 4 patients with narrowly excised lesions more than 1 mm in thickness, it is premature to conclude that narrow margins are the standard of care for melanomas 1.1 mm–2 mm in thickness, despite the fact that it is unknown whether wider margins of excision would have modified outcome in these 4 individuals.—J.S. Dover, M.D.

The Relationship Between Risk of Death From Clinical Stage 1 Cutaneous Melanoma and Thickness of Primary Tumour: No Evidence for Steps in Risk

Keefe M, Mackie RM (Univ of Glasgow, Scotland; Royal South Hants Hosp, Southampton, England)

Br J Cancer 64:598–602, 1991 12–6

Introduction.—Studies have shown that the most important independent predictor of survival from clinical stage I cutaneous malignant melanoma is the thickness of the primary tumor. Various breakpoints have been suggested for purposes of patient stratification. Data from the Scottish Melanoma Group database were examined to determine whether the relationship between thickness and survival is smooth or stepped.

Methods.—Included in the study sample were 1,100 cases of clinical stage I primary cutaneous malignant melanomas of Clark level II or more that were excised between 1979 and 1983; the cases available for follow-up evaluation numbered 997. Thickness was categorized into 8 levels. The male to female ratio of the patients was 296:701; mean patient age was 56 years, and the mean thickness of the lesions was 2.5 mm.

Results.—There were 233 deaths from melanoma and 101 deaths from other causes. Among the variables tested, age, sex, thickness, and site were significant predictors of survival in adjusted analyses. A lower survival rate was associated with males, lesions on the trunk, volar, or subungual sites, increasing age, and increasing thickness. After entering thickness into a model either as a regressor or as a factored variable, it was determined that a step effect was unlikely.

Conclusion.—Although the presence of breakpoints was not unequivocally excluded, the findings of this study suggest that, for melanomas less than 9.75 mm in thickness, there is a continuous, probably linear relationship between survival and thickness adjusted for sex, age, and site. There does not appear to be a biological reason to assume natural breakpoints.

▶ These results throw a monkey wrench into the extensively used, straightforward "breakpoint" approach to predicting melanoma prognosis. Balch first separated survival into breakpoints at thicknesses of .76 mm and 4 mm in 1978 (1). Since the Massachusetts General Hospital/New York University collaborative study extended the breakpoints to .85 mm, 1.7 mm, and 3.6 mm in 1981, the concept of biologically occurring breakpoints in melanoma survival has become well established (2). Keefe and Mackie's study from the Scottish Melanoma Group's national registry, the largest study to look at the concept of breakpoints, found that the risk of death from melanoma is probably a linear (not stepwise) function of tumor thickness. The proponents of biological breakpoints must readdress the concept. In the meantime, although clinicians may be comfortable in grouping patients for prognostic purposes, it is probably safe to assume that there is linearity to melanoma outcome and that, for example, a melanoma .2 mm in thickness probably has a better prognosis than one that is .8 mm in thickness, despite the fact that they are in the same breakpoint group.—J.S. Dover, M.D.

Reference

1. Balch CM, et al: *Ann Surg* 188:732, 1978.
2. Day CL, et al: *N Engl J Med* 325:1155, 1981.

Observer Variation in the Measurement of Breslow Depth and Clark's Level in Thin Cutaneous Malignant Melanoma

Colloby PS, West KP, Fletcher A (Leicester Royal Infirmary, England)

J Pathol 163:245–250, 1991 12–7

Introduction.—Patient management in thin cutaneous malignant melanoma is affected by the depth of invasion. The 2 most common indicators for measuring depth, Breslow depth and Clark's level, were evaluated for intraobserver and interobserver variations in thin cutaneous malignant melanomas.

Methods.—Fifty cases of invasive cutaneous malignant melanomas had depth determined by Breslow depth and Clark's level, and the degrees of observer variation were assessed. For each case, a total of 6 depth measurements and 6 Clark's level assessments were done.

Results.—Clark's level was more difficult to assess in thin melanomas, whereas Breslow depth was more reproducible. The interobserver and intraobserver variation was significant; in some cases it was as much as .86 mm. After 1 assessment, interobserver agreement produced similar levels of agreement, and after 2 measurements and calculation of the mean, it generally improved.

Conclusion.—Because prognosis and disease management depend on accurate measurement of the depth of invasion, it is recommended that several measurements be taken at the point of deepest invasion at different times; these measurements should be reviewed by different observers. The methods must be consistent and accurate, and major discrepancies should be identified and discussed.

▶ The findings of this study are extremely bothersome. Because the prognosis of a melanoma depends so heavily on its thickness, inaccurate thickness measurements are intolerable. The interobserver and intraobserver differences, which were as great as ±.86 mm in some of the cases reviewed in this study, are staggering. If these findings are reproducible, then pathologists will be required to reevaluate the manner in which melanoma specimens are evaluated.—J.S. Dover, M.D.

Uveal Melanoma: Development of Metastases After Helium Ion Irradiation

Nowakowski VA, Ivery G, Castro JR, Char DH, Linstadt DE, Ahn D, Phillips TL, Quivey JM, Decker M, Petti PL, Collier JM (Univ of California, San Francisco; Univ of California Lawrence Berkeley Lab; Northern California Cancer Ctr, Belmont)

Radiology 178:277–280, 1991 12–8

Background.—Although there are therapeutic alternatives to enucleation for uveal melanoma, distant metastases develop in many patients. The natural history of these metastases was reviewed to identify the prognostic factors for their development.

Methods.—The records of 261 patients treated with helium ions for ocular melanoma during a 9-year period were reviewed. All but 1 patient was followed for at least 24 months, and 116 were followed for 5 years or more. The radiation doses ranged from 50 to 80 Gy-equivalent in 5 fractions for 7–12 days. Patient, disease, and treatment variables were compared. The analytical endpoints were metastasis and death.

Results.—The median time between the start of treatment and the finding of metastases was 27 months. Metastases developed in 42 patients, all of whom died. The mean pretreatment tumor height was 7.7 mm. Patients survived a median of 5 months after metastasis, the longest survival being 49 months. Thirty-four of the metastases were to the liver, and 4 metastases were accompanied by local recurrence. The variables that independently predicted metastasis and death were anterior tumor location, a tumor height of more than 5 mm, and a tumor diameter of more than 10 mm.

Conclusion.—In uveal melanoma, helium ion therapy appears to offer tumor control and survival rates similar to those of enucleation and other therapies. Almost 20% of patients have metastases, and there is no effective salvage therapy. Large tumor size and anterior location are poor prognostic factors.

▶ Efforts to save the eye affected with uveal melanoma still appear to be worthwhile. Nonetheless, there is a finite risk of dissemination. This study shows that the location, tumor height, and tumor diameter are important factors in predicting dissemination after helium ion irradiation of the melanomatous eye.—E. Glatstein, M.D.

The Effect of Palliative Radiation Therapy on Epidural Compression Due to Metastatic Malignant Melanoma

Herbert SH, Solin LJ, Rate WR, Schultz DJ, Hanks GE (Univ of Pennsylvania, Philadelphia)

Cancer 67:2472–2476, 1991 12–9

Background.—Little information is available on the use of palliative radiation therapy for spinal cord compression in metastatic malignant melanoma. The outcomes of patients who received this treatment during a 20-year period were evaluated.

Patients.—Thirty-eight sites were treated in 35 patients, all of whom had radiographically documented spinal cord or cauda equina compression and symptoms of cord or nerve root compression. All but 3 patients were also given steroids. Palliative radiation therapy was started within 24 hours of the detection of epidural compression. Daily radiation fractions ranging from 200 to 800 cGy were given (median dose, 2,850 cGy).

Outcome.—One month after treatment, 28 sites in 26 patients were evaluable. In 39% of sites, the symptoms responded completely, and in another 46% of sites, the symptoms responded partially. Of the patients who received a dose of 3,000 cGy or more, 62% achieved a complete response, compared with 20% of those who received less than 3,000 cGy. This difference was significant on both univariate and multivariate analysis.

Conclusions.—In patients with epidural compression caused by metastatic malignant melanoma, treatment with radiation therapy and corticosteroids can effectively palliate symptoms. An accelerated course of radiation (to 3,000 cGy or more without exceeding spinal cord tolerance) should be used. No factor other than radiation dose was predictive of response.

▶ Spinal cord compression secondary to metastatic melanoma is, unfortunately, a common problem. No treatment is optimal for this kind of problem. The value of radiation therapy is well established in this particular series, despite melanoma's reputation for being "radioresistant." Regardless of what various individuals mean by that term, cord compression usually can be alleviated by radiation therapy; in the majority of patients, it can be controlled for the duration of the patient's life. Obviously, there are many factors that influence outcome, including performance status, previous treatment, and the extent of involvement at the time of cord compression. The smaller the amount of disease that is present, the more aggressive the treatment generally becomes (in terms of dose or the use of concomitant surgery).

The actual outcome of patients who have cord compression depends less on the treatment than on the time of diagnosis. When the diagnosis can be made early, the results of treatment—almost regardless of type—are vastly better than if the treatment is delayed until the patient paralysis actually manifests. In that setting, there is little benefit from almost any treatment.—E. Glatstein, M.D.

Squamous Cell

Nonmelanoma Skin Cancer Mortality: A Population-Based Study

Weinstock MA, Bogaars HA, Ashley M, Litle V, Bilodeau E, Kimmel S (VA Med Ctr; Roger Williams Med Ctr; and Brown Univ, Providence, RI)

Arch Dermatol 127:1194–1197, 1991 12–10

Background.—Nonmelanoma skin cancer (NMSC) is common, but its mortality is not well understood. The magnitude of NMSC mortality and its parameters were investigated through a population-based study.

Methods.—All deaths among Rhode Island residents that occurred during a 9-year period and were certified as resulting from NMSC were studied. Kaposi's sarcoma associated with AIDS was excluded, as were cancers of the skin of the scrotum and genitals and cutaneous lymphomas. The population estimates were derived from census figures.

Results.—Fifty-one deaths resulting from NMSC were confirmed, which was one fourth the number of reported melanoma deaths. When adjusted for age, mortality from NMSC was .44/10^5/year. Death resulted from squamous cell carcinoma in 59% of the cases and basal cell carcinoma in 20%. The majority seemed to be actinically induced. The mean age was 73 years among those patients who died of squamous cell carcinoma; at least 80% of these tumors metastasized, and 47% originated on the ear. None of these deaths appeared to result from refusal of treatment. The mean patient age was 85 years among patients who died from basal cell carcinoma; 40% of these patients had refused surgical intervention.

Conclusions.—Prevention, early detection, and treatment of NMSC originating on the ears appear to be particularly important.

▶ With all the attention that melanoma has been receiving during the past several years, squamous cell carcinoma has taken a back seat. This study should, however, perk up a few unattentive, burnt ears. Squamous cell carcinoma accounts for more morbidity and far more mortality than one would expect: one fourth as many deaths as melanoma per year. The lips and especially the ears are the areas of greatest risk for metastasizing lesions.—J.S. Dover, M.D., F.R.C.P.C.

A Management Approach to Incompletely Excised Basal Cell Carcinomas of Skin

Liu F-F, Maki E, Warde P, Payne D, Fitzpatrick P (Princess Margaret Hosp, Toronto)

Int J Radiat Oncol Biol Phys 20:423–428, 1991 12–11

Introduction.—The management of incompletely excised basal cell carcinoma (BCC) of the skin, without gross residual disease, has ranged from expectant observation to immediate treatment. Two approaches were compared with regard to medical outcome and relative costs.

Methods.—In 1970–1985, 187 patients with incompletely resected BCC of the skin were referred to the study institution. The median patient age was 62 years, and most (93%) of the lesions were located in the head and neck region. Of the 120 lesions that were treated immediately, 119 were irradiated and 1 was excised. The remaining patients were managed expectantly.

Results.—At a median follow-up of 32 months, the immediately treated and expectantly observed groups had significantly different 5- and 10-year relapse-free rates (RFR). Both the 5- and 10-year RFRs for the group that was immediately treated were 91%. The observed lesions, however, had 5- and 10-year RFRs of 61% and 40%, respectively. Once relapse occurred in patients treated expectantly, most (85%) of these relapses were salvaged by radiation or surgery. Thus, the 10-year actuarial probability of local control was 92% with immediate treatment and 90% with observation. Although immediate radiation therapy saves approximately $233 per patient, such therapy results in acute morbidity and a potential for long-term morbidity.

Conclusion.—Given the fact that most of these lesions occur in elderly patients, observation is recommended for incompletely excised BCC of skin with no gross residual disease. Lesions that have previously recurred or that have deep and lateral margins may require immediate radiation or surgery.

▶ With rationing of health care dollars becoming more of a reality in the United States, studies that look both at the medical outcome and the relative costs of treatment are of great importance. Despite the difficulty that most Americans have with the concept of rationing health services, it is practiced worldwide, and it must (and will) play a role in our everyday decision-making in the future.

Those incompletely excised BCCs without gross evidence of disease that were simply observed and not treated immediately had a 10-year RFR of only 40% compared with 91% in those lesions that were treated immediately. However, the salvage rates were very high; if the basal cell carcinoma was treated upon recurrence, then the 10-year actuarial probability of local control was virtually the same as in those patients who were treated initially. The authors' suggestion that microscopic recurrences of BCC in elderly individuals be observed and not immediately irradiated or excised is worth consideration.—J.S. Dover, M.D.

The Subsequent Risk of Internal Cancer With Bowen's Disease: A Population-Based Study

Chute CG, Chuang T-Y, Bergstralh EJ, Su W-PD (Mayo Clinic and Found, Rochester, Minn; Wright State Univ, Dayton, Ohio)

JAMA 266:816–819, 1991 12–12

Introduction.—Bowen's disease has often been reported to be predictive of internal cancer, but most of these studies were uncontrolled or had methodologic flaws. Patients with Bowen's disease were evaluated to address the subsequent risk of internal cancer.

Methods.—The study was based on the permanent population of a single city during a 9-year-period. Within this population of 57,906 residents, incident patients with skin cancers (excluding malignant melanoma) were categorized as having basal cell carcinoma, squamous cell carcinoma, or Bowen's disease. All patients were followed up for development of internal cancer until they either died or moved from the study area, or until the end of the study. After computation of the incidence rates of skin and subsequent cancer, the rate of internal cancer was compared with the prevailing rate in the community.

Results.—There were 657 patients with basal cell carcinoma, 169 with squamous cell carcinoma, and 71 with Bowen's disease. Compared with the population base, patients with Bowen's disease had a relative risk of subsequent internal cancer of 1.1. When adjusted to the white population in the United States, the annual incidence rates were 14.9 per 100,000 for Bowen's disease compared with 38.8 for squamous cell carcinoma and 146 for basal cell carcinoma. For patients with the latter 2 skin cancers, the estimated risk of subsequent cancer was .9 for squamous cell carcinoma and 1 for basal cell carcinoma. Considering the various durations of follow-up and the sun exposure of different sites, the risks were not significantly different.

Conclusion.—Bowen's disease, as well as other forms of nonmelanomatous skin cancer, does not appear to be associated with increased risk of subsequent internal cancer. Therefore, an exhaustive work-up will probably not be of benefit in young patients with Bowen's disease.

▶ Yet again, no association could be found between Bowen's disease and an underlying malignancy.—J.S. Dover, M.D.

Relation Between Skin Cancer and HLA Antigens in Renal-Transplant Recipients

Bavinck JNB, Vermeer BJ, van der Woude FJ, Vandenbroucke JP, Schreuder GMT, Thorogood J, Persijn GG, Claas FHJ (University Hosp Leiden; Eurotransplant Found; Leiden; The Netherlands)

N Engl J Med 325:843–848, 1991 12–13

Background.—Renal allograft recipients have an increased risk for skin cancer. Recipients who are homozygous for HLA antigens and those who are mismatched with their donors for these antigens have an increased risk for certain kinds of cancer. The relationship between skin cancer in renal-transplant recipients and HLA homozygosity and mismatching was investigated in a case-control study.

Methods.—Between 1966 and 1988, 764 patients received renal transplants. Sixty-six had squamous cell carcinoma or basal cell carcinoma of the skin after transplantation. Homozygosity of HLA was assessed in all 66 patients, and HLA mismatching was assessed in 39. The results of these assessments were compared with those of 124 recipients without skin cancer. In addition, the relationship between skin cancer and immunosuppressive drug use was studied. The effect of exposure to the sun and keratotic skin lesions on the risk of skin cancer was investigated in a separate case-control study.

Results.—Recipients who were mismatched for HLA-B antigens had an increased risk of squamous cell carcinoma. The relative risks were 2.6 with mismatching for 1 antigen and 5 with mismatching for 2 antigens, compared with no mismatching. Antigen mismatching of HLA-A and HLA-DR had no influence on the risk of squamous cell carcinoma. In addition, there was no association between mismatches at any of the HLA loci and occurrence of basal cell carcinoma. The total doses of azathioprine and prednisone were unassociated with occurrence of skin cancer or HLA matching. Exposure to sunlight and keratotic skin lesions were strongly related to skin cancer but not to HLA mismatching. Homozygosity for HLA-DR occurred more often among patients with squamous cell carcinoma and those patients with 100 or more keratotic skin lesions.

Conclusions.—Both HLA-B mismatching and HLA-DR homozygosity ware significantly associated with the risk of squamous cell carcinoma in renal transplant recipients. These findings cannot be explained by an indirect effect on the level of immunosuppression, by exposure to sunlight, or by the number of keratotic skin lesions.

▶ Why some renal transplant patients get squamous cell carcinoma of the skin and others do not is a mystery. Squamous cell carcinoma in renal transplant patients has usually been attributed to the amount of sun exposure, to human papillomavirus (HPV) infection, or to longstanding immunosuppression. These Dutch authors have ruled out at least 2 of these explanations. Both HLA-B mismatching and HLA-DR homozygosity appear to be the most important factors in determining whether squamous cell carcinoma will develop in a patient, whereas the level of immunosuppression and exposure to sunlight do not appear to play a significant role. Whether HPV plays a role in tumorigenesis in these individuals remains unclear.—J.S. Dover, M.D.

Presence of Human Papilloma Virus Type 16 DNA Sequences in Human Nonmelanoma Skin Cancers

Pierceall WE, Goldberg LH, Ananthaswamy HN (Univ of Texas; Baylor College of Medicine, Houston)

J Invest Dermatol 97:880–884, 1991 12–14

Background.—There is an association between the human papillomaviruses (HPV) and the development and progression of invasive genital tract, skin, and head and neck cancers. Various lesions and tumors have yielded HPV types 1, 3, 4, 5, 8, 14, 16, 37, and 38, but the importance of types 6, 11, 16, and 18 is not well understood. The presence of these HPV types in nonmelanoma human skin cancers was evaluated.

Methods.—Twenty-one squamous cell carcinomas (SCC) and 16 basal cell carcinomas (BCC) occurring on sun-exposed areas in white patients were studied. The tumors were analyzed by a highly sensitive polymerase chain reaction (PCR) technique using primers designated to amplify DNA encoding the E6-E7 region and the 6b/11, 16, and 18 HPV types.

Results.—None of the tumors contained HPV type 6b/11 and 18 sequences. However, agarose gel electrophoresis showed a single specific DNA band of the predicted 98 base-pair length, which indicated the presence of HPV type 16 sequences, in 19% of the SCC and 19% of the BCC. Analysis of normal skin from these 7 patients did not show HPV type 16 sequences. The PCR-amplified material demonstrated dot blot hybridization to ^{32}P-labeled HPV type 16, but not to probes specific for HPV type 6b/11 or 18.

Conclusions.—The HPV type 16 appears to be associated with some nonmelanoma skin cancers in humans, but types 6b/11 and 18 do not. The finding of this HPV type in tumor (but not in normal skin) suggests that it plays some role in the pathogenesis of some sunlight-induced tumors. This might be ultraviolet (UV) activation of papillomavirus DNA sequences or cooperation between the effects of papillomavirus gene products and a separate, UV-induced change.

▶ Whether HPV is associated with nongenital SCC remains unclear. Several recent studies have isolated HPV type 16 from warty SCC of the finger; however, others have found little or no evidence of HPV in skin cancers in other nongenital skin locations, thereby suggesting that SCC of the finger may be a unique tumor type.

The presence of HPV type 16 in 19% of the SCC and BCC occurring on varied sun-exposed skin sites in the group of patients studied suggests at least 2 possibilities: (1) HPV 16 is involved in skin tumorigenesis; therefore, the reason that more tumors were not positive for HPV 16 is because of the disappearance of the antigen as tumor development occurs; and (2) HPV 16 was found in only a fraction of the tumors evaluated because it is a bystander to the neoplastic process. Further study is needed.—J.S. Dover, M.D.

PUVA and Cancer: A Large-Scale Epidemiological Study

Lindelöf B, Sigurgeirsson B, Tegner E, Larkö O, Johannesson A, Berne B, Christensen OB, Andersson T, Törngren M, Molin L, Nylander-Lundqvist E, Emtestam L (Karolinska Hosp, Stockholm; Univ Hosp, Lund, Sweden; Sahlgrenska Hosp, Gothenburg, Sweden; Swedish Psoriasis Assoc, Stockholm; Univ Hosp, Uppsala, Sweden; et al)

Lancet 338:91–93, 1991 12–15

Introduction.—Psoralen and ultraviolet A radiation (PUVA) therapy is used to treat various skin disorders—most commonly, psoriasis. The risk of cutaneous cancer in patients who receive such therapy was examined by a review of almost all patients treated with PUVA in Sweden during an 11-year period.

Methods.—A total of 4,799 patients (2,343 males and 2,456 females) who had received PUVA treatment for skin disorders was studied. Average follow-up was 6.9 years for male patients and 7.2 years for female patients; 1,038 patients were followed up for more than 10 years.

Results.—A dose-dependent increase in the risk of squamous cell cancer of the skin was demonstrated in the study population. In male patients who had received more than 200 treatments, the incidence of squamous cell cancer was more than 30 times greater than that in the general population. Statistically significant increases were also noted in respiratory cancer in male and female patients, pancreatic cancer in male patients, and kidney and colon cancer in female patients. Patients who received treatment with trimethoxypsoralen—as opposed to 8-methoxypsoralen—did not demonstrate increased risk of any type of cancer.

Discussion.—By decreasing the intensity and total dose of PUVA, the risk of skin cancer may possibly be reduced. Those patients with long-term exposure to PUVA should be monitored carefully for early detection of tumors or skin cancer, or both.

▶ For years, Europeans have contended that PUVA therapy does not increase the risk of skin cancer, despite the fact that meticulous 10-year follow-up studies done by R.S. Stern et al. in the United States have found a substantial increase in the incidence of squamous cell carcinoma in patients receiving long-term PUVA (1). This large Swedish study seems to have finally established that the risk from PUVA, at least when it concerns skin cancer, is no different, regardless of on which side of the Atlantic one receives therapy. The surprising finding in this study was the significant increase in cancers of the respiratory tract, pancreas, kidney, and colon in patients treated with PUVA; these findings were never before detected in the large United States studies.—J.S. Dover, M.D.

Reference

1. Stern RS, et al: *N Engl J Med* 322:1093, 1990.

Mycosis Fungoides

Total Skin Electron Beam and Total Nodal Irradiation of Cutaneous T-Cell Lymphoma

Micaily B, Campbell O, Moser C, Vonderheid EC, Brady LW (Hahnemann Univ, Philadelphia, Pa)

Int J Radiat Oncol Biol Phys 20:809–813, 1991 12–16

Background.—Total skin electron beam radiation (TSEB) has been the most effective treatment for cutaneous T-cell lymphoma (CTCL); approximately 40% of patients with early-stage disease attain long-term durable remissions. Combined TSEB and total nodal irradiation (TNI) was tried because clinical and autopsy evidence showed that extracutaneous involvement first occurs in the lymph nodes.

Methods.—Nineteen patients with CTCL limited to the skin and/or lymph nodes were treated with a TSEB + TNI. The patients were categorized by disease stages Ib, IIa, IIb, and IVa. The acute effects of TSEB + TNI were well tolerated. The patients with stage Ib, IIa, and IIb had a 100% response to treatment, and the patients with stage IVa disease had a 60% complete response rate. The patients with stage Ib and IIa disease had 100% survival and a disease-free survival of 44% at 6 years. Of the 5 patients with stage IIb CTCL, 4 relapsed within 3 months of completing TSEB + TNI, with an overall 5 years survival of 40%. The 5 patients with stage IVa disease all relapsed within 7 months of completing treatment and died of disease within 50 months.

Conclusion.—Although CTCL response has been achieved with many different modalities, the durability of complete response has been limited. The benefits of TSEB + TNI may be related to the additional radiation delivered to the skin, which receives low-dose radiation from TSEB. Therapy with TSEB + TNI resulted in significant tumor reduction and complete response in patients with CTCL. More effective chemotherapeutic agents and earlier detection of extracutaneous involvement will aid in treating advanced CTCL.

▶ Mycosis fungoides represents a particularly difficult problem. Electron beam treatment is an excellent palliative tool that has limited curative potential beyond stage I. In this small series of patients, adding total nodal irradiation suggests some modest benefit in the stage IIa patients. Because these numbers are small, it is hard to know how solid this conclusion really is. Certainly, in more advanced patients, there does not appear to be any curative potential. This is an enormous amount of treatment; however, this is a disease that is extraordinarily difficult to control, despite its remarkable sensitivity to both radiation and chemotherapy. I believe that future treatment in this area probably rests largely on biologicals, because these cells are most unusual compared with other lymphoma cells. The fact that this appears to be a lymphoma should not suggest that it must be approached as a typical lymphoma. Responses are very easy to achieve with almost any modality in this condition, but the durability of most complete responses has been extraordinarily limited.—E. Glatstein, M.D.

13 Brain Tumors

Introduction

There is little exciting to report in brain tumor therapy from the literature of the past year. These tumors remain remarkably difficult to treat because their location limits surgical approaches, because they have a basic resistance to radiation and chemotherapy, and because of the serious side effects that can result from overly aggressive therapeutic intervention. I have selected several papers that indicate the state-of-the-art techniques in this field and provide some glimmers of hope for the future.

J.V. Simone, M.D.

A Population-Based Study on the Incidence and Survival Rates of 3857 Glioma Patients Diagnosed From 1953 to 1984

Kallio M, Sankila R, Jääskeläinen J, Karjalainen S, Hakulinen T (Univ of Helsinki, Finland; Finnish Cancer Registry, Helsinki, Finland)

Cancer 68:1394–1400, 1991 13–1

Objective.—Using data from the Finnish Cancer Registry, a population-based study was conducted to determine the incidence of intracranial gliomas diagnosed during patients' lives. The survival rates were calculated and compared with the expected rates in a matched general population. The effect of age at diagnosis, sex, calendar period of diagnosis, surgery, radiation therapy, and length of follow-up on survival rates were assessed using regression modeling.

Patients/Treatment.—Between 1953 and 1984, intracranial glioma was histologically verified in 3,857 patients. The patients were followed until either death or the end of 1987, and the follow-up was complete. Treatment consisted of surgery in 1,193 patients, radiation in 459, and both operation and radiation in 1,486; the remaining 719 patients had neither surgery nor radiation therapy.

Outcome.—The age-adjusted annual incidence rate of gliomas increased during the study period, from 1.4 in 1953–1957 to 3.6 per 100,000 in 1980–1984 among women, and from 1.9 in 1953–1957 to 4.6 per 100,000 in 1980–1984 among men, possibly because of improved diagnosis. The cumulative relative survival rate was 53% in the first year, 29% in the fifth year, 20% in the tenth year, and 18% in the 15th year. The youngest patients (newborn to age 14 years) lost 56% of their life expectancy compared with 91% for the oldest patients (age, 65–99 years). The relative excess risk of death was more than fourfold in the oldest patients in the first year of follow-up and almost sixfold dur-

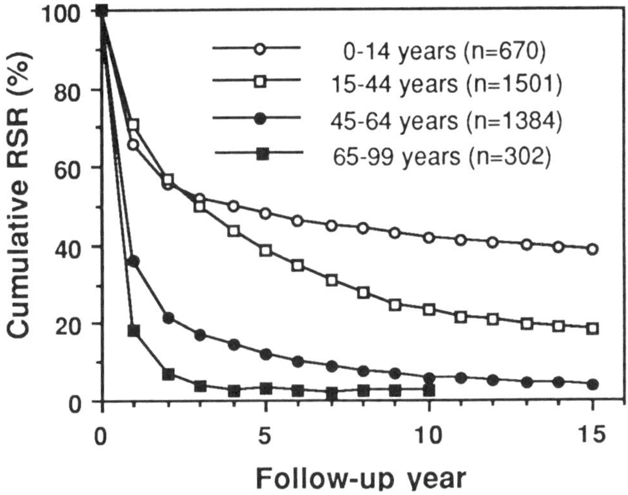

Fig 13–1.—Cumulative relative survival rates (RSR) according to age. (Courtesy of Kallio M, Sankila R, Jääskeläinen J, et al: *Cancer* 68:1394–1400, 1991.)

ing the 2nd to 15th year of follow-up, compared with the youngest patients (Fig 13–1). There was a trend toward better prognosis by period of analysis (Fig 13–2). In the first follow-up year, the relative excess risk of death was least among patients who had both surgery and radiation (Fig 13–3), whereas in the second to 15th follow-up year, it was highest among patients who had radiation and the oldest patients, irrespective of treatment (Fig 13–4).

Conclusion.—In patients with intracranial glioma, the prognosis is sig-

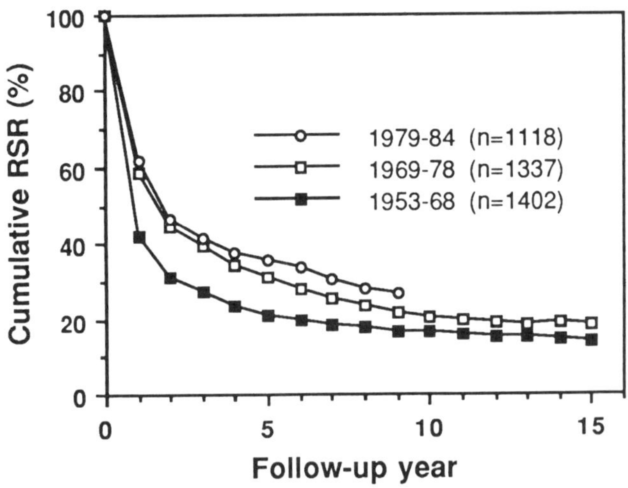

Fig 13–2.—Cumulative relative survival rates (RSR) according to calendar period of diagnosis. (Courtesy of Kallio M, Sankila R, Jääskeläinen J, et al: *Cancer* 68:1394–1400, 1991.)

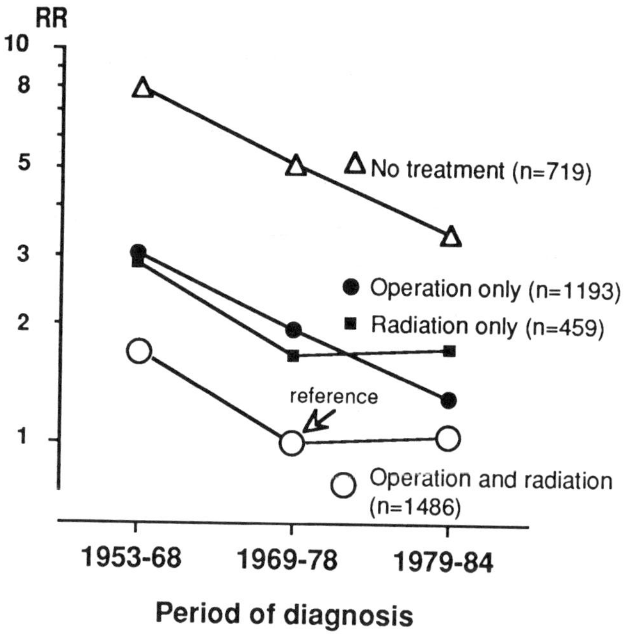

Fig 13–3.—Relative excess risk of death (RR) in the first follow-up year for the 3,857 patients (according to treatment and period of diagnosis). The reference value is 1. (Courtesy of Kallio M, Sankila R, Jääskeläinen J, et al: *Cancer* 68:1394–1400, 1991.)

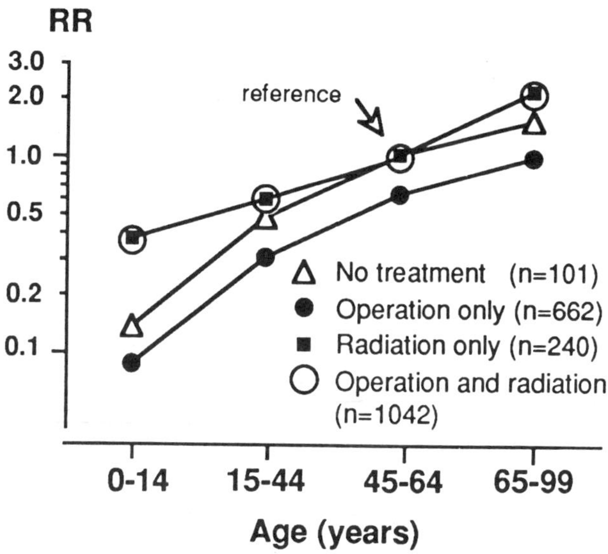

Fig 13–4.—Relative excess risk of death (RR) in the second to 15th follow-up year for the 2,045 patients surviving the first follow-up year according to age and treatment. The reference value is 1. The values for the group given radiation only and for the group treated by operation and radiation are almost identical. (Courtesy of Kallio M, Sankila R, Jääskeläinen J, et al: *Cancer* 68:1394–1400, 1991.)

nificantly better among young patients who have received a recent diagnosis and who have undergone both operation and radiation.

▶ This large study from Finland is included because it is 1 of the few articles that includes an entire national population. The authors state that the observed increase in the frequency of gliomas, which was more than doubled in both men and women, was probably a result of improved diagnosis. However, there have also been reported increases in glioma in this country in the past 2 decades, and one wonders whether better diagnosis is the only explanation. The figures included in this article and reproduced for the YEAR BOOK provide an encapsulated summary of the "natural" history of this difficult tumor. One must keep in mind, however, that approximately 18% of the 3,857 patients received no therapy, and the remainder received surgery alone, radiation alone, or a combination of surgery and radiation. Figure 13–1 demonstrates very clearly that age is an important prognostic feature in this tumor. Figure 13–2 is the most depressing, demonstrating little improvement in survival during a 30-year period. The slight improvement observed may have been a result of the differences shown in Figure 13–3, indicating that the risk of death in the first year was certainly lowest in patients treated with both surgery and radiation. However, after the first year (as shown in Figure 13–4), the relative risk of death was not very different among the treatment groups except, perhaps, in the pediatric age group.

Rather than view these results with pessimism for future progress, I believe that the ability to segregate any positive effects is very useful for interpreting modern treatment regimens. For example, anything done in the first year (other than no treatment) improves the outcome during that period and moves the survival curve to the better. On the other hand, as new modalities or agents are tried in the first year after diagnosis, one should not be dazzled by slight improvements after only a few years follow-up.—J.V. Simone, M.D.

Long-Term Outcome of 89 Low-Grade Brain-Stem Gliomas After Interstitial Radiation Therapy

Mundinger F, Braus DF, Krauss JK, Birg W (Neurosurgical Hosp, Freiburg, Germany)

J Neurosurg 75:740–746, 1991 13–2

Background.—The management of low-grade brain stem gliomas remains controversial. Between 1974 and 1985, 89 patients with brain stem lesions underwent stereotactic biopsy aided by CT, and all had low-grade brain stem astrocytomas. Twenty-six patients were treated interstitially with iridium-192 (^{192}Ir) and 29 were treated with iodine-125 (^{125}I). The long-term results of this treatment modality were evaluated.

Pathological features.—For the radiation therapy group, CT showed that 78% of the tumors were located predominantly in the mesencephalic region, 70% were circumscribed, and 78% were contrast-enhanced. For the 34 patients who underwent biopsy alone, 70% of the tumors were

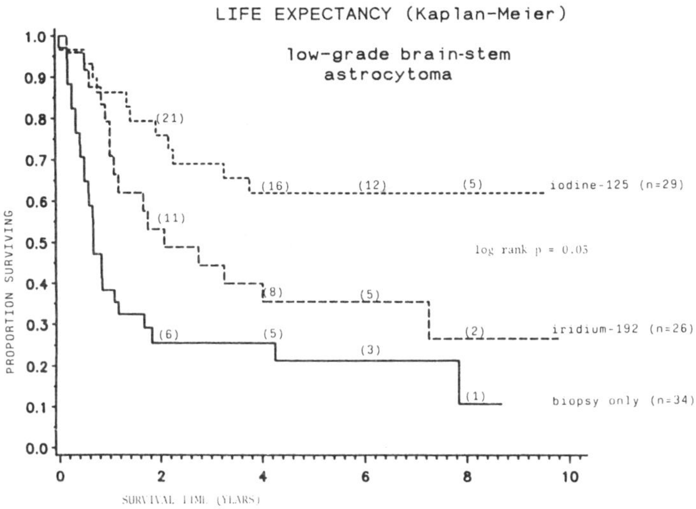

Fig 13–5.—An actuarial representation of the proportion of 89 patients with brain stem astrocytoma surviving, grouped by treatment modality as "biopsy only," "iridium-192," and "iodine-125." (From Kaplan EL, Meier P: *J Am Stat Assoc* 53:457–481, 1958.) The number of surviving patients at each interval is shown in parentheses. N = the number of patients in each treatment group. (Courtesy of Mundinger F, Braus DF, Krauss JK, et al: *J Neurosurg* 75:740–746, 1991.)

located predominantly in the pons, 74% were diffuse, and 59% were hypodense or isodense on contrast enhancement.

Outcome.—During an average catamnestic period of 40.8 months (range, 1–167 months), 30 patients were alive, including 19 treated with ^{125}I, 6 treated with ^{192}Ir, and 5 treated with biopsy only. The actual survival rate at 5 years was 54.8% in the ^{125}I group, 26.9% in the ^{192}Ir group, and 14.7% in the biopsy group. The life expectancy curve, using the Kaplan-Meier method, showed a marginal statistically significant difference between the ^{125}I group and the ^{192}Ir group (Fig 13–5). Life expectancy did not differ significantly between patients with grade I and II brain stem gliomas.

Conclusion.—Stereotactic radiation therapy with interstitial ^{125}I appears to be an appropriate and effective treatment for slowly proliferating, differentiated, well-delineated, nonresectable gliomas of the brain stem. There is a trend toward improved life expectancy when compared with ^{192}Ir implantation.

▶ Interstitial radiation therapy is 1 of the more attractive options for the treatment of gliomas. Implantation of a radiation source directly in the tumor makes it possible to deliver substantially higher tumor doses of radiation while sparing a larger bulk of normal tissue. Although the number of patients is not large, the results shown in the figure certainly suggest that interstitial therapy with ^{125}I is a promising alternative to conventional therapy. The newer technology that allows stereotactic placement of radiation sources may make this approach far more common in the near future.—J.V. Simone, M.D.

Outcome and Patterns of Failure Following Limited-Volume Irradiation for Malignant Astrocytomas

Garden AS, Maor MH, Yung WKA, Bruner JM, Woo SY, Moser RP, Lee Y-Y
(Univ of Texas, Houston)

Radiother Oncol 20:99–110, 1991 13–3

Introduction.—Whole-brain irradiation has been the accepted radiation treatment for high-grade astrocytomas. The advent of CT and MRI permit superior tumor localization. A trial of limited volume irradiation was conducted in 60 patients with high-grade astrocytomas, 39 of whom had glioblastoma multiforme (GBM) and 21 of whom had anaplastic astrocytoma (AA). Paresis, headache, and seizure were the most common symptoms, and the frontal lobe was the most common tumor site.

Methods.—In 13 patients, radiation was administered after biopsy; in 47, resection was performed before radiation. In 7 patients, whole-brain irradiation was performed because of multiple primary tumors, tumor invasion of the ventricular system, or large tumors; the other 53 patients had limited volume irradiation determined from the presurgical CT scan. The patients received a mean tumor dose of 65.4 Gy.

Results.—For patients with GBM, the 1-year survival rate was 40% and the 2-year survival rate was 14%. For patients with AA, the 1-year survival rate was 76% and the 2-year survival was 52%. At 1 year, 13% of patients with GBM and 29% of patients with AA were progression free (Fig 13–6). Postirradiation CT scans showed evidence of progression in 34 of 48 patients who had limited-volume irradiation. A new intracranial metastatic site was seen in 6 patients; this site was within the irradiated volume in 3 patients. All 6 patients also had progression of their primary tumor. Recurrent masses necessitated at least 1 reoperation

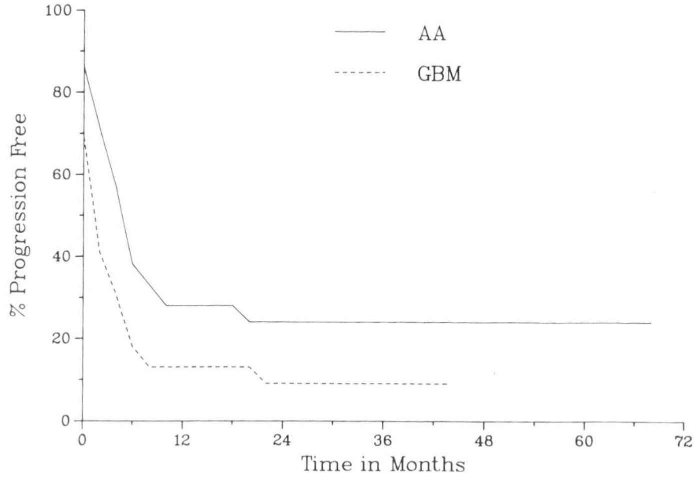

Fig 13–6.—Freedom from progression (percent) of patients with glioblastoma or anaplastic astrocytoma. (Courtesy of Garden AS, Maor MH, Yung WKA, et al: *Radiother Oncol* 20:99–110, 1991.)

in 21 patients. Tumors recurred in the primary site in 19 patients, and there was necrosis without tumor in 2.

Conclusion.—Survival appears to be the same for patients who receive limited volume irradiation for high-grade astrocytomas as for those who receive whole-brain irradiation. The outcome is better for patients who have reoperation for suspected recurrence; thus, reoperation appears to be justified for such recurrences.

▶ This careful study by good investigators demonstrates conclusively that, with the improved imaging that has been developed during the last decade and a half, there is no benefit to be obtained from whole-brain irradiation in the treatment of high-grade malignant gliomas. The revolution in CT and MRI that has taken place makes it unnecessary to treat the whole brain any more. In addition, the use of limited-volume techniques generally implies that one can use higher dose. Even so, photon irradiation by itself does not appear to be adequate, except in a modest minority of patients with AA. With today's imaging technology, there is no further indication for whole-branch irradiation in primary gliomas.—E. Glatstein, M.D.

Improved Survival With the Use of Adjuvant Chemotherapy in the Treatment of Medulloblastoma

Packer RJ, Sutton LN, Goldwein JW, Perilongo G, Bunin G, Ryan J, Cohen BH, D'Angio G, Kramer ED, Zimmerman RA, Rorke LB, Evans AE, Schut L (Children's Hosp of Philadelphia, Pa)

J Neurosurg 74:433–440, 1991 13–4

Background.—The value of adjuvant chemotherapy was examined in a series of 108 children treated between 1975 and 1989 for newly diagnosed medulloblastoma/primitive neuroectodermal tumor (MB/PNET) of the posterior fossa. Starting in 1983, standard-risk patients received craniospinal radiotherapy alone, whereas those assigned to a poor-risk group received adjuvant chemotherapy as well.

Management.—When possible, posterior fossa decompression was done within 48 hours of diagnosis. Total resection of the tumor was attempted in all cases. Most patients received craniospinal radiotherapy first, followed by a local tumor boost. Adjuvant chemotherapy included CCNU, vincristine, and cisplatin, starting 6 weeks after radiotherapy was completed.

Results.—Those patients treated from 1975 to 1982 had an actuarial 5-year disease-free survival rate of 68%. When patients dying within 2 weeks of surgery were excluded, the rate increased to 73%. Survival improved subsequently with adjuvant chemotherapy in poor-risk patients (Fig 13–7), but the prognosis did not change significantly for children with standard-risk factors. Before 1983, younger patients had a poorer outlook.

Conclusions.—At present, children with MB/PNET have a relatively

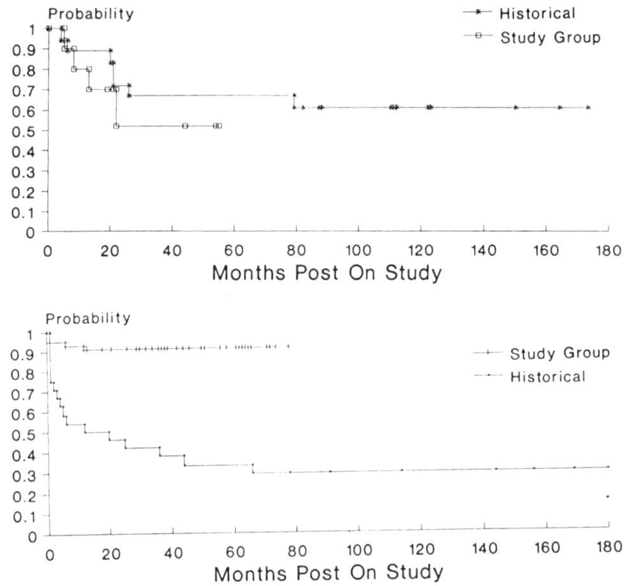

Fig 13–7.—Five-year actuarial disease-free survival rate for children with MB/PNET treated between 1983 and 1989. **Top,** the rate for children with standard-risk disease. The historical group (18 cases) includes those treated between 1975 and 1982, and the study group (10 cases) includes those treated with radiation therapy alone. **Bottom,** the rate for children with poor-risk MB-PNET. The historical group (18 cases) includes those treated between 1975 and 1982, and the study group (42 patients) includes all poor-risk patients treated with both radiation therapy and chemotherapy. (Courtesy of Packer RJ, Sutton LN, Goldwein JW, et al: *J Neurosurg* 74:433–440, 1991.)

encouraging outlook when managed by aggressive resection followed by both radiotherapy and chemotherapy. The side-effects from cisplatin have generally been transient.

▶ Medulloblastoma is one of the brain tumors with significant hope for long-term, disease-free survival. The authors demonstrate that, since 1983, the results of therapy have improved in an interesting manner. The outcome using aggressive adjuvant chemotherapy after surgery and radiotherapy in patients thought to be at poor risk improved substantially, as is shown in Figure 13–7. In the more favorable group, the results not only failed to improve, but were not as good as those seen in the poor-risk group in the early follow-up period. There are a variety of ways of interpreting this data, but the simplest interpretation is that therapy is a more important prognostic feature than whatever pretherapeutic parameters the authors had chosen. Perhaps the more aggressive chemotherapy should be used in all patients, allowing for a reduction in radiation therapy that is responsible for many of the undesirable late effects on brain function. The authors have indicated that they had already reduced the standard radiation dosage from 2,400 to 1,800 cGy for children younger than 5 years of age, with no apparent loss of effectiveness. If that result persists, therapy for this tumor may rely more heavily on chemotherapy and less on radiation therapy.—J.V. Simone, M.D.

Experimental Therapy of Human Glioma by Means of a Genetically Engineered Virus Mutant

Martuza RL, Malick A, Markert JM, Ruffner KL, Coen DM (Harvard Med School, Boston; Massachusetts Gen Hosp-East, Charlestown, Mass)
Science 252:854–856, 1991 13–5

Introduction.—A large percentage of brain tumors in the United States are gliomas. Glioblastomas are almost always fatal, and no present therapeutic modality has changed the outcome for patients with this type of cancer. The use of a genetically engineered virus found to destroy glioma cells and spare normal brain cells was examined.

Methods.—Twenty nude mice were inoculated with cell inoculum that caused 100% mortality within 1.5 months in a pilot study. The mice were then divided into 3 groups. One group received 10^3 pfu of *dl*sptk, a thymidine kinase-negative mutant of herpes simplex virus-1; group 2 received 10^5 pfu of *dl*sptk; and a control group received DME+ alonc.

Outcomes.—Growth inhibition of the tumor was noted in mice with subrenal U87 human gliomas given *dl*sptk. In mice with intracranial U87 gliomas given *dl*sptk, the survival was longer. In cell culture, human glioblastoma cells were destroyed.

Conclusions.—Genetically engineered viruses may play an important role in the treatment of some resistant tumors, such as malignant human gliomas. These viruses merit evaluation as new antineoplastic agents and should be further investigated.

▶ I couldn't resist including this paper, because it takes an entirely different approach to the treatment of gliomas. Talk about a magic bullet! This type of study has a long way to go, but with the dismal results we obtain in treating gliomas in humans, we could do a lot worse than introduce mutant viruses that are specifically toxic for the brain tumor cells.—J.V. Simone, M.D.

14 Head and Neck Tumors

Diagnosis of Nasopharyngeal Carcinoma by DNA Amplification of Tissue Obtained by Fine-Needle Aspiration

Feinmesser R, Miyazaki I, Cheung R, Freeman JL, Noyek AM, Dosch H-M (Hosp for Sick Children, Toronto, Ont, Canada; Mount Sinai Hosp, Toronto, Ont, Canada; Beilinson Med Ctr, Tel Aviv, Israel)

N Engl J Med 326:17–21, 1992 14–1

Objective.—In patients with nasopharyngeal carcinoma, it may be difficult to detect the primary lesion from metastases. The nasopharyngeal carcinoma cells carry the viral genoma of the Epstein-Barr virus (EBV). The relationship between EBV and nasopharyngeal carcinoma with metastasis to the neck was evaluated.

Methods.—Tumor samples from 41 patients with metastatic squamous cell carcinoma of the neck were tested by polymerase chain reaction to assess the presence of EBV genomes. Fifteen samples were obtained by fine-needle aspiration, and 26 were obtained by lymph node biopsy. The tumors were sampled at various stages. A variety of controls were also tested: disease-free nodes from 10 patients with various neck tumors; tonsillar tissue from 46 subjects; blood from EBV-seropositive blood donors; and mononuclear cells from 8 patients with fatal lymphoproliferative lesions.

Findings.—The EBV genomes were found only in the 9 nasopharyngeal carcinomas—1 primary tumor and 8 metastases. No EBV could be detected in the 20 nodes with other types of cancer, the 10 disease-free nodes, or any of the 105 normal controls. On the basis of the presence of EBV, 2 patients with suspected metastases from occult primary tumors were predicted to have nasopharyngeal carcinoma—this tumor developed in both within 1 year.

Conclusion.—The DNA amplification of EBV genomes can be diagnostic of nasopharyngeal carcinoma; tissue for diagnosis can be obtained by fine-needle aspiration biopsy. When EBV is found in metastases from an occult primary tumor, the development of overt nasopharyngeal carcinoma can be predicted. A large, prospective study of this conclusion is underway.

▶ The diagnosis of nasopharyngeal cancer can be difficult because of both inadequate visualization of the nasopharynx and the tendency of primary tumors to infiltrate submucosally, which can produce false negative superficial biopsy specimens. Even when neck metastases are obvious, the diagnosis can still be difficult, because the nasopharynx can appear normal. This is of more than academic interest, because treatment decisions are based on histopathology. Nasopharyngeal tumors are treated with radiation both for the primary tumor and for neck metastases, whereas other squamous cell tumors of the head and neck are treated surgically. An association between EBV and nasopharyngeal carcinoma has been well recognized. This study concludes that fine-needle aspirations of neck metastases provide sufficient tumor for diagnosis (using the polymerase chain reaction) of nasopharyngeal carcinoma by DNA amplification of the EBV genome. This should help in the diagnosis of nasopharyngeal carcinomas in patients with occult tumors of the head and neck, and it can also be used to help select specific forms of treatment.—R.F. Ozols, M.D., Ph.D.

Nasopharyngeal Carcinoma: CT Evaluation of Patterns of Tumor Spread

Sham JST, Cheung YK, Choy D, Chan FL, Leong L (Queen Mary Hosp, Pokfulam, Hong Kong)

AJNR 12:265–270, 1991 14–2

Objective.—In a prospective study, 262 patients with newly diagnosed nasopharyngeal carcinoma were examined to assess the role of CT in the evaluation of tumor spread at initial presentation, with special emphasis on the qualitative assessment of paranasopharyngeal extension of tumor.

Methods.—The involvement of the paranasopharyngeal space is evaluated with reference to 3 anatomical lines (Fig 14–1). The first line extends from the medial pterygoid plate to the carotid artery; the second line extends from the scaphoid fossa to the styloid process; and the third

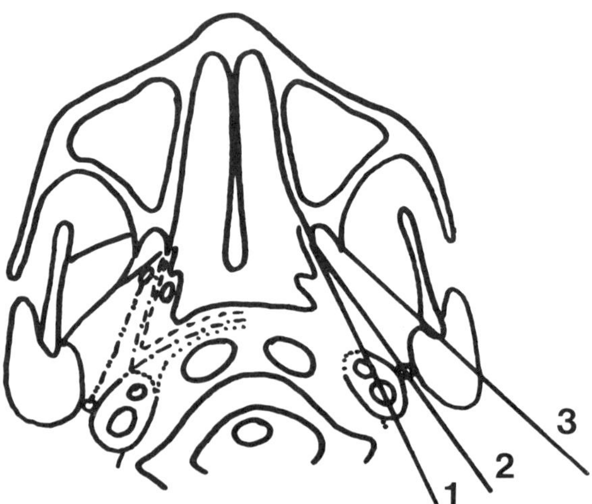

Fig 14–1.—Schematic drawing outlines pharyngobasilar fascia *(dashed line)*, buccopharyngeal fascia *(dot-dash line)*, prevertebral fascia *(dotted line)*, and tensor palatini fascia *(dash-dot-dot line)*, on the right side. The 3 lines for evaluating the degree of paranasopharyngeal extension are on the left side: 1 = into the retrostyloid space; 2 = into the prestyloid space; 3 = into the anterior part of masticator space. (Courtesy of Sham JST, Cheung YK, Choy D, et al: *AJNR* 12:265–270, 1991.)

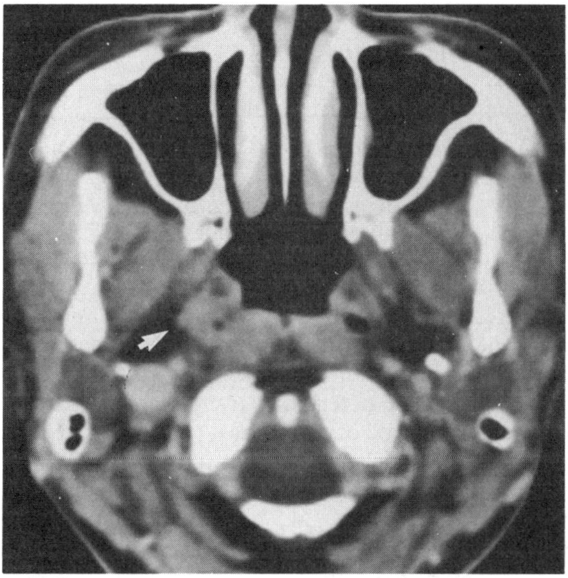

Fig 14–2.—Type 1 paranasopharyngeal extension on the right side. Tumor *(arrow)* has extended beyond line joining medial pterygoid plate and lateral border of carotid artery. Note the absence of paranasopharyngeal extension on the left side. (Courtesy of Sham JST, Cheung YK, Choy D, et al: *AJNR* 12:265–270, 1991.)

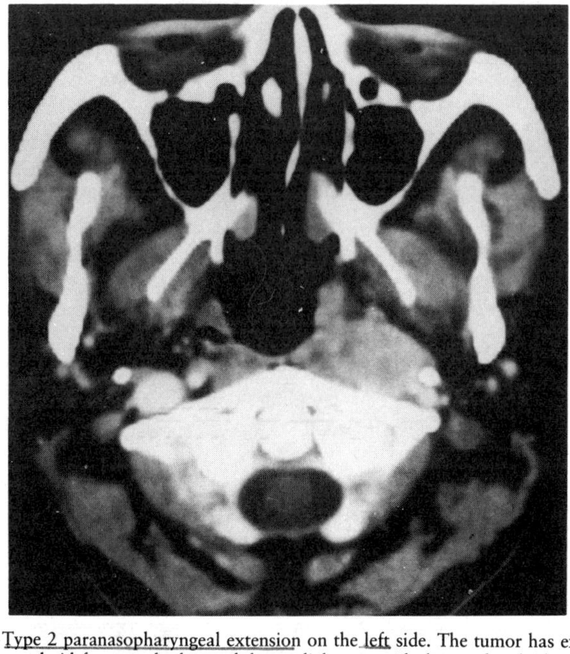

Fig 14–3.—Type 2 paranasopharyngeal extension on the left side. The tumor has extended beyond line, joining the scaphoid fossa at the base of the medial pterygoid plate and styloid process. Note the absence of paranasopharyngeal extension on the right side. (Courtesy of Sham JST, Cheung YK, Choy D, et al: *AJNR* 12:265–270, 1991.)

line extends from the lateral pterygoid plate to the ascending ramus of the mandible. The tumors, by reaching or extending beyond these lines, were ranked as types 1–3, respectively (Figs 14–2, 14–3, and 14–4).

Findings.—Tumor spread most commonly involved the paranasopharyngeal space (84.4%), both unilaterally and bilaterally, followed by the sphenoid sinus (26.7%), nasal fossa (21.8%), and ethmoid sinus (18.3%). Erosions of the base of the skull (31.3%) and intracranial extensions (12.2%) were also common. The primary tumor in the nasopharynx was contiguous with the metastatic upper cervical nodes indirectly through paranasopharyngeal extension of the tumor in 13.4% of the patients. The extent of paranasopharyngeal extension correlated significantly with other attributes of tumor extent, namely, nasal or oropharyngeal extension (T3-level tumor) and erosion of the base of the skull or orbit (T4-level tumor). The extent of paranasopharyngeal extension also correlated with local control of the tumor. At a median follow-up of 27 months, nasopharyngeal relapse occurred in only 3 (7.9%) of 38 patients with no paranasopharyngeal extension, compared with 12 (11.2%) of 107 patients with type 1 and 17 (34.7%) of 49 patients with type 2 paranasopharyngeal extensions.

Conclusions.—Computed tomography has a definitive role in the evaluation of patients with nasopharyngeal carcinoma. It provides accurate assessment of the extent of the tumor, (e.g., erosion of the base of the

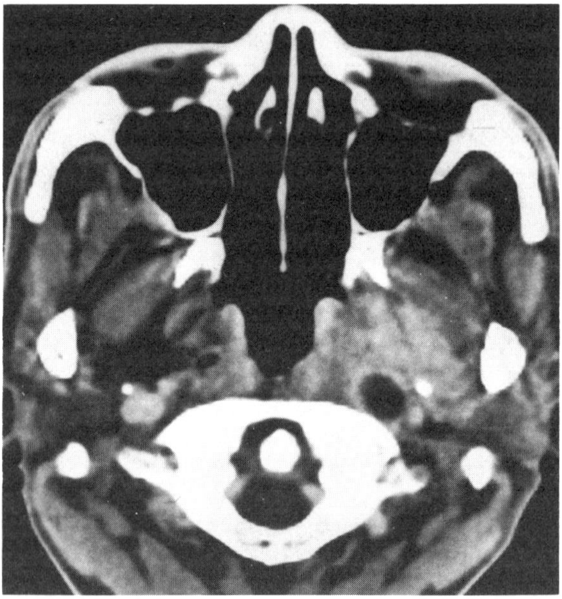

Fig 14–4.—Type 3 paranasopharyngeal extension on the left side. The tumor has extended beyond line, joining the lateral pterygoid plate and posterior border of the ascending ramus of the mandible. Note central necrosis of the node in the left paranasopharyngeal space and the absence of paranasopharyngeal extension on the right side. (Courtesy of Sham JST, Cheung YK, Choy D, et al: *AJNR* 12:265–270, 1991.)

skull and intracranial extension of the tumor), evaluation of the lateral extension of the tumor to the paranasopharyngeal space, and documentation of the extensive posterolateral extension of tumor contiguous with metastatic cervical nodes.

▶ This is an excellent radiologic evaluation of the interpretation of CT in assessing the patterns of spread of carcinoma of the nasopharynx. An extremely high frequency of the involvement of the paranasopharyngeal space was recognized, as were erosion of the base of the skull and extension into the middle cranial fossa. To accurately assess individual patients and define appropriate radiotherapy (including an accurate tumor volume), these patterns should be studied by the physicians caring for such patients.—E. Glatstein, M.D.

Incisional or Excisional Neck-Node Biopsy Before Definitive Radiotherapy, Alone or Followed by Neck Dissection

Ellis ER, Mendenhall WM, Rao PV, McCarty PJ, Parsons JT, Stringer SP, Cassisi NJ, Million RR (Univ of Florida, Gainesville)

Head Neck 13:177–183, 1991 14–3

Methods.—The effect of open neck-node biopsy before definitive treatment of squamous cell carcinoma of the head and neck remains controversial. Therefore, the influence of pretreatment incisional or excisional neck-node biopsy in patients treated either with radiotherapy alone or with planned neck dissection was studied in 508 patients with head and neck squamous cell carcinoma and clinically positive neck nodes. Treatment consisted of radiotherapy alone to the primary lesion, with or without neck dissection. The probability of neck disease control, the risk of distant metastasis, and the cause-specific survival rates were established. A control group of 442 patients who did not have a neck-node biopsy served as the comparison group.

Results.—The biopsy had no detrimental effect on neck control, distant metastasis, or cause-specific survival. Biopsy status was not among the first 4 factors for any of the outcome variables analyzed in a multivariate analysis, which included N stage, neck treatment, node mobility, node location, T stage, primary site, control of disease above the clavicles, and biopsy status of the neck. The 4 most important factors in neck recurrence were increasing N stage, treatment of the neck with radiotherapy alone, fixed nodes, and T stage.

Conclusion.—When radiotherapy is the next stage of treatment, there appears to be no adverse effect of violating the neck before definitive treatment. Open neck-node biopsy is not recommended, because it may complicate subsequent management and is often unnecessary. A needle biopsy of the suspicious neck node is the usual procedure when a careful search for a mucosal head and neck primary lesion is not successful.

▶ The traditional surgical teaching in head and neck cancer is that performing open biopsy for diagnostic purposes leads to a decreased chance for a cure.

Although this may be true for patients whose cancer is managed with surgery alone, this paper presents an interesting analysis from thorough investigators in head and neck cancer. They demonstrate that performing biopsy on a neck node for diagnosis, either incisionally or excisionally, does not imply a poor survival if the next step is radiation therapy. All too often, patients with this problem are managed with a radical neck dissection to avoid the impact of the open biopsy. This study lends support to those who would recommend such a procedure before radiotherapy. It is implied that the spread that may result from the biopsy procedure can still be sterilized by adequate doses of radiation therapy. Even so, it is not usually necessary to recommend an open biopsy of the neck, especially if a diagnosis can be obtained from the primary site or if needle biopsy of a suspicious neck node can be obtained. If an open biopsy has been performed in the neck and a diagnosis of cancer has been established, then the authors recommend radiotherapy as the next step in the patient's management, either with definitive radiation or preoperative radiotherapy. In any event, this is an important paper for those involved in the management of patients with head and neck cancer.—E. Glatstein, M.D.

Elapsed Treatment Days: A Critical Item for Radiotherapy Quality Control Review in Head and Neck Trials: RTOG Report

Pajak TF, for the Radiation Therapy Oncology Group (American College of Radiology, Philadelphia, Pa)

Int J Radiat Oncol Biol Phys 20:13–20, 1991 14–4

Introduction.—Radiation Therapy Oncology Group studies usually include a review of patient treatment that checks for compliance in terms of borders, total dose, fraction, and total elapsed time. In 2 head and neck studies in patients, prolonged elapsed treatment was not used to qualify treatment as unacceptable.

Methods.—Data from these 2 studies of 426 patients were reevaluated to assess the relationship between prolonged elapsed treatment time and outcome.

Results.—Those patients with treatment prolonged by 14 days or more had significantly worse locoregional control and absolute survival than those treated promptly. Even after adjustment for other prognostic factors, these differences remained significant.

Conclusion.—Prolonging elapsed radiotherapy treatment time results in significantly poorer outcome in patients with head and neck carcinoma. Therefore, sequential treatment with chemotherapy and radiotherapy should be compared with simultaneous treatment, which would not increase the overall treatment time.

▶ This is an important paper that documents the importance of the timing of radiotherapy treatment. As treatment becomes extensively protracted, it can allow repopulation to occur, thereby defeating the purpose of the treatment. There is some point beyond which things cannot be protracted realistically. This may vary from patient to patient; however, the authors demonstrate quite nicely that breaks in treatment can potentially harm a patient with head and neck cancer. This kind of insight represents a stimulus to those who argue for treatment with accelerated hyperfractionation (i.e., twice a day or three times a day) to shorten the overall treatment time.—E. Glatstein, M.D.

Randomized Study of Preoperative Versus Postoperative Radiation Therapy in Advanced Head and Neck Carcinoma: Long-Term Follow-up of RTOG Study 73-03

Tupchong L, for the Radiation Therapy Oncology Group (Thomas Jefferson Univ Hosp, Philadelphia, Pa)

Int J Radiat Oncol Biol Phys 20:21–28, 1991 14–5

Introduction.—In May 1973, the Radiation Therapy Oncology Group (RTOG) began a phase III study comparing preoperative radiation therapy with postoperative radiation therapy for supraglottic larynx and hypopharynx primary tumors. The results after a 10-year median follow-up period were reviewed.

Results.—Of the 277 patients who were initially enrolled in the study, approximately 7% were unavailable for follow-up. Among the remaining patients, locoregional control was significantly better for the postoperative radiation group than for the preoperative radiation group. However, absolute survival was not significantly different between the 2 groups. When only the supraglottic larynx tumors were considered, the difference in control was even more significant, but survival was still not significantly different. The rate of complications from treatment was similar in the 2 groups. By 2 years after therapy, distant metastases and second primary tumors were the predominant failure pattern in both groups.

Conclusion.—Although there was no difference in survival between the pre- and postoperative radiation groups, there appears to be an advantage in control in the postoperative group. However, to increase survival significantly, additional therapeutic intervention is required to decrease the incidence of distant metastases and second primary tumors.

▶ These are the results of a 10-year median follow-up of patients with advanced head and neck cancer, comparing preoperative radiotherapy with postoperative radiotherapy. In terms of survival, there was no difference. Local control was statistically significantly improved with postoperative radiotherapy compared with preoperative radiotherapy. It appeared to be especially improved with the supraglottic larynx receiving postoperative radiation; however, these kinds of subpopulation analyses can be misleading. It is important to note that, even in these supraglottic subpopulations, no survival gain was seen. One wonders what the survival outcomes would look like if they were compared with radiation therapy alone (with curative intent) and a surgical salvage. Unfortunately, that type of treatment was not administered in this prospective study.—E. Glatstein, M.D.

Cisplatin and Fluorouracil Chemotherapy Does Not Yield Long-Term Benefit in Locally Advanced Head and Neck Cancer: Results From a Single Institution

Vokes EE, Mick R, Lester EP, Panje WR, Weichselbaum RR (Univ of Chicago, Ill)

J Clin Oncol 9:1376–1384, 1991 14–6

Objective.—Fifty-one patients with locally advanced head-neck squamous cell carcinoma without evident distant disease received 3 cycles of cisplatin and fluorouracil (5-FU) as induction treatment. None of the patients had been treated previously.

Treatment Plan.—A dose of cisplatin, 100 mg/m^2, was followed by a 5-day continuous infusion of 5-FU in a daily dose of 1,000 mg/m^2. Surgery ensued when possible, and the patients also were irradiated. Those patients who responded at least partially to induction treatment received 3 cycles of adjuvant chemotherapy.

Outcome.—Clinical complete remission was noted in 22 patients (43%) and was confirmed pathologically in 12 (24%) (table). Another 24 patients (47%) had a partial remission. Twenty-four patients had surgery, and 22 had radiation therapy alone as local treatment. Adjuvant chemotherapy, often in a much reduced dosage, was given to 32 patients. At a median follow-up of 90 months for the 9 patients who were alive at last contact, the median survival was estimated to be 22 months, and the 5-year survival rate was 25% (Fig 14–5). The median time to progression was 14 months. Eight patients had a progressive second neoplasm.

Conclusions.—Despite high initial response rates, the overall survival of patients with locally advanced head-neck cancer who receive cisplatin and 5-FU chemotherapy is not encouraging. This regimen should not be routinely used in the community setting.

Response by Tumor Stage, Node Stage, and Overall Stage

Stage	CR (%)	No CR (%)	*P*
Tumor			
T_1	0 (0)	2 (100)	
T_2	1 (50)	1 (50)	
T_3	13 (57)	10 (43)	
T_4	8 (35)	15 (65)	.30
Node			
N_0	8 (53)	7 (47)	
N_1	7 (44)	9 (56)	
N_2	3 (43)	4 (57)	
N_3	4 (33)	8 (67)	.76
Overall			
III	11 (65)	6 (35)	
IV	11 (33)	22 (67)	.04

(Courtesy of Vokes EE, Mick R, Lester EP, et al: *J Clin Oncol* 9:1376–1384, 1991.)

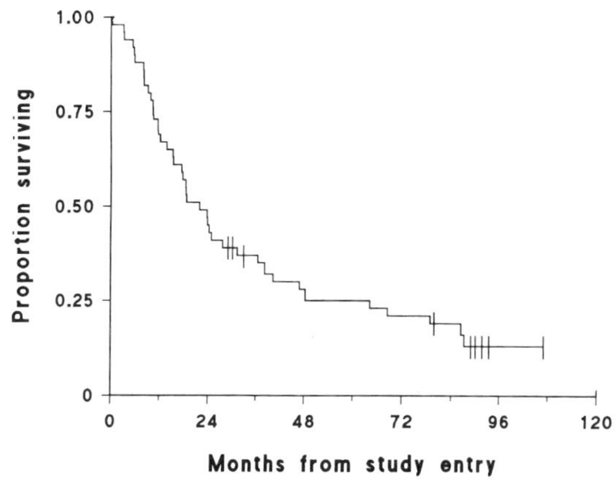

Fig 14–5.—Overall survival. Tick marks indicate patients alive. (Courtesy of Vokes EE, Mick R, Lester EP, et al: *J Clin Oncol* 9:1376–1384, 1991.)

▶ This is an interesting and important study done by thorough investigators interested in the use of combined-modality treatment for head and neck cancer. The important observations they make focus on the fact that, despite the known responsiveness of head and neck cancer to chemotherapy, the long-term follow-up shows no real gain in survival or disease-free status compared with what is expected from radiation therapy/surgery alone. The essential point is that patients with advanced head and neck cancer who are at high risk for dissemination show no evidence that the adjuvant or neoadjuvant cisplatinum and 5-FU treatment can sterilize micrometastatic disease. The local control figures are approximately what is expected with local treatments alone in advanced head and neck treatments. Although there clearly is a need to deliver effective systemic treatment to these patients, caution should be used at all times when interpreting data with short follow-up in such difficult problems. At this time, chemotherapy has no clearly established role in advanced head and neck cancer, and further studies will require careful controls from a randomized investigation.—E. Glatstein, M.D.

Concomitant Boost Radiotherapy Schedules in the Treatment of Carcinoma of the Oropharynx and Nasopharynx

Ang KK, Peters LJ, Weber RS, Maor MH, Morrison WH, Wendt CD, Brown BW (Univ of Texas, Houston)

Int J Radiat Oncol Biol Phys 19:1339–1345, 1991 14–7

Background.—Tumor clonogen proliferation during conventional fractionated irradiation may be overcome by shortening the overall duration of treatment. To shorten the treatment duration without increasing the size of dose per fraction, 2 or more fractions can be delivered each day, separated by sufficient interfraction interval. The concomitant boost, a variant of accelerated treatment, can deliver the boost (10–12 fractions) as second daily treatments during, rather than after, the basic wide-field irradiations.

Method.—The radiotherapy boost is delivered during the basic wide field treatment as a second daily dose to a reduced "field-within-a-field." Seventy-nine patients with T2–T4 carcinomas of the oropharynx or nasopharynx were treated with 1 of 3 variants of the concomitant boost technique.

Results.—Optimal timing for the concomitant boost is during the last 2–2½ weeks of the basic treatment. The severity of acute reactions in patients receiving this schedule of treatments was similar to that occurring after a boost given twice a week, but less than that occurring after a boost administered at the beginning of treatment. Tumor control on this schedule appeared to be superior both to the other schedules and to the historical control group. Acute mucosal reactions were more severe than those observed with conventional fractionation, but there were few late complications.

Conclusions.—A concomitant boost schedule of twice-a-day radiotherapy for patients with head and neck cancer produced better results than conventional radiotherapy. The accelerated fractionation may eliminate tumor regeneration during therapy.

▶ This provocative paper from another group of excellent investigators suggests that the twice-a-day approach has significant value in moderate-to-advanced stage head and neck cancer. A prospectively randomized trial will be required to prove this conclusively, but the data look good. The essential advantages of the twice-a-day approach revolve around the use of the second daily dose to decrease tumor repopulation during the treatment. In addition, there may be some significant gain in the area of reassortment of the tumor cells' inherent radiosensitivity through the cell cycle, because partial synchronization may result from the first fraction. In addition, simply reducing the size of each exposure should have some biological advantage in reducing normal tissue damage, but shortening the overall treatment time and increasing the number of exposures should be critically important in eliminating tumor repopulation during the course of the treatment to make the treatment more effective.—E. Glatstein, M.D.

Expression of Epidermal Growth Factor Receptor in Glottic Carcinoma and Its Relation to Recurrence After Radiotherapy

Miyaguchi M, Olofsson J, Hellquist HB (Kagawa Med School, Kagawa, Japan; University Hosp, Bergen, Norway; Örebro Med Center, Örebro, Sweden)

Clin Otolaryngol 16:466–469, 1991 14–8

Background.—Epidermal growth factor receptor (EGFR) is expressed in laryngeal squamous cell carcinoma but not in normal epithelia. After a full course of radiotherapy, expression of EGFR was immunohistochemically determined in small glottic carcinomas with and without recurrences to investigate whether the amount and distribution of EGFR in these tumors affected recurrence rates.

Methods.—Two groups of patients were studied. Group 1 consisted of 15 patients with recurrent disease after a full course of radiation therapy; group 2 included 18 patients without recurrences. All patients had T_1 glottic and small T_2 glottic-subglottic carcinoma. A 4-graded scale, in which tumors were rated as −, +, ++, or +++, was used.

Results.—Of the recurrent carcinomas, 80% had a staining intensity and stained cell proportion of ++ or +++. By contrast, only 39% of the nonrecurrent carcinomas were rated as ++ or +++. These proportions were significantly different.

Conclusions.—Increased expression of EGFR is a significant prognostic factor for T_1 and small T_2 glottic-subglottic laryngeal squamous cell carcinoma after radiotherapy. Elevated expression may affect the rate of recurrence of glottic squamous cell carcinoma after this treatment.

▶ This is a small, but very provocative series of patients with carcinoma of the glottis, that suggests that the risk of recurrence after radiotherapy is highly correlated with the expression of EGFR. If so, this needs to be confirmed, because it may be very important in the selection of appropriate treatment for an individual patient. Other studies of this nature are obviously of considerable interest.—E. Glatstein, M.D.

Larynx Preservation With Combined Chemotherapy and Radiation Therapy in Advanced but Resectable Head and Neck Cancer

Pfister DG, Strong E, Harrison L, Haines IE, Pfister DA, Sessions R, Spiro R, Shah J, Gerold F, McLure T, Vikram B, Fass D, Armstrong J, Bosl GJ (Mem Sloan-Kettering Cancer Ctr; Cornell Univ, New York)

J Clin Oncol 9:850–859, 1991 14–9

Introduction.—Most previously untreated patients with advanced squamous cell carcinoma of the head and neck (SCHN) respond to combination chemotherapy. However, attempts to combine chemotherapy with radiation therapy and standard surgery have shown no clear survival advantage. A group of 40 patients with resectable stage III and IV SCHN underwent chemotherapy followed by radiotherapy to preserve the larynx. The results of this treatment were reviewed.

Methods.—All of the patients had advanced but resectable squamous cell carcinoma of the larynx, oropharynx, or hypopharynx and would have required total laryngectomy as surgical treatment. The patients received 1–3 cycles of chemotherapy, the first 11 patients with cisplatin-vinblastine and the remainder with very high dose cisplatin/bleomycin. The patients were then reevaluated; those with a complete or partial response at the primary site received radiation therapy with or without neck dissection, and those with less than a partial response received appropriate surgery.

Results.—There was at least a partial response in 65% of the patients (table); 37 patients were referred for radiation therapy. Overall, 78% of

Clinical Response to Chemotherapy

Variable	Total Patients	Clinical Response CR	PR	< PR	CR + PR	%
Primary site only						
T_2/T_3	32	13	13	6	26	81
T_4	8	4	1	3	5	63
Neck only						
N_0	15	—	—	—	—	—
N_1/N_2	10	5	3	2	8	80
N_3	15	8	2	5	10	67
Overall						
Stage						
II/III	18	8	5	5	13	72
IV	22	7	6	9	13	59
Site						
Larynx	13	5	6	2	11	85
Oropharynx	18	9	3	6	12	67
Hypopharynx	9	1	2	6	3	33
Total	40	15	11	14	26	65

(Courtesy of Pfister DG, Strong E, Harrison L, et al: *J Clin Oncol* 9:850–859, 1991.)

the patients had no evidence of disease at a median follow-up of 49 months; the survival rate was 58% at 2 years and 33% at 5 years. The 2-year failure-free survival rate was 42%, and the 5-year rate was 33% (Fig 14–6). Survival may have been affected adversely by 7 patients who refused recommended total laryngectomy. A greater percentage of patients in whom remission was achieved after chemotherapy remained free of disease compared with those in whom less than partial remission was achieved. The larynx was actually preserved in 85% of patients; including those who refused total laryngectomy, the expected rate was 68%.

Conclusion.—In patients with advanced, resectable SCHN, combined treatment with chemotherapy and radiation, with the goal of larynx preservation, appears to be a feasible and effective treatment approach. The patient must be motivated and requires careful monitoring, and the oncologists must cooperate closely.

▶ In today's combined-modality world, this study is an example of what is going on in the area of head and neck cancer treatment. Efforts to take advanced but resectable patients with laryngeal, pharyngeal, and hypopharyngeal lesions resulted in a program for chemotherapy followed by radiation therapy for responsive lesions. The study actually looks impressive, especially if one deletes reference to the hypopharyngeal lesions, which had a very poor rate of regression compared with the other primary sites. This kind of effort to preserve organs will continue as investigators empirically try to match chemotherapy, radiation, and surgery in a way that makes the most sense for the individual patient.—E. Glatstein, M.D.

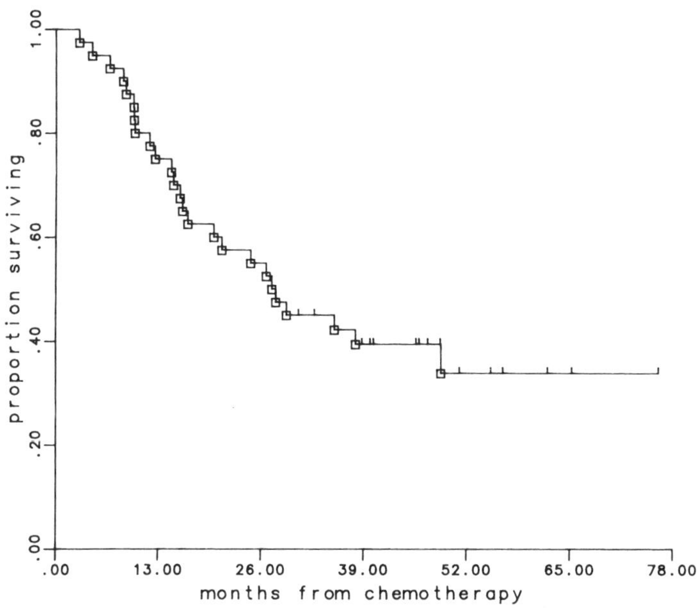

Fig 14–6.—Overall survival measured in months from the first day of chemotherapy. (Courtesy of Pfister DG, Strong E, Harrison L, et al: *J Clin Oncol* 9:850–859, 1991.)

Photon Irradiation of Unresectable Carcinomas of Salivary Glands

Wang CC, Goodman M (Massachusetts Gen Hosp, Boston; Massachusetts Eye & Ear Infirmary, Boston)

Int J Radiat Oncol Biol Phys 21:569–576, 1991 14–10

Objective.—Resection remains the treatment of choice for salivary gland carcinoma. High-dose irradiation is the best option for obtaining locoregional control if a lesion is unresectable. Data were reviewed on 24 patients with unresectable cancers who received photon irradiation from 1980 to 1989.

Patients.—The mean age of the 10 men and 14 women was 71 years. Nine patients had advanced parotid carcinomas and 15 had lesions of the minor salivary glands of the oral cavity or oropharynx.

Management.—Megavoltage irradiation was delivered by using various boost techniques. In patients with high-grade or poorly differentiated lesions, the primary site and regional nodes were comprehensively treated to a median dose of 68 Gy.

Results.—The 5-year overall, actuarial local control rate was 85%, and actuarial survival was 83% (Fig 14–7). All 9 patients with unresectable parotid lesions achieved local control; 65% of them lived 5 years. The respective figures for patients with oral cavity and oropharyngeal lesions were 78% and 93%. Complications from radiation therapy were insignificant. Osteoradionecrosis, soft tissue ulceration, and radiation myelitis were not found in any patient.

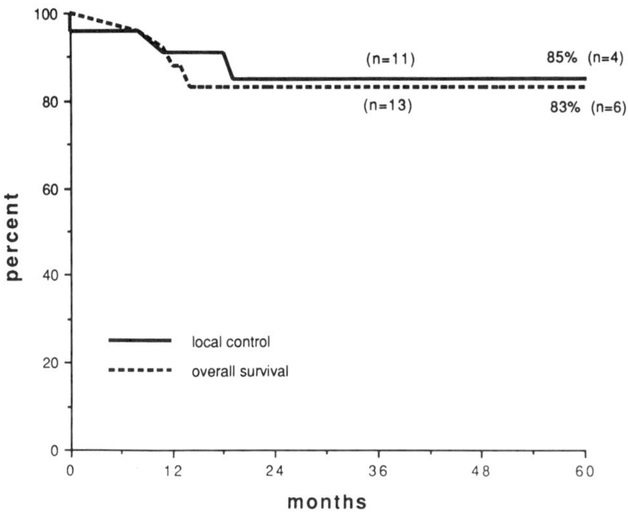

Fig 14–7.—Diagram showing the 5-year actuarial local control and survival rates of 24 patients after radiation therapy. (Courtesy of Wang CC, Goodman M: *Int J Radiat Oncol Biol Phys* 21:569–576, 1991.)

Conclusions.—Modern photon radiation therapy can yield good local control of unresectable salivary gland tumors. Other measures such as adjuvant chemotherapy may help control distant disease in patients whose primary tumor is controlled.

▶ This very interesting paper by careful investigators deals with the relatively neglected problem of inoperable salivary gland tumors treated by photon irradiation. The results in this relatively small series are surprisingly good, with a local control rate of 100% at 5 years and a survival rate of 65%. This is considerably better than what is generally reported in the literature; however, one has to question how aggressively the patients in the literature were treated, because this tumor has been reputed to be a "radioresistant" neoplasm. These investigators used accelerated hyperfractionation. The results are good enough to call into question the results achieved by neutron irradiation.—E. Glatstein, M.D.

15 Endocrine Tumors

Survival and Causes of Death in Thyroid Cancer: A Population-Based Study of 2479 Cases From Norway

Akslen LA, Haldorsen T, Thoresen SØ, Glattre E (Univ of Bergen, Norway; The Cancer Registry of Norway, Oslo)

Cancer Res 51:1234–1241, 1991 15–1

Introduction.—Several previous studies have reported prognostic factors of thyroid cancer (TC), however, methodological problems, such as differences in patient selection criteria between series and changes in therapy over time, plagued most of them. In a population-based study, the major prognostic factors of TC were determined using data collected by a single institution.

Methods.—From 1970 to 1986, 2,479 patients with clinically identified TC were reported to the Norwegian Cancer Registry. Those patients in whom TC was first diagnosed at autopsy were excluded. The 1,977 women and 648 men were observed from the time of diagnosis through 1985. The maximum follow-up was 16 years, and the median follow-up was 48 months.

Findings.—Of the patients with diagnosed TC, 714 (28.8%) died during follow-up. Thyroid cancer was the main cause of death in 498 (69.7%) of these patients. Among the 216 patients who died of other main causes, TC was a contributing factor in 80 (11.2%). When only deaths from TC were considered, there were no sex differences in patient survival for any of the histologic subtypes. The proportion of TC deaths increased with age, except in those patients with anaplastic TC. Only 5 of the 498 patients who died of TC were younger than 35 years. Although none of these 5 patients had papillary TC, survival decreased significantly in patients with papillary TC older than 55 years of age. Marked differences were also observed between various histologic types, even between papillary and follicular TCs when interactions were included. Tumor stage was the third strong predictor of TC death. Regional tumor spread, distant metastases, and lymph node metastases were associated with reduced survival.

Conclusion.—Age, histologic type, and tumor stage are the 3 major prognostic factors in patients with TC.

▶ This study by Akslen et al. is a good, 16-year population-based study of TC in a homogenous population. The strength of this study is that the relatively short period of accrual may prevent the drift in biological characteristics of the cancer that can occur with longer periods of accrual. The authors studied 2,479 cancers that originated during this time, and they came to a number of conclusions that are somewhat provocative when compared with those from studies of similar size in which data was collected for a longer period of time. First, there was a fairly high incidence of second primary cancers (12%). This is unusual, and it was not explained by the authors. The second controversial finding is that there was no benefit in survival for women. It is generally considered that women have a better outcome for TC; however, in this study, women were found to have a rate of disease progression similar to that in men. Finally, the authors found that the stage of disease had a significant impact on survival, and that involvement of regional lymph nodes and extrathyroidal spread of the primary cancer were both poor prognostic factors. This latter observation is quite important, because other series, including the series in Abstract 15–2, suggested that metastasis to the lymph nodes is not a poor prognostic sign at the time of diagnosis.

This series is important because the patients were accrued during a short period of time, without the drift in biological characteristics of TC that may occur in studies that accrue patients during a longer period of time. Thus, the finding that the stage of disease at presentation impacts on survival may be quite important. It will be of interest to determine whether population-based studies of similar magnitude, accrued for 1–2 decades, will match the findings of this series.—J.M. Jessup, M.D.

Prognostic Indices for Tumor Relapse and Tumor Mortality in Follicular Thyroid Carcinoma

Mueller-Gaertner H-W, Brzac HT, Rehpenning W (University Hosp, Hamburg-Eppendorf, Germany)

Cancer 67:1903–1911, 1991 15–2

Objective.—To establish an objective basis for treating follicular thyroid cancer, a prognostic scoring system quantifying clinical, histologic, and therapeutic parameters was developed.

Methods.—The prognostic implications of 9 parameters were examined by multivariate analysis of 149 patients with follicular carcinoma of the thyroid. Prognostic indices conveying the individual risk levels for tumor relapse and tumor mortality were derived. These indices categorized patients into low-, medium-, and high-risk groups.

Observations.—Follow-up (mean, 7.1 years) showed that the risk of relapse increased nearly sevenfold in the presence of a moderate degree, compared with a high degree, of tumor differentiation. The risk increased with advancing age at the time of diagnosis, and was decreased by both neck dissection and percutaneous radiotherapy delivered to the neck (Fig 15–1). The risk of death increased tenfold in the absence of a tumor capsule and sixfold with moderate (compared with high) histologic tumor differentiation. Distant metastasis increased the mortality risk by approximately threefold. Persistent and progressive initial disease leading to death occurred chiefly in older patients, those with higher-stage tumors, and those whose tumors lacked a capsule.

Conclusions.—Prognostic indices for relapse and death can help in selecting those patients who require aggressive treatment for follicular thyroid cancer. Prospective trials are needed to determine the role

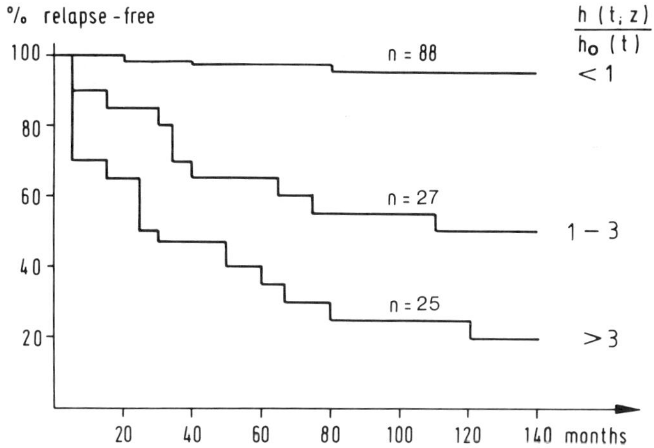

Fig 15–1.—Relapse-free interval (observed data) after initial therapy in the low-risk, medium-risk, and high-risk category of the IRR prognostic index for follicular thyroid carcinomas. The mean follow-up time was 7.1 years (*n* = the number of investigated patients; $h_{(t;z)} / ho_{(t)}$ = individual relative risk of tumor relapse). (Courtesy of Mueller-Gaertner HW, Brzac HT, Rehpenning W: *Cancer* 67:1903–1911, 1991).

of either radioiodine ablation of thyroid remnants or prophylactic radioiodine in low-risk patients.

▶ This study counterbalances the study in Abstract 15–1. In this institutional series, data on 149 patients seen during a 30-year period were analyzed. The authors examined their population for prognostic factors, and they found that age at diagnosis, degree of tumor differentiation (well-differentiated vs. moderately differentiated tumors), and either performance of neck dissection or administration of radiotherapy are significant prognostic factors in a multivariant analysis. Unlike the study in Abstract 15–1, stage was not a significant factor in determining prognosis. Although this study is a careful analysis of 1 type of thyroid carcinoma, it suffers from the difficulty of analyzing patients during a long period of accrual. The disease may have changed its biological characteristics during this time as a result of either changes in the referral patterns or the inherent capacity of the tumor to metastasize. Thus, although the study may reflect the prevailing opinion on the prognostic factors in thyroid cancer, it may well be that the larger, more tightly controlled population-based study in Abstract 15–1 reflects the current biology of the disease. Interestingly, sex did not have a significant impact on the disease. It is hoped that future research into the natural history of thyroid carcinoma will use large population-based studies that have a fairly short interval of accrual.—J.M. Jessup, M.D.

5-Fluorouracil, Doxorubicin, and Cisplatin as Treatment for Adrenal Cortical Carcinoma

Schlumberger M, Brugieres L, Gicquel C, Travagli J-P, Droz J-P, Parmentier C (Inst Gustave-Roussy, Villejuif, France)

Cancer 67:2997–3000, 1991 15–3

Introduction.—For some patients with carcinoma of the adrenal cortex, resection may control the disease; however, current treatments are largely ineffective in patients with local recurrence and metastatic disease. Data were reviewed on 14 patients who were treated during a 6-year period with combined 5-fluorouracil, doxorubicin, and cisplatin (FAP).

Methods.—All of the patients had large tumors with progressive distant metastases. Every 4 weeks, 5-fluorouracil (500 mg/m^2/day) was administered on days 1–3; doxorubicin (60 mg/m^2) was administered on day 2; and cisplatin (120 mg/m^2) was administered with hydration and mannitol diuresis on day 2. Of the patients with hormone-producing tumors; 5 received mitotaine because of its possible antihormonal effects. The final analysis included 13 patients.

Results.—A 23% response rate was achieved: 1 patient had complete remission for 42 months; 2 patients had partial remissions of 6 and 11 months; 1 patient had a minor response lasting 22 months; and 2 patients had disease stabilization for 4 and 6 months. There was cardiotoxicity in 3 patients, myelotoxicity in 4, and nephrotoxicity in 1.

Conclusion.—The FAP regimen appears to be an active combination for treatment of metastatic adrenal cortical carcinoma. Mitotaine and FAP do not appear to be cross-resistant; the 2 regimens might be combined, even if the tumor progresses during mitotaine treatment. Further study of cisplatin and cisplatin-based intensive combinations is warranted.

▶ Adrenal cortical adenocarcinoma is a very difficult tumor to treat because it is largely unresponsive to chemotherapy and metastasizes early and aggressively. Recently, the drug mitotaine has become the drug of choice, with objective tumor response rates of 14% to 23%. The drug may not improve survival, but it does decrease endocrine hypersection in 75% of patients. In this study, the authors show that FAP has a 23% objective response rate that is equivalent to mitotaine. Furthermore, the authors suggest that mitotaine might be combined with the FAP regimen. It is hoped that the FAP regimen will be shown to be an active regimen for adrenal cortical carcinoma.—J.M. Jessup, M.D.

16 Novel Cancer Treatment Techniques

Radiation Therapy

Technique of Photodynamic Therapy for Disseminated Intraperitoneal Malignant Neoplasms: Phase I Study

Sindelar WF, DeLaney TF, Tochner Z, Thomas GF, Dachoswki LJ, Smith PD, Friauf WS, Cole JW, Glatstein E (Natl Cancer Inst; Natl Ctr for Research Resources, Bethesda, Md)

Arch Surg 126:318–324, 1991 16–1

Background.—One goal of cancer treatment is to selectively destroy malignant cells while preserving normal tissue and function. Photodynamic therapy destroys malignant lesions through the uptake of photosensitizing compounds. These are then activated by light exposure of a specific intensity and wavelength. A phase I study of photodynamic treatment for disseminated intraperitoneal malignant neoplasms was evaluated.

Methods.—Twenty-three patients with disseminated intraperitoneal malignant disease underwent intra-abdominal photodynamic therapy. Thirteen had ovarian cancer, 8 had sarcoma, and 2 had pseudomyxoma peritoneii. The patients were given dihematoporphyrin ethers intravenously 48–72 hours before laparotomy. The doses ranged from 1.5 mg of dihematoporphyrin per kg to 3 mg of dihematoporphyrin per kg. As much tumor as possible was resected. Red light, 630 nm, was administered to all peritoneal surfaces from an argon-pumped dye laser in doses of .2 J/cm^2–3 J/cm^2 in an escalating manner. The viscera and peritoneal surfaces were isolated anatomically and exposed to light. Light was delivered to mesentery and bowel using a flat-cut optical fiber, and other areas were exposed to light through a diffusing wand.

Outcomes.—After treatment, 5 of 8 patients cleared positive peritoneal cytologies. Six patients remained clinically free of disease for as long as 18 months. Five patients had treatment-related complications, including postoperative hemorrhage, necrotizing pancreatitis, ureteral leak and urinoma, and intestinal fistula. Cutaneous photosensitivity reactions and abnormal liver function also occurred in 3 and 19 patients, respectively, but were resolved spontaneously.

Conclusions.—Photodynamic therapy can be delivered to the peritoneal cavity in doses that produce therapeutic effects in experimental models without limiting toxic effects. Research on this treatment should continue.

▶ Photodynamic therapy exploits a photosensitizer and visible light with a wavelength that is consistent with the absorption of that photosensitizer. For reasons that are not clear, the photosensitizer appears to localize for a much longer period of time either in or on malignant tumor cells than in normal tissues. Thus, this classic binary system has minimal effects on normal tissues. Because the process is dependent on the penetration of light, it is most appropriate for superficial problems. The National Cancer Institute has spent the last few years working on photodynamic therapy applied to intraperitoneal neoplasms. This paper represents the completion of a phase I study of patients with intraperitoneal neoplasms. Investigators hope to apply this kind of treatment to patients who were thought to have complete remission, but who were likely to relapse. For example, patients with ovarian cancer who have had a complete remission with chemotherapy would be an ideal group of patients. Whether this treatment effectively adds something is unclear at this time, but it does have the real advantage of having minimal side effects in terms of normal tissues. To apply the phototherapy, the patients undergo a major surgical exploration and gross disease is resected. The phototherapeutic part of the treatment is then applied at the operating table when the patient is under anesthesia. It adds approximately a 1½–2 hours to the surgical procedure itself. Controlled clinical trials are being planned to assess the objective benefit of such treatment.—E. Glatstein, M.D.

Tumor Hypoxia Can Be Exploited to Preferentially Sensitize Tumors to Fractionated Irradiation

Brown JM, Lemmon MJ (Stanford Univ, Stanford, Calif)

Int J Radiat Oncol Biol Phys 20:457–461, 1991 16–2

Background.—Drug-induced intermittent hypoxia might be a means of making tumors more sensitive to fractionated irradiation without altering the sensitivity of the surrounding normal tissues. A group of bioreductive cytotoxic drugs that are preferentially toxic to hypoxic cells includes 3-amino-1,2,4-benzotriazine 1,4-dioxide (SR 4233), which is very selectively toxic to hypoxic cells in vitro and in tumors in vivo.

Study Design.—The effects of SR 4233 were examined in mice with a transplantable squamous cell carcinoma. Treated animals received 8 sessions of 2.5 Gy, and SR 4233 or saline was given 30 minutes before or immediately after each dose. The dose of SR 4233 was .08 mM/kg.

Observations.—Administration of SR 4233 led to a significantly enhanced radiation response by the tumor and no change in the sensitivity of normal skin. The hypoxic cell radiosensitizer SR 2508 had no such effect.

Conclusions.—The hypoxic cytotoxin SR 4233 enhances the radiation response of murine squamous cell carcinoma when fractionated treatment is delivered. Normal skin does not become more sensitive to radiation. Human tumors probably undergo reoxygenation, implying that SR 4233 or a close analogue may be useful in conjunction with clinical radiotherapy.

▶ Hypoxia has been described as occurring intermittently in solid tumors, but not in normal tissues. This paper describes a new approach using the drug

SR4233, which, in hypoxic cells, is rapidly metabolized to a toxic product capable of killing those cells. Using this approach, the authors show that SR4233 added to a fractionated x-ray program yields a marked improvement in the radiation response of a model tumor system, without any worsening in the sensitivity of normal mouse skin. It appears to be a very interesting model for subsequent investigation and may potentially be an entirely new approach to tumor therapy. Of course, the relationship between this kind of model system and humans is a leap of faith that requires a lot more work.—E. Glatstein, M.D.

The Dose-Rate Effect Revisited: Radiobiological Considerations of Importance in Radiotherapy

Hall EJ, Brenner DJ (Columbia Univ)

Int J Radiat Oncol Biol Phys 21:1403–1414, 1991 16–3

Background.—A wide spectrum of dose-rates has been used in radiation biology and radiotherapy (Fig 16–1). Important radiobiological considerations in radiotherapy were reviewed.

Discussion.—In radiotherapy, the dose-rate range of importance extends from approximately .1 Gy per hour to several Gy per minute. In this dose range, the fraction of cells killed by a given dose declines as the dose-rate is decreased, primarily because the sublethal damage is repaired. However, in some cell lines, the dose-rate effect is inverse. Over a narrow range of dose-rates, the efficacy of a given dose increases with decreasing dose-rates if the cells move through the cycle and are arrested in G_2, a radiosensitive phase (Fig 16–2). The low dose-rate data for cells of human origin, together with radiobiological theory, can help clinicians select high dose-rate doses that may produce early effects equivalent to the low dose-rate doses. The data can also help identify cases in which the late effects may not be worse for high dose-rate treatments.

Conclusions.—In recent years, accumulating data have been analyzed for values of the survival curve parameters and the rate of repair of sublethal damage in radiotherapy. These data sets have been used to address

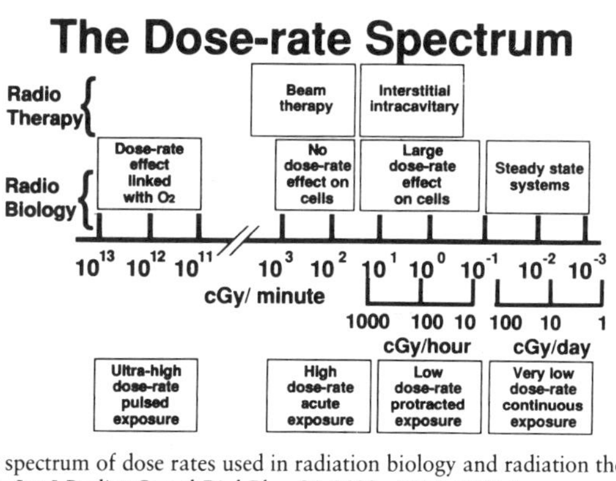

Fig 16–1.—The spectrum of dose rates used in radiation biology and radiation therapy. (Courtesy of Hall EJ, Brenner DJ: *Int J Radiat Oncol Biol Phys* 21:1403–1414, 1991.)

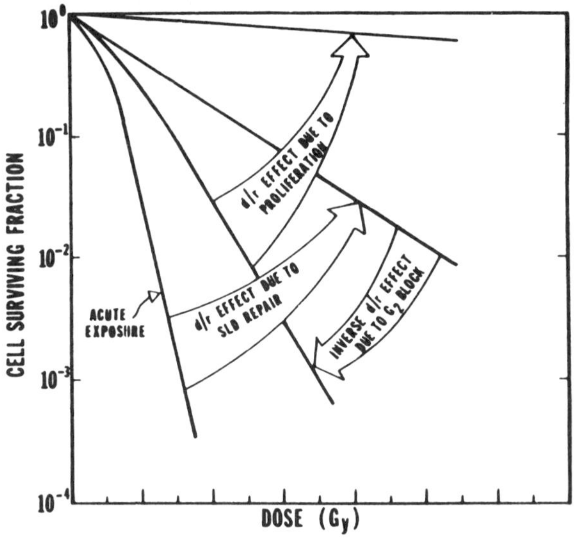

Fig 16–2.—Revised and updated illustration of the dose-rate effect caused by repair of sublethal damage, redistribution within the cycle, and cell proliferation. The dose-response curve for acute exposures is characterized by a broad initial shoulder. As the dose rate is reduced, the survival curve becomes progressively shallower as more and more sublethal damage is repaired; however, the cells are "frozen" in their positions within the cycle and do not progress. As the dose rate is lowered further, and for a limited range of dose rates, the survival curve steepens again as cells can progress through the cycle and pile up at a block in G_2, which is a radiosensitive phase but still cannot divide. A further lowering of the dose rate allows the cells to escape the G_2 block and divide; cell proliferation may then occur during the protracted exposure, and the survival curve becomes shallower as cell birth caused by mitosis offsets cell killing resulting from irradiation (redrawn from an idea by Joel Bedford). (Courtesy of Hall EJ, Brenner DJ: *Int J Radiat Oncol Biol Phys* 21:1403–1414, 1991.)

3 important questions: (1) the proposal to use pulsed irradiation rather than continuous irradiation in interstitial brachytherapy; (2) the equivalence of high dose-rate and low dose-rate intracavitary treatments for cervical carcinoma; and (3) an analysis of equivalent doses for a range of dose-rates in interstitial implants.

▶ The subject of dose-*rates* does not receive a great deal of attention in medical textbooks. This is a very scholarly review of dose-rates and their importance in clinical radiotherapy. It's a complicated subject because definitions of low dose-rate and high dose-rate are all relative. One can slow the dose-rate to a level below which the cells are capable of repairing the biological damage induced by radiation treatment during the period of exposure. Continuous low dose-rate radiotherapy is what is implied by interstitial brachytherapy. In the modern era, afterloading techniques, the computer, and the development of intracavitary treatments with high dose-rate brachytherapy have led to a reevaluation of the dose-rate. Hall and Brenner are among the foremost authorities on this subject, and this particular article is really a review of the state-of-the-art on this subject. There is an ongoing debate about high dose-rate brachytherapy and how well it can do against human neoplasms. There is no major biological advantage for high dose-rate over low dose-rate treatment. There may, in fact, be some modest advantage for low dose-rate over high dose-rate. The major advantage to the high dose-rate is one of convenience and reduced cost in terms of hospitalization. At the same time, one has to be careful that nothing is lost in shifting from continuous low dose-rate brachytherapy to high dose-rate intracavitary treatment. Hall and Brenner suggest that no major price will be paid. Early data appear to confirm that, but it will take a long time to achieve enough final information to be confident that that is the case.— E. Glatstein, M.D.

Improved Dose Distributions for 3D Conformal Boost Treatments in Carcinoma of the Nasopharynx

Leibel SA, Kutcher GJ, Harrison LB, Fass DE, Burman CM, Hunt MA, Mohan R, Brewster LJ, Ling CC, Fuks ZY (Mem Sloan-Kettering Cancer Ctr, New York)

Int J Radiat Oncol Biol Phys 20:823–833, 1991 16–4

Introduction.—Using 3-dimensional (3D) conformal radiation therapy, high radiation doses can be shaped to conform to the entire target volume while concomitantly reducing dose levels to normal tissues. The nasopharynx is an appropriate site for testing the feasibility and effects of this technique. Two-dimensional (2D) and 3D treatment planning were compared in 10 previously untreated patients with nasopharyngeal carcinomas and 5 patients with recurrent lesions.

Methods.—Planning of only the boost portion of treatment (19.8 Gy of a total 70.2-Gy treatment schedule) by both 2D and 3D approaches was compared qualitatively and quantitatively. The 3D images were reconstructed and displayed by means of beam's eye view techniques (Fig 16–3). Comparisons were made by dose-volume histograms, tumor control probabilities, normal tissue complication probabilities, and a figure describing the probability of control. No attempt was made to use the 3D approach throughout the treatment course.

Results.—For each endpoint, the 3D approach improved planning. When the 2D approach was used, 22% of the target volume was underdosed at the 95% isodose level, compared with 7% with 3D planning. The use of 3D planning increased the mean dose to the tumor volume by an average of 13%. The mandible, parotid glands, and other normal structures received a reduced dose, and the brain stem and spinal cord stayed within the limits of tolerance. The use of 3D planning increased the probability of tumor control by an average of 15%.

Conclusion.—Treatment of carcinoma of the nasopharynx might be improved by the use of 3D treatment planning. Because it can visualize the target volume in all dimensions, 3D planning can reduce the volume of tumor underdosed. Prospective studies are needed to establish the actual clinical advantages of 3D planning.

▶ A great deal of work is being done in the area of computerized treatment planning, with special attention being given to 3D treatment planning. This paper, carried out by some of the leaders in the area of treatment planning, sug-

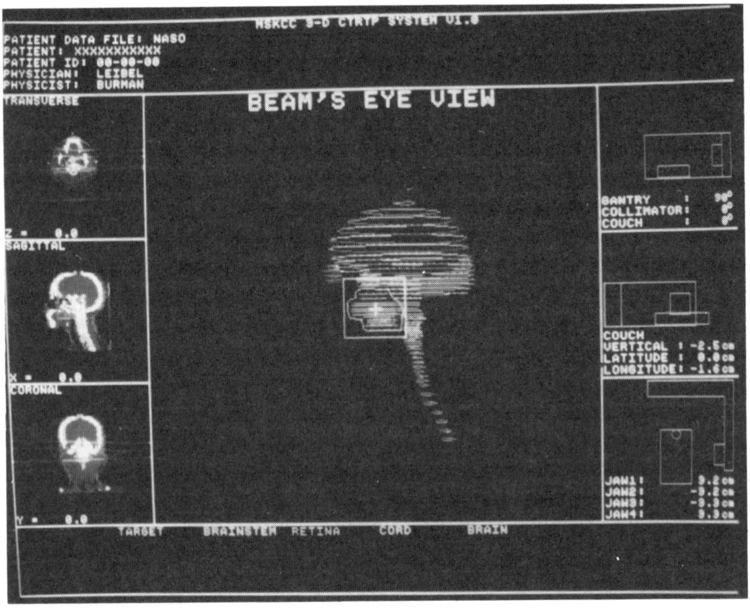

Fig 16–3.—Beam's eye view display of a patient with carcinoma of the nasopharynx showing the tumor and its surrounding structures as wire-frame surfaces using color to differentiate between structures. Reconstruction of the body surface outline, the tumor, retinas, and brain and spinal cord are shown in relation to the beam path of a lateral rectangular radiation field. In this field, a beam aperture, is drawn around the target volume. Shown on the left margin of this figure are 3 smaller sagittal, coronal, and axial CT images with the intersections of the displayed beam in each section. Parameters of the machine orientation for this field are displayed on the *right margin*. (Courtesy of Leibel SA, Kutcher GJ, Harrison LB, et al: *Int J Radiat Oncol Biol Phys* 20:823–833, 1991.)

gests that 3D plays a major role. In reality, it will require a prospective study of some sort to demonstrate conclusively that 3D treatment planning is a significant improvement over a combination of 2D treatments. After all, the basis of 3D treatment planning is an integration of 2D treatments. One must question how much better the 3D treatment is, and how much it costs. We can talk about probabilities, but the essential point has to do with individual patients. This work will obviously continue, and hopefully, the questions will be answered by some investigators.—E. Glatstein, M.D.

Radiation Induction of Drug Resistance in RIF-1: Correlation of Tumor and Cell Culture Results

Moulder JE, Hopwood LE, Volk DM, Davies BM (Med College of Wisconsin, Milwaukee)

Int J Radiat Oncol Biol Phys 20:213–216, 1991 16–5

Introduction.—Radiotherapy and chemotherapy have been used in combination to treat tumors. However, there is a concern that radiation may increase tumor drug resistance.

Methods.—Radiation-induced drug resistance was studied in both tumors and cultures of RIF-1 cells, which contain cells that are resistant to antineoplastic drugs.

Results.—The frequency of drug-resistant cells was higher in cells derived from tumors than in cells derived from cultures. When cell cultures were irradiated with 5 Gy, there was a significant increase in drug resistance. When tumors were irradiated with as much as 12 Gy, which gave a similar cell kill, the long-term drug resistance appeared to be unrelated to radiation dosage.

Conclusion.—There can be significant differences in drug-resistance frequencies between tumors and original cell lines. Drug resistance induced by radiation varies, depending on whether tumors or cell cultures are used. Theories about the induction of drug resistance that are based on cell culture studies may not be easily extrapolated to the induction of drug resistance in tumors.

▶ This is a very provocative paper by a group of thorough investigators who have an unusual hypothesis concerning the role of radiation in inducing drug resistance. Their careful observations raise questions about applying the results of the induction of drug resistance *in vitro* to an *in vivo* situation. Those who are interested in this subject would do well to read this paper.

In medical oncology, when cells are called "resistant," what is meant is "refractory" (i.e., increasing doses of drug show *no* killing of cells at all, and the survival curve is parallel to the horizontal axis [or even increasing]). By contrast, in radiation oncology, every mammalian cell line (tumor or normal tissue) shows a decrease in survival with each increasing dose. The rate of decline may not necessarily be great, but survival does decrease. Thus, in radiation oncology, resistance is a *relative* rather than an absolute, phenomenon. Also, sensitivity and resistance are probably best viewed as a continuum. Precise definitions of resistance in radiation oncology depend *entirely* on parameters derived from in vitro cell survival curves (i.e., the Do and the extrapolation numbers); however, the exact numerical cut-off is essentially arbitrary.

The difference between the medical and radiation concepts probably reflect the importance of the cell membrane to drug entry. Ionizing radiation, which is physical process, experiences no barrier at the membrane level. The only thing that's clear to me concerning the prediction of radiation resistance for cells that are chemoresistant (or vice versa) is that, at the present time, there is *no* reliable way to predict this. Presuming radioresistance when cells are chemoresistant clinically, or vice versa clinically, is simply unreliable—regardless of who has made *ex cathedra* pronouncements.—E. Glatstein, M.D.

Development of Scanned Focussed Ultrasound Hyperthermia: Clinical Response Evaluation

Harari PM, Hynynen KH, Roemer RB, Anhalt DP, Shimm DS, Stea B, Cassady JR (Univ of Wisconsin; Madison; Univ of Arizona; Arizona Cancer Ctr, Tucson)

Int J Radiat Oncol Biol Phys 21:831–840, 1991 16–6

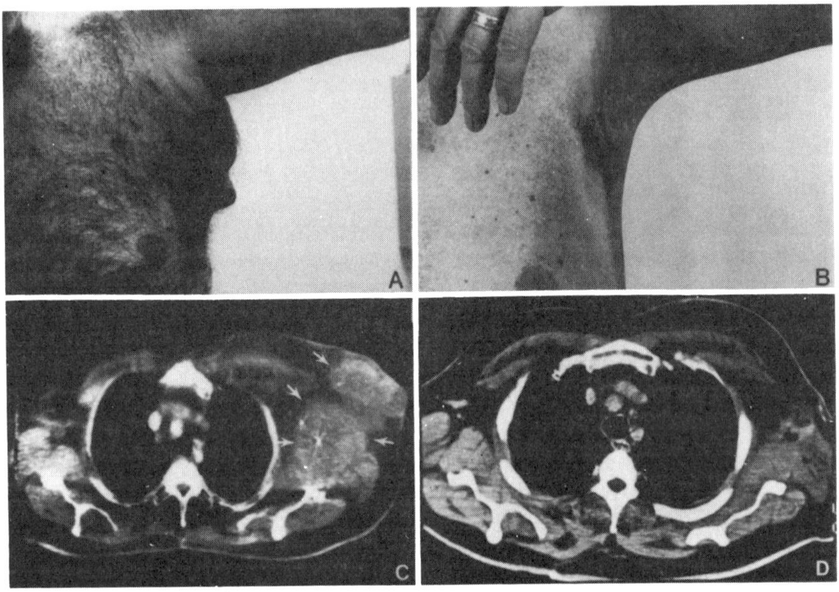

Fig 16–4.—An SFUS hyperthermia response. Photograph and CT scan slice of a man, 50, with a 455-cc axillary melanoma before (A and C) and 2 months after (B and D) SFUS hyperthermia plus 4,000-cGy photon irradiation. Four SFUS hyperthermia treatments were delivered, and the patient had complete disappearance of local tumor, pain, bleeding, and limitation of motion. The tumor was scored as a complete response. (Courtesy of Harari PM, Hynynen KH, Roemer RB, et al: *Int J Radiat Oncol Biol Phys* 21:831–840, 1991.)

Introduction.—The selectively heating of irregularly shaped tumors at depth can now be done through focusing and controlled scanning of energy deposition patterns by ultrasound. A scanned focused ultrasound (SFUS) hyperthermia system was used to deliver 220 treatments to 87 tumors in 71 patients with extracranial malignancies in 1986–1990.

Methods.—The patients were given an average of 3 SFUS hyperthermia treatments, spaced weekly, during ongoing fractionated radiotherapy. The pelvis was treated in 22 patients, the chest wall or breast in 14, the neck in 8, and the axilla in 7. The most common histologies were adenocarcinoma, squamous cell carcinoma, and melanoma. Concurrent radiotherapy at a mean dose of 4,320 cGy was given to 67 patients, and 4 received concomitant chemotherapy. The tumor volumes were 1–2,100 cm^3, and 75% were at depths greater than 3 cm from skin.

Results.—The overall response rate was 62%; 22% of the tumors treated completely responded, and 40% partially responded. Local pain was reduced dramatically in 42% of the tumors treated. Acute tolerance of SFUS hyperthermia was good. Chronic toxicities, which occured in 2 patients, consisted of persistent skin blisters and burns (Fig 16–4).

Conclusion.—Thus far, the successes achieved with this system warrant assessment of the study protocols that incorporate ultrasound hyperthermia in the frontline therapy of advanced locoregional malignancies.

▶ Hyperthermia remains a treatment of great promise; however, in the immortal words of Charlie Brown and Charles Schultz: "A great potential is man's heaviest burden." Although the laboratory basis for hyperthermia shows unequivocal biology to exploit, the major problem has been technical limitations on such exploitations. There are 2 major facets of the problem that have to be overcome. One facet is how to control the heat distribution so that heat can be put where one wants it. The second problem is how to monitor the temperature distribution accurately so that one knows that one is delivering and controlling the amount of heat desired. Both of these problems remain to be solved, although the monitoring can apparently be solved (expensively) by MRI.

This is an important paper by an excellent team of investigators trying new approaches of controlling the heat distribution by means of scanning focused ultrasound. It appears to be promising, but it is still in its infancy. It is unfortunate that industry has not made a real commitment to developing basic equipment to try and overcome these problems. Until the technology improves, hyperthermia treatment will continue to be considered "of great potential."—E. Glatstein, M.D.

Two or Six Hyperthermia Treatments as an Adjunct to Radiation Therapy Yield Similar Tumor Responses: Results of a Randomized Trial

Kapp DS, Petersen IA, Cox RS, Hahn GM, Fessenden P, Prionas SD, Lee ER, Meyer JL, Samulski TV, Bagshaw MA (Stanford Univ, Stanford, Calif)

Int J Radiat Oncol Biol Phys 19:1481–1495, 1990 16–7

Background.—Nonrandomized studies have suggested that response rates improve with locoregional hyperthermia (HT) in conjunction with radiation therapy for locally advanced, recurrent, or metastatic superficial malignancies. Retrospective studies have suggested that the use of more than 2 HT treatments for superficial tumors may have no added benefit. A prospective study was done to assess the effects of repeated HT treatments.

Methods.—The study included 165 fields in 64 patients treated during a 4-year period. All had recurrent or metastatic malignancies located less than 3 cm from the surface. The patients were stratified according to tumor size, histology, and previous radiation treatment. Radiation therapy was standardized according to the same criteria, and the patients were randomized to receive either 2 or 6 courses of HT.

Results.—For all fields, the mean minimum temperature was 40.2°C, the mean maximum temperature was 44.8°C, and the average intratumoral temperature was 42.5°C. These temperatures were not significantly different between the 2 groups. Hyperthermia was well tolerated, and complications were acceptable. All measurable tumor disappeared in 52% of the fields. Tumor was reduced by at least 50% in 7% of fields, and by less than 50% in 21%; continuing regression was observed in 20% at 3 weeks after therapy. Tumor response and duration of local control were not significantly different between the 2-treatment and 6-treatment groups (Fig 16–5). The factors that correlated with the du-

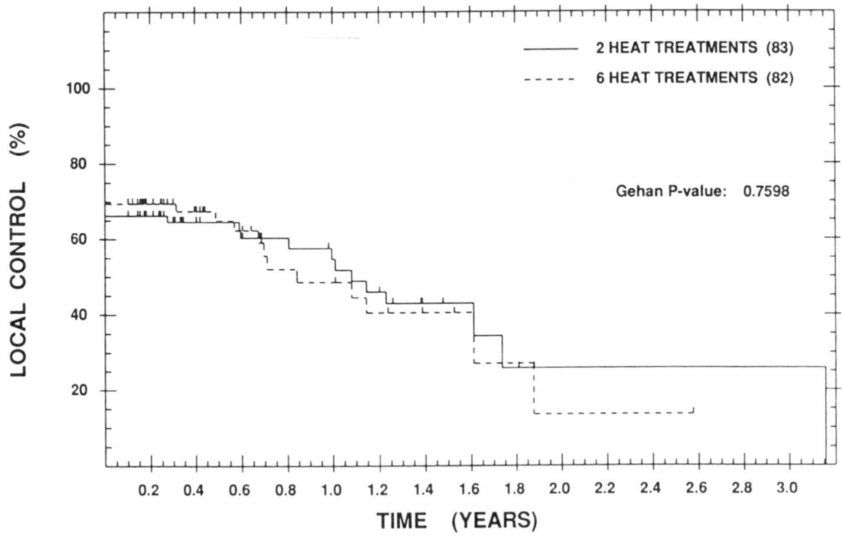

Fig 16–5.—The duration of local control for all analyzed fields (165) randomized to either 2 hyperthermia treatments *(solid line)* or 6 hyperthermia treatments *(dashed line)*. (Courtesy of Kapp DS, Petersen IA, Cox RS, et al: *Int J Radiat Oncol Biol Phys* 19:1481–1495, 1990.)

ration of local control were tumor histology, concurrent radiation dose, and tumor volume (Fig 16–6). On univariate analysis, the mean of the minimum intratumoral temperatures had borderline prognostic significance and added power to the best three covariate models.

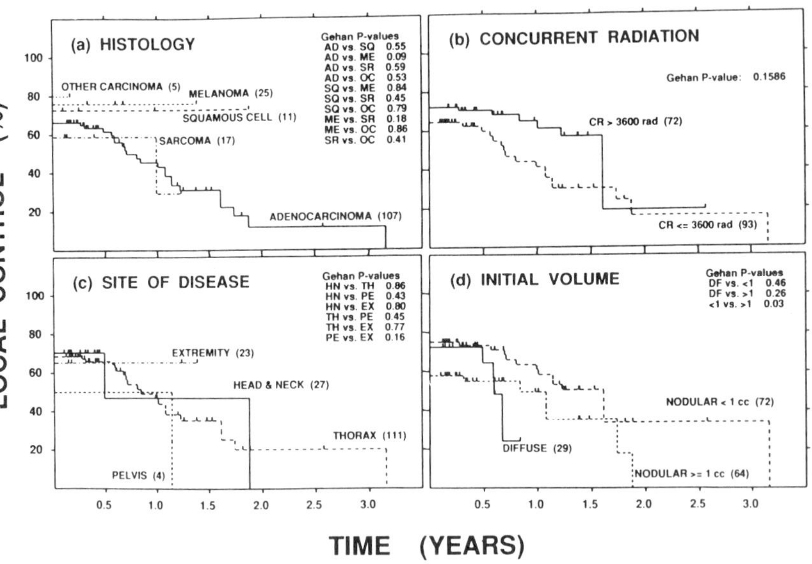

Fig 16–6.—Duration of local control by histology, radiation dose, site of disease, and initial tumor volume. (Courtesy of Kapp DS, Petersen IA, Cox RS, et al: *Int J Radiat Oncol Biol Phys* 19:1481–1495, 1990.)

Conclusions.—The choice of 2 or 6 HT treatments appears to have no significant effect on the response rate or duration of local control. Thermotolerance may limit the effectiveness of multiple closely spaced HT treatments.

▶ This is a well-performed clinical trial carried out by an excellent team of investigators in the field of hyperthermia. The trial quite nicely shows that the number of hyperthermia treatments had little impact on the outcome, i.e., 2 treatments were as effective as 6. The thing that makes this particular study of high quality is the attention directed toward monitoring of the maximum, minimum, and average intratumoral temperatures. Monitoring the temperatures has become as much a challenge to the investigator as actually delivering the heat itself.

The laboratory basis for hyperthermia demonstrates quite conclusively that there's real biology to exploit with such treatment. In the past, the big hang-up has simply been that the technology for delivering and monitoring hyperthermia has not been optimal. A great deal of further basic investigation is required in this area, but it's too soon to dismiss hyperthermia in the treatment of cancer.—E. Glatstein, M.D.

Estimates of Radiation Absorbed Dose for Intraperitoneally Administered Iodine-131 Radiolabeled B72.3 Monoclonal Antibody in Patients With Peritoneal Carcinomatoses

Larson SM, Carrasquillo JA, Colcher DC, Yokoyama K, Reynolds JC, Bacharach SA, Raubitchek A, Pace L, Finn RD, Rotman M, Stabin M, Neumann RD, Sugarbaker P, Schlom J (Sloan-Kettering Mem Cancer Ctr, New York; Natl Inst of Health; Natl Cancer Inst, Bethesda, Md; Oak Ridge Associated Univ, Oak Ridge, Tenn)

J Nucl Med 32:1661–1667, 1991 16–8

Introduction.—Colorectal and ovarian cancers spread locally in the peritoneum and may remain confined there for a long time before spreading to distant sites. A newly developed model for determining estimates of radiation-absorbed doses of radioisotopes administered intraperitoneally was used to calculate absorbed dose to tumor and normal tissue based on a surgically controlled study of radiolabeled antibody distribution.

Methods.—Ten patients with peritoneal carcinomatosis were injected intraperitoneally with the murine monoclonal antibody B72.3 radiolabeled with ^{131}I. Biodistribution studies were performed using nuclear medicine techniques until laparotomy was performed 4–14 days after the injection. Surgical biopsy specimens of normal tissue and tumor were obtained.

Results.—The critical organ was predicted to be the marrow, with the maximum-tolerated dose expected at approximately 200 mCi. In patients with large intraperitoneal tumor deposits, the tumor was an important source of radiation exposure to normal tissue. Local hot spots for the tumor-absorbed dose were noted. The maximum tumor-absorbed dose was calculated to be 11,000 rad per 100 mCi administered intraperitoneally. However, the tumor rad dose varied markedly, which could pose serious problems for curative treatment, particularly in patients with large tumor burdens.

Conclusion.—Clearance rates vary substantially, which will have a major impact on the actual radiation dose to individual organs. To correlate toxicity observed with computed radiation-absorbed doses, individual estimates of absorbed dose should be computed on the basis of the clearance values obtained for each patient.

▶ These investigators have worked very hard to estimate the radiation-absorbed dose from radiolabeled antibody therapy in patients with peritoneal carcinomatosis. Their work should be reviewed very carefully. Nonetheless, I have to question the actual numerical values. I believe that what we have in this instance is a fundamental difference in the concepts of dose between nuclear medicine and radiation oncology. As far as the tumor itself is concerned, these estimates given by the authors are basically determined by some of the imaging studies they have done, along with determinations of the biological and isotopic half-life. These can be measured from the patient, and I can understand the desirability of calculating them. However, when we talk about dosimetry in radiation oncology, we have to begin with a target for our tumor volume. We have to define the tumor in advance and then figure out how to encompass it with a certain distribution of radiation. With isotope therapy, the dose-rate is actually variable over time (unless the half-life is very long); many of the individual disintegrations measured by nuclear medicine techniques do not actually strike the tumor and, therefore, they do not represent absorbed dose or rad to the predefined tumor volume. Those disintegrations that do not strike the tumor volume are of no help in tumor control but, rather, strike other tissues.

There is an enormous need for investigation of microdosimetry to determine the true dose that is striking the actual tumor volume itself, and to determine the homogeneity (or lack thereof) of that dose distribution. Until then, I believe that many of the calculations that are attempted in good faith simply cannot be taken at face value. This has to be construed as my own opinion, but I believe many physicists would agree.—E. Glatstein, M.D.

Radioimmunology: Imaging and Therapy

Larson SM (Mem Sloan Kettering Cancer Ctr, New York)

Cancer 67:1253–1260, 1991 16–9

Background.—Several clinical trials have affirmed the principle of immune-specific targeting of radiolabeled antibodies against human tumors. Research in these methods is being pursued for diagnosis and therapy, despite current limitations.

Discussion.—Kohler and Milstein's development of the hybridoma technique probably is the most important contribution to the field of radioimmunology. Since 1978, there have been 110 clinical trials in which monoclonal antibodies against human tumors have been created and labeled with radioisotopes. Some conclusions about the benefits of certain combinations of antibodies and isotopes are beginning to emerge. Radiolabeled antibodies have been used to demonstrate melanomas, lymphomas, neuroblastomas, and colorectal malignancies that could not be demonstrated by conventional methods. Lasting remissions have been achieved in patients with malignant lymphoma in whom conventional therapy has failed.

Recent Developments.—Slow but steady progress has been made by applying the principles of immunocytochemistry, imaging physics, and tumor immunology. A few "magic bullets" have been developed. Cheung's introduction of iodine ^{131}I, 3-F8, and IgG3 against the GD2 antigen of neuroblastoma and Royston's use of indium ^{111}I T-101 against the CD5 antigen of T cells have been highly consistent and have delivered high concentrations of radioactivity to tumors in clinical trials. In the future, "humanized" antibodies may be produced by genetic engineering, the range of available isotopes will expand, and new imaging methods will detect smaller lesions and allow quantitative imaging for dosimetry. Improved computerized work stations may also broaden the applications of fusion imaging.

Conclusion.—Many practical techniques for diagnosis and treatment are expected to result from technological advances in radioimmunology.

▶ This is a nice review of a complicated subject. The author is obviously enthusiastic about the subject, but there are some things that he overlooks. Proteins, including antibodies, are designed to stay inside the vascular system to maintain osmotic pressure, and their ability to get outside vessels is quite limited. Moreover, the proportion of the injected dose absorbed by human tumors is several logarithms less than the uptake in rodent tumor systems. There appears to be little question that antibodies labeled with isotope will be useful diagnostically. However, it remains to be seen whether enough dose can be delivered to the neoplastic cells to sterilize them in humans. This is a much different question than simply increasing the administered dose by a factor of 10 or even 100.

Those who embrace radioimmunotherapy (or antibodies labeled with toxins) must realize that neoplastic cells are not simply passive receptacles of antigen waiting to be destroyed by antibody that has been armed. The cells are very adaptive and remarkably capable of adjusting to a variety of environmental maneuvers. Indeed, some of us are beginning to believe that the neoplastic cells actually have Ph.D.s in immunology!—E. Glatstein, M.D.

Planning of Radiotherapy for Patients with Hip Prosthesis

Erlanson M, Franzén L, Henriksson R, Littbrand B, Löfroth P-O (Univ of Umeå, Umeå, Sweden)

Int J Radiat Oncol Biol Phys 20:1093–1098, 1991 16–10

Introduction.—The number of patients with hip prostheses undergoing radiotherapy for pelvic cancer is increasing. Depending on the materials used, this might present a problem for radiotherapy. Therefore, the effects of a hip prosthesis on the dose distribution used in the treatment of pelvic cancer were evaluated.

Methods.—A titanium alloy prosthesis in a water phantom was used as a model. Photon radiation beams with energies of 6, 20, and 50 mV and a focus phantom distance of 100 cm were directed against the prosthesis. The dose profiles were measured with the RFA-7 radiation field analyzer system.

Results.—The sphere of the prosthesis was not homogenous. The dose in a beam behind the prosthesis was reduced from 10% to 40%, with the largest distortion behind the shaft. Using an opposed 4-field technique with a 50% weight on the lateral fields, the dose reduction was only 4% to 8% of the average dose. The local increase of dosage close to the prosthesis seemed to be of little practical concern, even at the highest dosages.

Conclusion.—Dose distribution is not homogenous; therefore, a treatment technique not including the prosthesis is preferred. When necessary, isocentric 3- and 4-field techniques can help to reduce distortion.

▶ It is not uncommon in today's world to treat a patient with pelvic neoplasm who has already had a hip prosthesis inserted. The impact of this prosthesis on dose distribution is a continuing problem for the radiotherapist. This is a very nice analysis and evaluation of the problem, demonstrating a significant dose reduction behind the prosthesis with AP-PA fields and a minimizing of this with 4-field techniques. The impact of such altered dose distribution could affect the curability of certain types of neoplasms, but have very little to do with others, depending on the kind of cancer being treated, its location, and its probability pattern of spread.—E. Glatstein, M.D.

Radiosurgery of Acoustic Neurinomas

Flickinger JC, Lunsford LD, Coffey RJ, Linskey ME, Bissonette DJ, Maitz AH, Kondziolka D (Univ of Pittsburgh, Pa; Pittsburgh Cancer Inst, Pa)

Cancer 67:345–353, 1991 16–11

Introduction.—Previous studies of radiosurgery have not adequately analyzed the rate of tumor control and the risk of delayed onset of cranial nerve dysfunction after radiosurgery. These factors were analyzed after 30 months of experience in treating acoustic neurinomas with a 201-source cobalt 60 (^{60}Co) gamma unit.

Methods.—Stereotactic radiosurgery with the gamma unit was used to treat 85 patients with acoustic neurinomas during its first 30 months of operation. Neuroimaging studies were performed.

Results.—In the 40 patients who were followed up for longer than 1 year, tumors were smaller in 55%, unchanged in 43%, and larger in 2%. The 2-year actuarial rate was 46% for preserving useful hearing and 62% for preserving any hearing. Previously undetected neuropathies of the trigeminal nerve in 12 patients and of the facial nerve in 14 patients were noted 1 week to 1 year after radiosurgery; these improved at median intervals of 13 and 8 months, respectively, after onset. Hearing loss and an increasing average tumor diameter were significantly related. There was no deterioration of any cranial nerve function in 7 patients with average tumor diameters of less than 10 mm.

Conclusion.—Although surgical resection is still the standard treatment for most patients with acoustic neurinomas, stereotactic radiosurgery will probably play an increasing role in the treatment of these tumors in selected patients. The treatment is an attractive alternative for patients who are unwilling to accept the risks of permanent facial nerve damage from surgical resection. In addition, radiosurgery is associated with a 40% to 70% reduction in hospital charges compared with microsurgery.

▶ Stereotactic radiosurgery has become a very popular (and expensive) technique for treating certain problems. The gamma knife is a particularly expensive piece of equipment that is designed to use sophisticated dosimetry from multiple cobalt sources to treat small volumes in the brain.

The volume is the key in this kind of treatment. Apparently, there is enough follow-up reported from experience in other countries to suggest that small lesions (less than 2 cm) can tolerate large single doses of radiation in the CNS. This is exactly the opposite of findings resulting from all the years of experience and empiricism that have gone into radiation therapy except that empiricism is generally based on larger volumes.

Fractionation studies have shown rather convincingly that repeated small doses of radiation take advantage of differential repopulation, redistribution, reoxygenation, and repair characteristics between tumors and normal tissues. None of these can be exploited with 1 single dose. In addition, although the effects of increasing the dose on the tumors remain relatively unpredictable, the effects of increasing the dose on normal tissues are highly predictable.

These authors report on the first series of patients with acoustic neuromas who have undergone such treatment. Their results look relatively good, but the maximum follow-up is only 30 months, and there is a relatively small proportion of patients who are beyond 1 year. If the lesion is small enough, it appears that no real damage will be done. I remain very cautious and skeptical of the long-term safety of this kind of modality for lesions greater than 2 cm. Future analyses will have to distinguish the sizes of the radiation fields very carefully; I would be very unwilling to subject a patient with a lesion larger than 2 cm to this kind of treatment at this time. Moreover, why (and if) this form of treatment is reputedly superior to conventional fractionated therapy for the same problem remains unclear to me, because reducing the number of treatments generally correlates with reducing the likelihood of local control. This treatment is certainly more expensive, and what can be achieved with fractionated radiotherapy in the long haul may actually be as good—or possibly even better.—E. Glatstein, M.D.

Chemotherapy

Studies With RP 56976 (Taxotere): A Semisynthetic Analogue of Taxol

Ringel I, Horwitz SB (The Hebrew Univ, Jerusalem, Israel; Albert Einstein College of Medicine, Bronx, NY)

J Natl Cancer Inst 83:288–291, 1991 16–12

Introduction.—Taxol, a diterpenoid isolated from the bark of the Pacific yew, is an antimitotic agent and a potent inhibitor of cell replication. It promotes the assembly of tubulin and stabilizes the formed polymers against depolymerization by Ca^{++} and low temperature. Efforts are being directed at the total synthesis of taxol, both because the Pacific yew is an extremely slow-growing species, and because even the low yield of taxol isolated from its bark kills the tree. A promising taxol analogue prepared in France is active against cancer, and its precursor can be prepared from leaves that regenerate. The properties of RP 56976 (taxotere), a taxol analogue, were reviewed.

Discussion.—Verification of the same mechanism of action as the parent drug is important in testing any analogue. Like taxol, RP 56976 promotes the in vitro assembly of stable microtubules in the absence of guanosine triphosphate and induces microtubule-bundle formation in cells (Fig 16–7). Compared with taxol, RP 56976 is slightly more active as a promoter of tubulin polymerization. It is 2.5 times more potent as an inhibitor of cell replication in J774.2 and P388 cells and 5 times more potent in taxol-resistant cells.

Conclusion.—The taxol analogue RP 56976 is a potent inhibitor of cell replication that promotes the in vitro assembly of stable microtubules in the absence of guanosine triphosphate and induces microtubule bundle formation in cells. Clinical studies of the activity and toxicity of RP 56976 are under way.

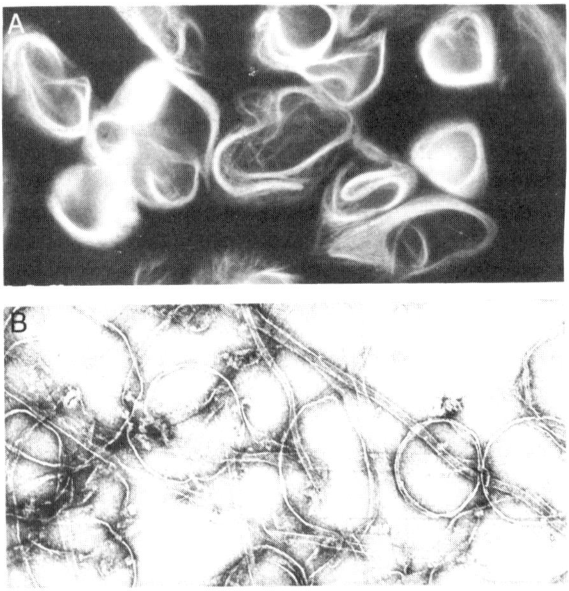

Fig 16–7.—Effect of RP 56976 on microtubule bundle formation in CHO cells and on microtubule protein assembly in vitro. **A,** immunofluorescence of CHO cells after incubation with 10 μM of RP 56976 for 6 hours. **B,** microtubule protein was assembled in the presence of 10 μm of RP 56976; at steady state (before mixing), a sample was taken for electron microscopy. (Courtesy of Ringel I, Horwitz SB: *J Natl Cancer Inst* 83:288–291, 1991.)

▶ Taxol has generated a great deal of excitement and interest, both in the medical community and in the general public. Environmentalists, loggers, pharmacists, oncologists, and patients with cancer have all been interested parties to the development of this drug. There is little doubt that taxol has great clinical potential. It has already been shown to have significant clinical activity against cisplatin-resistant ovarian cancer as well as Adriamycin-refractory breast cancer. It may have activity in lung cancer and other tumors as well. Until taxol is synthesized, supply looms as a potential major problem—particularly if it turns out to have meaningful clinical activity in common tumors. Consequently, there is now great interest in taxotere, which may have the same exciting clinical potential, but for which supply is not a problem. Whereas taxotere is in phase I–II trials, taxol appears to be almost ready for approval by the Food and Drug Administration, because pivotal phase III trials are nearing completion.—R.F. Ozols, M.D., Ph.D.

Antisense-Mediated Reductin in Thrombospondin Reverses the Malignant Phenotype of a Human Squamous Carcinoma

Castle V, Varani J, Fligiel S, Prochownik EV, Dixit V (Univ of Michigan, Ann Arbor; VA Med Ctr, Allen Park, Mich)

J Clin Invest 87:1883–1888, 1991 16–13

Background.—Production of thrombospondin (TSP), a homotrimeric protein made by a wide range of normal and transformed cells, has been related to proliferation of squamous epithelial cells. Functionally, TSP acts as a growth-supportive matrix component. It facilitates cell attachment and serves as an adhesion factor for many cell types.

Methods.—The role of TSP in tumor cell growth and tumor spread was studied using a human squamous carcinoma cell line exhibiting high TSP production and an invasive phenotype (UM-SCC-11B). The cells were transfected with a TSP complementary DNA antisense expression vector.

Observations.—Five unique transfected clones were obtained that exhibited reduced TSP production. Expression of the transfected antisense sequence was confirmed using a ribonuclease protection assay. The clones showed reduced rates of growth in vitro compared with a vector-transfected control clone. Athymic mice inoculated subcutaneously with antisense clones either formed no tumors or formed slow-growing, highly differentiated tumors. The control clone produced rapidly growing, poorly differentiated, invasive tumors.

Conclusions.—Thrombospondin may have a direct role in determining the malignant phenotype of some human tumors. It may help modulate the growth of both ectodermal and mesodermal cells. Altered synthesis of TSP might disrupt the capacity of cells to interact properly with their matrix, and to receive and process growth-controlling signals.

▶ Thrombospondin is a component of the extracellular matrix, which provides the required support for cells to adhere and attach. Adhesion factors have been shown to alter cell growth in vitro and in vivo by influencing cellular proliferation, presumably by altering the capacity of the cells to interact with the extracellular matrix and thereby altering their ability to receive and process growth-controlling signals. This study uses the antisense messenger RNA technique to provide direct evidence of the role of TSP in both the control of cell proliferation and the development of the malignant phenotype. The extracellular matrix and cell adhesion molecules may be novel therapeutic targets for interfering with malignant cell proliferation.—R.F. Ozols, M.D., Ph.D.

Topoisomerase II-Reactive Chemotherapeutic Drugs Induce Apoptosis in Thymocytes

Walker PR, Smith C, Youdale T, Leblanc J, Whitfield JF, Sikorska M (Natl Research Council of Canada, Ottawa, Ont)

Cancer Res 51:1078–1085, 1991 16–14

Introduction.—Chemotherapy for some cancers can be aided by drugs that interact with the enzyme topoisomerase II. The role of topoisomerase II in biological processes, especially its role in determining and modulating chromosome structure, can also be established by such drugs.

Methods.—The epipodophyllotoxins etoposide and teniposide, as well as amsacrine, were investigated for their effects on the viability of thymocytes in primary culture.

Results.—In experiments using rat thymocytes, all 3 drugs produced DNA cleavage, as detected by resolving DNA by pulsed field agarose gel electrophoresis. A 2-part process of DNA cleavage was noted. The first component resulted from interaction of the drugs with topoisomerase II, and the second was caused by endonuclease cleavage resulting from drug-induced entry of thymocytes into programmed cell death or apoptosis. The latter phenomenon was also noted in thymocytes that underwent apoptosis after being exposed to the glucocorticoid analog dexamethasone. The effect of the drugs on programmed cell death depended on new protein and RNA synthesis, suggesting that topoisomerase II plays a part in the initial stages of the process.

Conclusion.—The thymocyte responses to glucocorticoids and to drugs that interact with topoisomerase II appear to be similar, if not identical. Drugs that are active toward topoisomerase II yield the same reaction with the same kinetics; thus, they too may trigger apoptosis in thymocytes. The progress of apoptosis may be conveniently measured by flow cytometry.

▶ Apoptosis is a "suicide" process by which unwanted cells activate or induce an endonuclease that leads to DNA fragmentation and cleavage of chromatin. Apoptosis is important in regulating normal development as well as in determining levels of precursor cells in hematopoietic pathways to balance the production of various cell types. This programmed cell death has become a potential antitumor strategy for obvious reasons. If this process could be induced or activated selectively in tumor cells, then toxicity to normal tissues would be minimal. Topoisomerase II-reactive drugs appear to be involved in apoptosis.

However, the mechanism(s) by which drugs such as VP-16 induce the entry of cells into apoptosis is not understood and may be a result of the interaction of these drugs with topoisomerase II or some other target. In either case, more effective stimulus of the apoptosis process in tumor cells is a novel therapeutic approach.—R.F. Ozols, M.D., Ph.D.

Suppression of Dexamethasone-Induced Metallothionein Expression and *cis*-Diamminedichloroplatinum(II) Resistance by v-*Mos*[1]

Basu A, Lazo JS (Univ of Pittsburgh, Pa; Pittsburgh Cancer Inst)

Cancer Res 51:893–896, 1991 16–15

Introduction.—The role of metallothionein (MT) in resistance to anticancer drugs is not completely known. The effect of v-*mos* expression, both on the inducibility by dexamethasone of MT protein and on cellular resistance to *cis*-diamminedichloroplatinum (*cis*-DDP), was investigated.

Methods.—Whether the transient induction of MT by dexamethasone causes resistance to *cis*-DDP in malignant and nonmalignant cells was examined. Dexamethasone was selected because it is widely used as an antiemetic and as a palliative management of some malignancies, and also because it is a strong inducer of MT. Normal rat kidney cells were infected with a modified v-*mos* construct in which expression of v-*mos* and, consequently, transformation were temperature sensitive.

Results.—Temperature-sensitive oncogenic transformation by v-*mos* attenuated induction of MT by dexamethasone. There was no induction of MT in a revertant cell line that expressed v-*mos* and was transformed at a nonpermissive temperature of 37°C. Nontransformed cells displayed resistance to *cis*-DDP after dexamethasone pretreatment for 24 hours. Both MT levels and resistance to *cis*-DDP decreased significantly when cells were pretreated with dexamethasone and then incubated in dexamethasone-free medium for 24 hours.

Conclusion.—Transient resistant to *cis*-DDP was produced by a nonmetal inducer of MT in nontransformed cells. Glucocorticoid-induced protection is suppressed in cells expressing v-*mos*. Future treatment strategies for tumors with v-*mos* or other oncogenes may therapeutically exploit the selective difference in glucocorticoid induction of MT.

▶ Metallothioneins are the major intracellular protein thiols that are involved in heavy metal detoxification. As such, they also have been studied for their potential to protect drug-resistant tumor cells from cisplatin and bifunctional alkylating agents. However, their role in acquired, clinical drug resistance remains to be determined, because conflicting experimental results have been reported (1). This study demonstrates that, although glucocorticoids induce metallothioneins in nontransformed cells, they do not significantly do so in transformed cells expressing the v-*mos* oncogene. If this difference exists in human tumors, it provides a new therapeutic strategy: use high-dose steroids to induce metallothioneins in normal cells, thereby protecting them from cisplatin toxicity without inducing this protective protein in tumor cells expressing certain oncogenes.—R.F. Ozols, M.D., Ph.D.

Reference

1. Schilder R, et al: *Int J Cancer* 45:416, 1990.

Expression of the c-Ha-*ras* Oncogene in Mouse NIH 3T3 Cells Induces Resistance to Cisplatin

Isonishi S, Hom DK, Thiebaut FB, Mann SC, Andrews PA, Basu A, Lazo JS, Eastman A, Howell SB (Univ of California, San Diego, La Jolla; Univ of Pittsburgh, Pa; Dartmouth Medicine School, Hanover NH)

Cancer Res 51:5903–5909, 1991 16–16

Introduction.—The authors recently showed that sensitivity to *cis*-diamminedichloroplatinum(II) (DDP) can be modulated by signal transduction pathways. One signal transduction pathway includes the c-Ha-*ras* protein as a component, but it is not well understood. Using an NIH 3T3 cell containing a hormone-inducible form of c-Ha-*ras* oncogene, the mechanism of DDP resistance by the c-Ha-*ras* signal transduction pathway was studied.

Methods and Findings.—The cells were prepared by transfection with a construct containing c-Ha-*ras* oncogene linked to the dexamethasone (DEX)-inducible mouse mammary tumor virus long terminal repeat (LTR). These LTR H-*ras*(A) cells were treated for 24 hours with 5 μm of DEX, which induced c-Ha-*ras* expression and increased DDP resistance by a factor of 8.2, as measured by clonogenic assay. On induction of the c-Ha-*ras* oncogene, DDP accumulation was reduced by 40% and intrastrand adduct formation was reduced by 17%. Dexamethasone neither induced DDP resistance nor decreased DDP accumulation in nontransfected wild-type NIH 3T3 cells. In LTR H-*ras*(A) cells, the cellular glutathione content and glutathione-*S*-transferase activity were unchanged by induction of c-Ha-*ras* expression. The cellular metallothionnen content was increased by DEX 1.6 times in NIH 3T3 cells and 3.3 times in LTR H-*ras*(A) cells.

Conclusions.—Overexpression of a mutant c-Ha-*ras* gene resulting from DEX treatment appears to confer a significant degree of DDP resistance. This resistance is associated with impaired cellular DDP accumulation and increased metallothionen content. These results identify elements of the signal transduction pathways to target in preventing or reversing DDP resistance.

▶ Resistance to cisplatin is multifactorial, and its commonly identified mechanisms include: (1) a decrease in drug accumulation; (2) increased levels of glutathione or metallothionein, and (3) an increased repair of DNA crosslinks. This report adds to the growing evidence that resistance to cisplatin is also associated with the expression of certain oncogenes. In particular, those oncogenes involved in signal transduction appear to be involved in decreased sensitivity to cisplatin. Cyclosporine can prevent expression of these oncogenes and will restore sensitivity to cisplatin in some experimental systems (1). This observation has formed the basis of an ongoing clinical trial of cyclosporine plus cisplatin in drug-resistant patients.—R.F. Ozols, M.D., Ph.D.

Reference

1. Kacinski BM, Chambers SK: *Curr Opinion Oncol* 3:889, 1991.

An Unexpected Biotransformation Pathway for Tetrachloro-*(d,l-trans)*-1,2-diaminocyclohexaneplatinum(IV) (Tetraplatin) in the L1210 Cell Line

Chaney SG, Gibbons GR, Wyrick SD, Podhasky P (Univ of North Carolina, Chapel Hill)

Cancer Res 51:969–973, 1991 16–17

Introduction.—Tetraplatin has been considered a prodrug. Based on previous model reactions, it was expected that intracellular biotransformations of tetraplatin in the L1210 cell line would simply have reduced the tetraplatin to $PtCl_2$(dach). However, the tetraplatin taken up directly by the cell appeared to be metabolized by an alternative and unexpected pathway. Therefore, the biotransformations of tetraplatin were reviewed.

Methods.—The intracellular biotransformations of tetraplatin and $PtCl_2$(dach) in the L1210 cell line were followed with a 2-step high-performance liquid chromatography separation procedure. At early times, the biotransformation pathways in tetraplatin- and $PtCl_2$(dach)-treated cells are very different. In $PtCl_2$(dach)-treated cells, macromolecular-bound platinum and $PtCl_2$(dach) were the major platinum complexes in the cell through the first hour. In the tetraplatin-treated cells, almost all of the tetraplatin initially taken up by the cell was converted to the biotransformation products d_1 and d_2, and $PtCl_2$(dach) was a very minor biotransformation product at all times (Fig 16–8).

Conclusion.—There are unique features of tetraplatin metabolism that are observed only when tetraplatin is taken up directly by the cell without prior reduction. The reaction products do not react with DNA, and they may represent an inactivation pathway. The formation of d_1 and d_2 appears to be a side reaction, because most of the tetraplatin appears to be converted to $PtCl_2$(dach) extracellularly. The intracellular $PtCl_2$(dach) biotransformations are probably responsible for most of the therapeutic and toxic effects of tetraplatin.

► Platinum analogue development has had 2 separate goals: (1) to identify platinum drugs that have equal efficacy but less toxicity than cisplatin; and (2) to develop platinum compounds with clinical activity in cisplatin-resistant tumors. Carboplatin is a product of the first goal, and it clearly is a less toxic alternative to cisplatin; however, cisplatin is essentially totally cross-resistant to the parent compound.

On the other hand, tetraplatin is currently in phase I clinical trials based upon its effectiveness in a variety of cisplatin-resistant cell lines. The significance of the unexpected biotransformation pathway for tetraplatin described in this re-

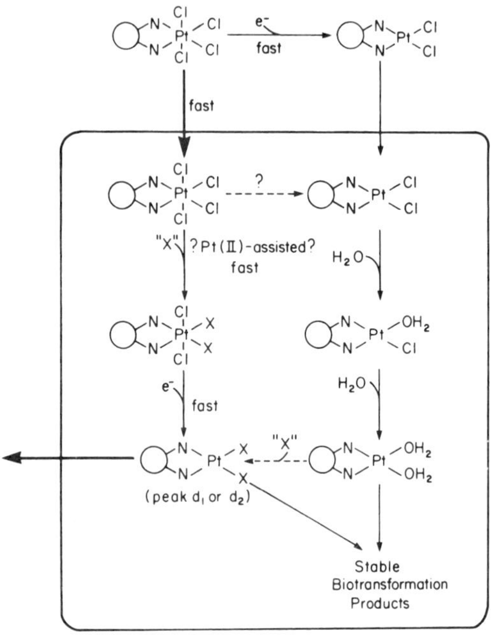

Fig 16–8.—A model for tetraplatin biotransformations in the L1210 cell line. The *(d,1-trans)*-1,2-diaminocyclohexane carrier ligand is drawn schematically. (Courtesy of Chaney SG, Gibbons GR, Wyrick SD, et al: *Cancer Res* 51:969–973, 1991.)

port is unclear. Although it may account for its cytotoxicity, it will not account for its lack of cross-resistance with cisplatin.—R.F. Ozols, M.D., Ph.D.

Complete Growth Inhibition of Human Cancer Xenografts in Nude Mice by Treatment With 20-*(S)* Camptothecin

Giovanella BC, Hinz HR, Kozielski AJ, Stehlin JS Jr, Silber R, Potmesil M (St Joseph Hosp, Houston; New York Univ)

Cancer Res 51:3052–3055, 1991 16–18

Introduction.—Water-soluble sodium salt (CAM-Na^+) derived from 20-*(S)*-camptothecin (CAM), a plant alkaloid, was tested for anticancer activity in clinical trials. Toxicities led to discontinuation of clinical applications of sodium salts. The efficacy of CAM in the treatment of various human cancer xenografts was evaluated, and the effects of CAM were compared with those of CAM-Na^+. Human tumor xenografts retain the histologic, biochemical, antigenic characteristics, and drug sensitivity pattern of original tumor tissue. Xenografts established as heterotransplants in nude mice have well-established predictive value in chemotherapy testing. Thirteen human cancer xenograft lines that are resistant to most chemotherapeutic agents were treated with CAM.

Results.—Treatment with CAM was more effective against the 13 human xenograft lines than any other clinically available drug tested. Intramuscular and oral administration were more effective than intravenous administration. In several of the lines, there was a pattern of emerging drug resistance. Analogues 9-AC and 10,11-MDC achieved the onset of complete response in a shorter time, with lower total dose compared with CAM. There was no sign of drug resistance at the second course of treatment.

Conclusion.—Although CAM-Na^+ showed low anticancer activity in clinical trials, 3 analogues of camptothecin showed unprecedented effectiveness against all human cancer xenograft lines. These analogues, 9-NC, 9-AC, and 10,11-MDC, are highly potent, and they may be tools with which to combat major therapy-resistant cancers.

▶ Camptothecin was dropped for clinical development in the early 1970s (despite documented cases of tumor response) because of an unfavorable toxicity profile (primarily severe urothelial damage). The subsequent discovery of a unique mechanism of action and the development of analogues of camptothecin has made these drugs a high priority for clinical development in the 1990s. These drugs stabilize a covalent complex between topoisomerase I and DNA that leads to enzyme-mediated DNA damage. This study demonstrates remarkable in vivo antitumor activity. Topotecan, a semisynthetic water soluble analogue of the more toxic CAM, is currently in phase II clinical trials after phase I studies demonstrated acceptable toxicity (primarily neutropenia).—R.F. Ozols, M.D., Ph.D.

Antibiotic Magainins Exert Cytolytic Activity Against Transformed Cell Lines Through Channel Formation

Cruciani RA, Barker JL, Zasloff M, Chen HC, Colamonici O (Natl Inst of Health, Bethesda, Md; Children's Hosp of Philadelphia, Pa; Univ of Chicago, Ill)

Proc Natl Acad Sci USA 88:3792–3796, 1991 16–19

Introduction.—Magainins belong to an ionophoric class of peptides that exhibit antibiotic activity against various microorganisms, and they were recently isolated from the vertebrate *Xenopus laevis.* Magainins can irreversibly lyse hematopoietic tumor and solid tumor cells with a relative cytotoxic potency that parallels their antibiotic activity with relatively little toxicity for peripheral blood lymphocytes (PBLs).

Results.—The peptides showed varying degrees of cytotoxic activity against various tumor targets. The relative antitumor activities of different structures similar to their relative antibiotic potencies. Magainin G was the most selective of the compounds tested, having virtually no cytotoxic effect on PBLs. Magainin B was the most potent of the structures; its lytic activity against PBLs and polymorphonuclear neutrophils was approximately 5 times the effective antitumor concentration. The magainins decreased bacterial membrane potential within minutes.

Conclusion.—Various magainin peptides are antitumor in vitro at concentrations that parallel their antibiotic activities. Their antitumor potency is less than antibiotic potency on a molar basis. Although magainins are selective for tumor targets over well-differentiated phenotypes, the degree of selectivity varies among analogues. Magainin G, the most selective peptide, should be tested for toxicity and antitumor efficacy in vivo.

▶ Magainins are naturally occurring antibiotic peptides. Zasloff isolated them from frog skin after he noted that skin infections did not develop in frogs after surgical procedures, even when the frogs were living in an environment filled with microorganisms (1). Magainins lyse bacteria by producing multimolecular channels in the cell wall. The observation that magainins also selectively lyse tumor cells in vitro represents a novel mechanism of cytotoxicity, and additional in vitro and in vivo studies are in progress. The basis for selectivity in magainin channel formation and lysis in tumor cells compared with normal cells is unclear, and it may represent differences in membrane potential or other physiochemical properties.—R.F. Ozols, M.D., Ph.D.

Reference

1. Zasloff M: *Proc Natl Acad Sci USA* 84:5449, 1987.

A Phase I Clinical Trial of Novobiocin, a Modulator of Alkylating Agent Cytotoxicity

Eder JP, Wheeler CA, Teicher BA, Schnipper LE (Charles A Dana Research Inst; Beth Israel Hosp; and Dana Farber Cancer Inst, Boston, Mass)
Cancer Res 51:510–513, 1991 16–20

Introduction.—Effective chemotherapy includes a combination of antineoplastic agents with individual activity against a particular tumor type. However, most adult cancers are either refractory to drug therapy at the initiation of treatment or become resistant after initial cytoreduction. Enhancing tumor cytotoxicity may potentially overcome drug resistance or enhance efficacy. Novobiocin increases the cytotoxicity of several alkylating agents in association with an increase in the formation of DNA-DNA cross-links.

Methods.—Because of a dose-response effect for novobiocin in murine tumors, an attempt was made to establish the maximum-tolerated dose of cyclophosphamide and novobiocin and the serum levels needed for a modulating effect in 34 patients with refractory cancer. In a phase I study, the patients received 65 courses of novobiocin. The dose-limiting toxicity of novobiocin was vomiting.

Results.—The maximum-tolerated dose of orally administered novobiocin was 6 g daily. Toxicity was mild to moderate, and novobiocin added very little toxicity to the cyclophosphamide. Partial responses were achieved in 2 of 30 evaluable patients. At daily doses of 4 g or greater, plasma levels of novobiocin achieved the in vitro concentration that resulted in synergistic cytotoxicity.

Conclusion.—Novobiocin achieved blood levels in the drug-potentiating range for patients with refractory cancer. It was well tolerated and did not potentiate cyclophosphamide toxicity. A phase II trial in patients with cyclophosphamide refractory will determine whether novobiocin can enhance the efficacy of chemotherapy.

▶ Alkylating agent resistance is multifactorial, and it includes alterations in drug accumulation, detoxification, and the repair of DNA adducts. Bifunctional alkylating agents produce lethal DNA-DNA interstrand adducts. A potential mechanism of resistance is the repair of the monoadduct between an alkylating agent and DNA before development of the lethal interstrand cross-link. The levels of topoisomerase II, a DNA gyrase enzyme that functions in part to remove such monoadducts, are elevated in drug-resistant tumors. Inhibition of this enzyme with novobiocin restores sensitivity to alkylating agents in experimental systems. It also led to the phase I trial described in this report. It was noteworthy that cyclophosphamide toxicity was not increased by novobiocin, suggesting at least the possibility of a specific effect on tumors. To determine whether drug resistance can be overcome will require a trial in which patients who are clearly resistant to an alkylating agent are treated with the same alkylating agent and novobiocin.—R.F. Ozols, M.D., Ph.D.

Specificity of Isozymes of Murine Hepatic Glutathione *S*-Transferase for the Conjugation of Glutathione With L-Phenylalanine Mustard

Bolton MG, Colvin OM, Hilton J (The Johns Hopkins Oncology Ctr, Baltimore, Md)

Cancer Res 51:2410–2415, 1991 16–21

Introduction.—Cancer cells exposed to chemotherapeutic drugs often acquire resistance to those drugs. Glutathione *S*-transferase (GST) isozymes protect cells from cytotoxic chemicals and may have a role in the intrinsic and acquired resistance of tumors to cytotoxic drugs. To determine whether isozymes of the α class of glutathione *S*-transferase are specifically involved in the detoxification of nitrogen mustard, GST isozymes were isolated and purified from mouse liver.

Methods.—The metabolic products of the reaction of L-phenylalanine mustard (L-PAM) with glutathione in the presence of GST isozymes were analyzed using reverse-phase high-performance liquid chromatography. A pH of 6.5 was optimal to study the effects of the presence of isozymes, because the nonenzymic conjugation of L-PAM and glutathione is suppressed, and the catalytic activity of the isozymes is more easily assessed. The presumed function of the glutathione *S*-transferases is enhancing the nucleophilicity of the sulfhydryl moiety of glutathione. The α class of GST isozymes is the principal form catalyzing the conjugation of glutathione with L-PAM.

Conclusion.—Increasing the amount of other isozymes in the reaction mixture had no effect on the metabolism of L-PAM. Only isozymes of the α GST class catalyzed the conjugation of L-PAM with glutathione. The cells may acquire resistance to nitrogen mustards by a mechanism involving increased levels of class α GST isozyme.

▶ The role of GST in clinical drug resistance to alkylating agents remains controversial. This study demonstrates that the α class of GST isozymes catalyzes the conjugation (and thereby inactivation) of glutathione (GSH) with melphalan. Previous transfection studies, however, failed to demonstrate a relationship between increased expression of the GST-π isozyme and resistance to anticancer agents. It is possible that the increase in GST-π that is often observed in drug-resistant tumors serves as a marker of neoplastic transformation rather than a specific mechanism of acquired drug resistance. Recently, O'Dwyer et al. (1) reported on the first clinical attempt to reverse alkylating agent resistance by inhibiting GST activity with ethacrynic acid. They showed that this inhibitor decreased GST activity in peripheral mononuclear cells. Additional trials are in progress to determine whether clinical resistance to alkylating agents is actually reversed by this diuretic.—R.F. Ozols, M.D., Ph.D.

Reference

1. O'Dwyer PJ, et al: *Cancer Res* 51:6059, 1991.

Biological Therapy

▶ ↓ Biological agents may exert antitumor effects indirectly or directly; they can also exert physiological effects that may not result in antitumor effects, but are deemed clinically beneficial. It is hardest to demonstrate the efficacy of an agent that exerts antitumor effects indirectly. Interleukin-2 was first reported to exert antitumor effects in melanoma and renal cell cancer in 1985, but it wasn't approved for use in renal cell cancer until more than 6 years later, and it has not yet been approved for use in melanoma. Interferon-α exerts direct antitumor effects and was approved for use based on its induction of responses in hairy cell leukemia and Kaposi's sarcoma. Tumor necrosis factor has not yet demonstrated sufficient activity to warrant approval. Also, most workers believe that cytokines will be most effective when used in combination and in the proper sequence.

On the other hand, evaluation and approval have been swift for agents used to exert physiologic endpoints other than tumor response. The colony-stimulating factors erythropoietin, G-CSF, and GM-CSF have been approved because, when given at pharmacologic doses, they exert their predicted physiologic effect. Erythropoietin induces red cell production, and G-CSF and GM-CSF stimulate production of granulocytes. When such changes are needed, these agents exert important positive effects. Nevertheless, it is not entirely clear how best to use colony-stimulating factors.—D.L. Longo, M.D., F.A.C.P.

Treatment of Established Renal Cancer by Tumor Cells Engineered to Secrete Interleukin-4

Golumbek PT, Lazenby AJ, Levitsky HI, Jaffee LM, Karasuyama H, Baker M, Pardoll DM (Johns Hopkins Univ, Baltimore, Md; Univ of Tokyo, Japan)

Science 254:713–716, 1991 16–22

Introduction.—Immunotherapy for cancer ultimately seeks to achieve antigen-specific antitumor immunity. Experiments were evaluated in mice in which a renal cell cancer was treated with tumor cells engineered to secrete the helper lymphokine interleukin-4 (IL-4).

Methods and Findings.—The tumor was a spontaneously occurring renal cell carcinoma from a BALB/c mouse. The cells of this tumor were transfected with murine IL-4 complementary DNA. Even at large doses, these cells were rejected completely when injected subcutaneously. The T cells appeared to play an important role in this rejection. Mice that rejected the IL-4–transfected tumors, however, demonstrated T-cell–dependent systemic immunity to the parental tumor. The immune response was found to be antigen specific, mediated mainly by $CD8^+$ T cells. In addition, this immune response was capable of curing established parental tumors.

Conclusion.—Poorly immunogenic, spontaneously occurring tumors that have been engineered to secrete high concentrations of Il-4 can generate tumor-specific $CD8^+$ cytotoxic T cells, which can produce systemic immunity against the parental tumor at distant sites. Thus, interleukin-4 may play an important role in recruiting antigen-presenting cells and enhancing tumor antigen presentation. Lymphokine gene-transduced cells are a promising technique for cancer therapy.

▶ The prospect of using gene therapy to treat human cancer is an appealing one. In this murine model, the tumor has been made more easily recognizable by the host through the introduction of a cytokine gene that presumably activates or attracts tumor antigen-specific T cells to the tumor in vivo. It must be acknowledged that the evidence for an effect against "established" tumor in this IL-4 model is pretty flimsy; the mice may have had only 10^4 or fewer cells as a tumor burden at the time of the treatment. In addition, IL-4 does not exert the same effects in man as it does in mice. Thus, IL-4 may not be the best cytokine to use in this setting. However, similar data have been generated with IL-2 (1), G-CSF (2), tumor necrosis factor (3), and interferon-γ (4). It appears feasible that a relatively nonimmunogenic tumor can be made more immunogenic by having it produce an appropriate cytokine. Initial human studies that are somewhat analogous to the one used in this report are under way.

The notion of applying the principle of vaccination, which has been so successful in the control of infectious diseases, to the treatment and prevention of cancer is not new; however, it has recently received additional impetus from a variety of experimental findings. First, Thierry Boon and his colleagues (5) have clearly demonstrated that patients with melanoma who express HLA-A1 share a melanoma-specific antigen that may be a target of vaccine attack. My colleague, Robert Fenton, has been able to prevent the development of *ras*-transformed tumors by giving vaccinations with the appropriate mutant *ras* protein. Similar work with the *bcr-abl* chimeric oncogene in chronic myelogenous leukemia is under way at the University of Washington. Larry Kwak and his colleagues (6) are developing vaccines in patients with B-cell lymphoma, using the monoclonal antibody on the tumor cells as the target of an anti-idiotype immune response; there has been some preliminary success in eliciting immunity in patients. Thus, the idea of eliciting and boosting a tumor-specific immune response is gathering significant momentum. The addition of an immunostimulating cytokine cofactor is 1 of many interesting approaches planned for clinical development.

Another application of gene therapy techniques would be to make bone marrow cells resistant to chemotherapy and radiation therapy. Such an experiment has been successfully performed in mice (7), and the ability to introduce genes into certain animals (such as cats [8]) that have a known susceptibility to retroviral infection has raised hopes for the application of this approach to humans. However, human marrow cells in general and stem cells in particular are not known to be natural targets for any retroviruses. Clearly, it will not be possible to use retroviral vectors for gene transfer if the target cell does not express receptors for the retrovirus. This technical barrier has not yet been addressed adequately by those who are developing retroviral vectors intended for human use.—D.L. Longo, M.D., F.A.C.P.

References

1. Fearon ER, et al: *Cell* 60:397, 1990.
2. Colombo MP, et al: *J Exp Med* 173:889, 1991.
3. Blankenstein T, et al: *J Exp Med* 173:1047, 1991.
4. Gansbacher B, et al: *Cancer Res* 50:7820, 1990.
5. Van der Bruggen P, et al: *Science* 254:1643, 1991.
6. Kwak LW, et al: *Blood* 78:2768, 1991.
7. Galski H, et al: *Mol Cell Biol* 9:4357, 1989.
8. Lothrop CD Jr, et al: *Blood* 78:237, 1991.

Corynebacterium parvum **Versus Bacille Calmette-Guérin Adjuvant Immunotherapy of Stage II Malignant Melanoma**

Lipton A, Harvey HA, Balch CM, Antle CE, Heckard R, Bartolucci AA (Milton S Hershey Med Ctr, Hershey, Pa; Pennsylvania State Univ, University Park, Pa; MD Anderson Hosp and Tumor Inst, Houston, Tex; Univ of Alabama at Birmingham)

J Clin Oncol 9:1151–1156, 1991 16–23

Background.—Animal experiments have suggested that *Corynebacterium parvum* might be superior to bacille Calmette-Guérin (BCG) as an immunostimulant in antitumor therapy. Two separate clinical trials have shown improvements in patients with stage II malignant melanoma treated with *C. parvum,* although the difference was significant in only one patient. The results of these studies were updated to determine if any conclusions can be drawn.

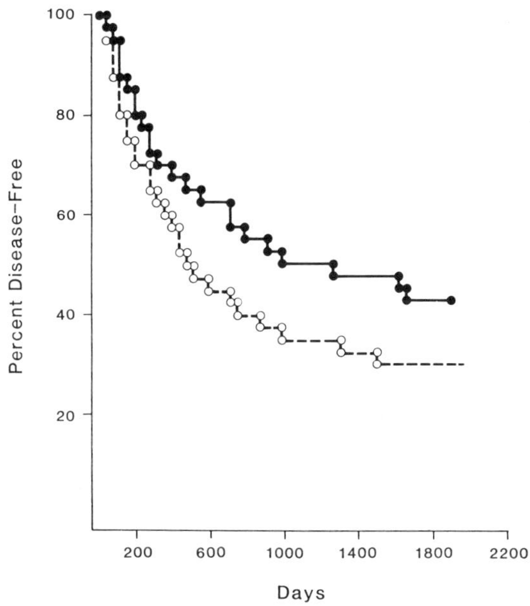

Fig 16–9.—Life-table analysis of disease-free survival of all stage II patients treated with *(filled circle) Corynebacterium parvum* or *(open circle)* bacille Calmette-Guérin; $P = .02$. (Courtesy of Lipton A, Harvey HA, Balch CM, et al: *J Clin Oncol* 9:1151–1156, 1991.)

Methods.—Forty-eight patients were treated at the Milton S. Hershey Medical Center, and 162 were treated by the Southeastern Cancer Study Group (SECSG). Because the 2 trials had similar patient selection criteria and drug treatment regimens, the data were pooled. Patients received either BCG, 3×10^8 live organisms per treatment by Tine technique, or *C. parvum*, 4 mg/m^2 in the SECSG trial and 5 μg/m^2 in the Hershey trial. Otherwise, the only difference was the frequency of immunization during the 2-year treatment period: 22 doses in the Hershey trial and 55 doses in the SECSG trial.

Results.—The estimated median disease-free survivals were 1,062 days for patients receiving *C. parvum* and 504 days for those receiving BCG. According to Kaplan-Meier life table analysis, the *C. parvum* group had a significantly prolonged disease-free interval (Fig 16–9). *Corynebacterium parvum*-treated patients had improved survival from all causes of death. Information on the number of positive nodes was available for 170 patients. According to a Cox analysis, which was stratified by nodes and used the covariates of place, treatment, age, and sex, the benefit of *C. parvum* on disease-free interval was .37. The benefit of *C. parvum* on survival time from all causes of death had a *P* value of .04. When the analysis was restricted to patients younger than 60 years of age, the benefit of *C. parvum* on disease-free interval had a *P* value of .08; the benefit on survival from all causes of death had a *P* value of .008.

Conclusions.—In the treatment of stage II malignant melanoma, *C. parvum* appears to offer benefits in terms of both disease-free interval and survival compared with BCG. The greatest benefit of C. *parvum* treatment may be seen in patients younger than 60 years of age. Other evaluations of C. *parvum* treatment are needed to determine whether it represents a therapeutic advance.

▶ Bacterial vaccines have a long and unclear history. However, a long-term follow-up of Southeastern Cancer Study Group patients suggests that patients with melanoma who received *C. parvum* adjuvant therapy had a lower rate of recurrence and superior survival compared with patients who received BCG. In light of concerns that BCG might reduce survival, it would be important for any future studies to include an untreated control group, because the results of this analysis are also compatible with the notion that *C. parvum* had no effect on natural history and that BCG made it worse.

Whole bacteria do have some theoretical advantages over isolated cytokines. Whole bacteria should elicit a panoply of host responses, whereas a particular cytokine may not elicit such a broad spectrum of responses. However, this theoretical advantage has not been clearly demonstrated, largely because of our lack of understanding of the best way to give either therapy to elicit maximal host responses. If we were trying to maximize the response to G-CSF, we would give it until the number of circulating granulocytes reached the target value. What do we measure for an immunotherapy? What do we try to maximize? What does the level of any activity measurable in the blood have to do with an immune response in the tissues? We are groping about empirically in our efforts to optimally activate the immune system. If we learn more about what our therapeutic endpoint should be, agents such as BCG and *C. parvum* may yet prove useful.—D.L. Longo, M.D., F.A.C.P.

Tumor Cell Invasion Inhibited by TIMP-2

Albini A, Melchiori A, Santi L, Liotta LA, Brown PD, Stetler-Stevenson WG (Istituto Nazionale per la Ricerca sul Cancro, Genoa, Italy; Natl Cancer Inst, Bethesda, Md)

J Natl Cancer Inst 83:775–779, 1991 16–24

Background.—Turnover and remodeling of the extracellular matrix are important events in many pathologic processes, including tumor invasion. The 72-kd type IV collagenase is 1 of the types of collagenase that is closely linked with an invasive phenotype of cancer cells. Normal cells and invasive tumor cells produce the 72-kd type IV procollagenase enzyme in a form complexed with TIMP-2, a tissue inhibitor of metalloproteinases.

Objective.—The balance between activated enzyme and available inhibitor may be a critical determinant of matrix proteolysis and, therefore, tumor invasion. The effects of adding exogenous TIMP-2 or antibody to 72-kd type IV collagenase on the invasiveness of human HT-1080 fibrosarcoma cells were studied. Invasiveness was assessed using a chemoinvasion assay.

Observations.—Addition of purified TIMP-2 altered the collagenase-inhibitor balance toward inhibition of cell invasion. Adding specific antiserum against 72-kd type IV collagenase inhibited cell invasion to the same extent. The HT-1080 cell line also produces 92-kd type IV collagenase, but it is specifically the 72-kd enzyme that has a role in tumor-cell invasion.

Conclusions.—Tumor-cell invasion is inhibited by TIMP-2 in this model. The fact that it is less widely distributed than TIMP-1 suggests that it may inhibit tumor-cell invasion in vivo more selectively than does TIMP-1. The therapeutic potential of TIMP-2 deserves further investigation.

▶ In vitro data are presented that indicate that TIMP-2 is a strong inhibitor of tumor cell invasion. These data are convincing, and the authors identify *in vivo* evaluation as an appropriate next step. It would also be appropriate to evaluate additional tumor cell lines in the in vitro assay. This would indicate whether certain classes of tumors were particularly susceptible to such a treatment strategy. For example, it would be exciting if TIMP-2 could be used chronically to inhibit reseeding of the peritoneal cavity by tumor cells in patients with ovarian cancer. A high percentage of these patients are destined to have recurrence, even if they achieve a pathologically documented complete response to intensive chemotherapy. Such patients are destined to die of the complications of extensive intraperitoneal disease that might be prevented or delayed by such adjuvant therapy.—T.C. Hamilton, Ph.D.

A Phase-I Study of Repeated Therapy With Radiolabelled Antibody to Carcinoembryonic Antigen Using Intermittent or Continuous Administration of Cyclosporin A to Suppress the Immune Response

Ledermann JA, Begent RHJ, Massof C, Kelly AMB, Adam T, Bagshawe KD (Charing Cross Hosp, London, England)

Int J Cancer 47:659–664, 1991 16–25

Background.—Limited uptake of radiolabeled antibody by human tumors has restricted the efficacy of targeted treatment of cancer. Attempts to increase the administered dose entail a risk of toxic effects of ^{131}I-labeled antibody on normal tissues. Repeat injections of small amounts of antibody might be safer, but formation of human anti-antibodies is a problem.

Study Design.—The efficacy of cyclosporine A was examined in patients given repeated intravenous injections of radiolabeled mouse monoclonal antibody to carcinoembryonic antigen (CEA). Patients received ^{131}I-labeled anti-CEA at 2-week intervals, with cyclosporine A given to suppress the antimouse antibody response. Cyclosporine was given either intermittently for 6 days with each course of anti-CEA or continuously.

Findings.—Both regimens of cyclosporine treatment suppressed the immune response, but continuous low-dose treatment was less toxic. Small amounts of antimouse antibody formed, but the rate of clearance of anti-CEA from the blood did not increase. No more than 2 courses of antibody were possible without cyclosporine A. The treatment-limiting side effect was thrombocytopenia, which delayed treatment in half the patients.

Discussion.—Cyclosporine A effectively suppresses the human anti-mouse antibody response. Improved radioimmunotherapy will require means of increasing both the absolute and relative amounts of antibody delivered to the tumor.

▶ One of the major obstacles limiting the development of monoclonal antibodies for use in human cancer therapy is the development of a host response to the murine antibodies. This paper makes an effort to suppress the host response to the antibody by using the general immunosuppressive agent, cyclosporine. In this study, a host antibody response occurred at a lower level than expected, but this response apparently made no impact on the clearance of the therapeutic antibody from the serum. Clearly, cyclosporine should be investigated further. In addition, deoxyspergualin and anti-CD4 antibody depletion of the $CD4^+$ helper T cells are 2 other strategies for preventing the development of a host antibody response that are being investigated.

An alternate strategy is to humanize the antibody. Antibody humanization is accomplished by cloning the regions determining murine antibody complementarity and inserting them into a human framework antibody. Studies of humanized antibodies are about to begin; however, there is no reason to think that the murine parts of the humanized receptor will fail to elicit a host response. The induction of a specific tolerance to the therapeutic antibody would be the best approach, and some preclinical data suggest that this may be possible in the next couple of years.

The strategy to link a radioisotope to the antibody is chiefly aimed at overcoming heterogeneity in expression of the target antigen. As long as some of the tumor cells express the target, and as long as the radioimmunoconjugate localizes to the tumor, the gamma irradiation can kill cells in the vicinity of the target-expressing cell without needing to be internalized, which is a requirement for immunotoxins and drug conjugates. However, this study and others with ^{131}I-labelled antibodies (1) have demonstrated that myelotoxicity is dose limiting, because the antibodies also localize to the marrow.

Why some investigators believe that CEA is a reasonable therapeutic target for antibodies puzzles me. It is not made by all colon cancers, is not made uniformly by those colon cancers that do make it, is not expressed on the cell surface, and is shed into the serum in large amounts. Serum levels of the target antigen have been demonstrated to distract an antibody from its tumor target. Even under ideal circumstances, the fraction of the labeled-antibody dose injection that ends up in tumor nodules is a disappointingly small fraction of a percent. Really good antibodies generally have the attribute of detecting some fraction of known sites of disease, and the fraction is always much lower than 1. In the absence of answers to these simple questions, it is not clear to me why CEA is a clever target.

In addition to radioisotope targets, the use of toxin and drug conjugates is being investigated. Another area of intense investigation is the use of antibodies to activate host cells to kill the tumor. Natural killer and LAK cells possess Fc receptors, as do granulocytes. Kushner and Cheung (2) recently demonstrated that granulocytes may efficiently kill tumor cells with the appropriate antibody attached to them. Full exploitation of the vast possibilities of monoclonal antibodies as cancer treatments awaits the removal of the host antibody response that limits the dose and duration of therapy.—D.L. Longo, M.D., F.A.C.P.

References

1. Goldenberg DM, et al: *J Clin Oncol* 9:548, 1991.
2. Kushner BH, Cheung N-KV: *Cancer Res* 51:4865, 1991.

Reversal of Adriamycin Resistance by Recombinant α-Interferon in Multidrug-Resistant Human Colon Carcinoma LoVo-Doxorubicin Cells

Scala S, Pacelli R, Iaffaioli RV, Normanno N, Pepe S, Frasci G, Genua G, Tsuruo T, Tagliaferri P, Bianco AR (Università di Napoli, Naples, Italy; Università di Cagliari, Cagliari, Italy; Univ of Tokyo, Japan)

Cancer Res 51:4898–4902, 1991 16–26

Background.—Agents that induce cell differentiation and reverse drug resistance phenotype provide a useful model for the study of chemoresistance. Alpha-interferon (IFN) causes phenotypical changes and modulates the growth of cancer cells in vitro. The effects of α-IFN on a human colon adenocarcinoma cell line and a multidrug-resistant subline were studied.

Methods.—The cell lines studied were the LoVo line and the subline LoVo/DX, which shows acquired resistance to Adriamycin. In the cytotoxicity assay, cells were grown for 48 hours in the presence or absence of 500 units of IFN-α per mL. Adriamycin was then added to final concentrations of 100–500 ng of Adriamycin per mL for 1 hour, after which both α-IFN and Adriamycin were removed. Monoclonal antibody analyses were done by flow cytometry.

Results.—The LoVo/DX cells showed increased sensitivity to low doses of Adriamycin after pretreatment with α-IFN. The parental LoVo line was unaffected by similar treatment. When the LoVo/DX cells were treated with α-IFN and 100 ng of Adriamycin per mL for 1 hour, 30% survived, compared with 100% of the untreated cells. The α-IFN–induced changes in cell cycle kinetics played no part in this effect, and variations in the expression of P-glycoprotein at the cell surface also played no part. Spectrofluorometric analysis suggested that α-IFN increased Adriamycin accumulation.

Conclusions.—Treatment with α-IFN appears to increase Adriamycin cytotoxicity in LoVo/DX cells. This effect results from modulation of the multidrug-resistance phenotype. Reproducing this effect clinically should become a major thrust of therapeutic strategies for optimizing α-IFN treatment of drug-resistant tumors.

▶ The potential uses of α-IFN combined with chemotherapy are just beginning to be explored. Alpha interferon potentiates the antitumor effects of 5-fluorouracil (1) and immunotoxins (2), and it also may reverse the multidrug resistance mediated by the *mdr* gene product, *p170* glycoprotein. A variety of agents are being tested for their effects on multidrug resistance. The calcium channel blocker, verapamil, has been shown to reverse *mdr*-mediated drug resistance in vitro, and it has been tested in several clinical trials in humans. Despite a poorly founded claim to the contrary (3), it appears that the levels of verapamil that are required to reverse drug resistance in vivo in humans are associated with complete heart block. There is some hope that the r-isomer of verapamil, which has very little effect on cardiac conduction but is effective at reversing *mdr* effects, will have a more favorable therapeutic index. A monoclonal antibody to the *p170* glycoprotein has also been shown to reverse *mdr* effects in vivo in mice bearing human tumor xenografts (4).

Progesterone has also been shown to inhibit the binding of drugs by the *p170* glycoprotein and to reverse *mdr* in vitro. Megestrol acetate is an orally active synthetic congener of progesterone that has been shown to reverse the *mdr* phenotype in vitro (5). It is in common use and can be safely administered to patients in rather large doses. Currently approved drugs such as IFN and megestrol acetate may be worth evaluating as drug reversal agents. Their effects should be readily assessable without the hurdles that often obstruct or delay the development of new chemical entities.—D.L. Longo, M.D., F.A.C.P.

References

1. Wadler S, et al: *Cancer Res* 50:2056, 1990.
2. Pearson JW, et al: *Cancer Res* 50:6379, 1990.
3. Miller TP, et al: *J Clin Oncol* 9:17, 1991.
4. Pearson JW, et al: *J Natl Cancer Inst* 83:1386, 1991.
5. Fleming GF, et al: *Cancer Chemother Pharmacol* 29:445, 1992.

Unproven Therapy

Survival and Quality of Life Among Patients Receiving Unproven as Compared With Conventional Cancer Therapy

Cassileth BR, Lusk EJ, Guerry D, Blake AD, Walsh WP, Kascius L, Schultz DJ (Univ of Pennsylvania, Philadelphia)
N Engl J Med 324:1180–1185, 1991 16–27

Background.—The popularity of unproved cancer treatments has reached new heights, particularly among well-educated patients. The length of survival and quality of life in patients at a prominent unorthodox cancer clinic who received treatments of unproved efficacy plus conventional therapy were compared with those of patients at an academic cancer center who received only the conventional treatment.

Methods.—Seventy-eight pairs of patients were matched for sex, race, age, diagnosis, and time from diagnosis of metastatic or recurrent disease. All had documented extensive malignant disease and a predicted median survival of less than 1 year. The patients were assessed approximately every 2 months until they died.

Results.—The length of survival did not differ between the 2 groups. Both had a median survival of 15 months. However, those patients treated conventionally from time of enrollment had consistently better quality-of-life scores.

Conclusions.—In this sample certain unorthodox treatments and conventional therapy produced similar results. The length of survival did not differ between the groups.

▶ These authors are to be congratulated for attempting to put some science into the murky world of unproven therapies. Although most physicians wish this subject would simply go away, previous studies have documented the common use of unproven therapies, particularly amongst the highly educated patient population. Indeed, a congressional subcommittee on quackery estimated that more than $10 billion is spent on unproven cancer treatments annually. In this study, survival and quality of life in patients treated with conventional therapy were compared with survival and quality of life in those receiving unorthodox cancer care such as immune-enhancing vaccines, vegetarian diets, and coffee enemas. Interestingly, the results of the study can be used by both proponents and opponents of unproven therapies to justify their prejudice. The study shows that the median survival is similar in the groups treated with conventional therapy and in those treated with unproven methods. Although this could be used as a argument for unorthodox cancer treatment, the patients were preselected to have extensive malignancies untreatable by conventional means. Thus, the equivalent survival is hardly unexpected. Surprisingly, quality of life was better in those patients receiving conventional treatment compared with whose those who were given unorthodox cancer treatment. Although this is not a randomized trial and patients with a variety of extensive cancers were included, the study does emphasize the toxic nature of unproven therapies. Given the widespread use of these therapies and their cost, more studies of this type should be performed.—R.C. Young, M.D., F.A.C.P.

Additional Reading

Steis RG, Smith JW II, Urba WJ, et al: Loss of interferon antibodies during prolonged continuous interferon-α2a therapy in hairy cell leukemia. *Blood* 77:792–798, 1991.

▶ The previously reported development of neutralizing antibodies to interferon were short-lived in the serum of patients who continued to receive interferon; neutralizing anti-interferon antibodies are produced only transiently.

Fossel ET, Fletcher JG, McDonagh J, et al: Selective cytotoxicity of low-density lipoprotein to helper T cells of cutaneous T-cell lymphoma after photperoxidation with 8-methoxypsoralen. *J Natl Cancer Inst* 83:1316–1321, 1991.

▶ It is proposed that the mechanism of action of extracorporeal ultraviolet light administered after oral 8-methoxypsoralen in patients with cutaneous T-cell lymphoma is the conversion of low-density lipoproteins into peroxidized carriers of free radicals that kill $CD4^+$ T cells in vivo.

Smith JW II, Longo DL, Urba WJ, et al: Prolonged continuous treatment of hairy cell leukemia patients with recombinant interferon-α2a. *Blood* 78:1664–1671, 1991.

▶ Typical short courses (12–14 months) of interferon are followed by relapse in the majority of hairy-cell leukemia patients; this series of 56 patients followed for a median of 5 years demonstrates that continuous therapy consisting of 3 megaunits of interferon given thrice weekly may keep the disease under control indefinitely, with continued improvement in response (decreasing soluble interleukin-2 receptor levels, improving blood counts) well beyond the first year of therapy.

Luger SM, Kirkwood JM, et al: High-dose cisplatin and dacarbazine in the treatment of metastatic melanoma. *JNCI* 82:1934–1937, 1990.

▶ A high dose of cisplatin plus dacarbazine (200 mg/m^2 per cycle) produced a 29% response rate in metastatic melanoma and could not confirm previous reports of higher response rates with high dose cisplatin.

O'Dwyer PJ, LaCreta F, et al: Phase I/pharmacokinetic reevaluation of thioTEPA. *Cancer Res* 51:3171–3176, 1991.

▶ The dose of thioTEPA was increased to 65 mg/m^2, with myelosuppression being dose limiting. The absence of other toxicities makes thioTEPA a potentially useful drug with colony stimulating factors.

Swinnen LJ, Ellis NK, et al: Inhibition of *cis*-diammine-1,1-cyclobutane dicarboxylatoplatinum(II)-induced DNA interstrand cross-link removal and potentiation of *cis*-diammine-1,1-cyclobutane dicarboxylatoplatinum(II) cytotoxicity by hydroxyurea and 1-β-D-arabinofuranosylcytosine. *Cancer Res* 51:1984–1989, 1991.

▶ Hydroxyurea plus *ara*-C modulates the repair of platinum-DNA adducts. Different schedules are required for carboplatin because of the slower formation of DNA adducts.

Teicher BA, Herman TS, et al: Lonidamine as a modulator of alkylating agent activity in vitro and in vivo. *Cancer Res* 51:780–784, 1991.

▶ Lonidamine inhibits oxygen consumption and potentiates the cytotoxicity of alkylating agents. The mechanism may be caused by inhibition of an energy-dependent repair process.

Smit EF, Willemse PHB, et al: Continuous infusion carboplatin on a 21-day schedule: A phase I and pharmacokinetic study. *J Clin Oncol* 9:100–110, 1991.

▶ Continuous infusion of carboplatin produced less hematologic toxicity than bolus administration. Because responses were observed in this phase I study, the authors propose a prospective comparison of a 21-day infusion schedule with standard bolus administration.

Sebti SM, Jani JP, et al: Metabolic inactivation: A mechanism of human tumor resistance to bleomycin. *Cancer Res* 51:227–232, 1991.

▶ The enzyme bleomycin hydrolase inactivates bleomycin. Inhibition of this reaction can increase the antitumor activity of bleomycin. It is unclear, however, whether inhibition of this hydrolase would also potentiate bleomycin toxicity.

La Rocca RV, Danesi R, et al: Effect of suramin on human prostate cancer cells in vitro. *J Urol* 145:393–398, 1991.

▶ Suramin has activity against prostate cancer by decreasing circulating androgens through its adrenocorticolytic effect, as well as by a direct inhibitory effect on cell proliferation. This latter effect may be a result of suramin's interference with the growth stimulatory effect of testosterone and growth factors.

Tilby MJ, Johnson C, et al: Sensitive detection of DNA modifications induced by cisplatin and carboplatin in vitro and in vivo using a monoclonal antibody. *Cancer Res* 51:123–129, 1991.

▶ The DNA adducts from carboplatin and cisplatin were similarly identified using a monoclonal antibody. This provides further confirmation of the almost complete cross resistance that exists clinically for these 2 platinum analogues.

Bissery M-C, Geunard D, et al: Experimental antitumor activity of Taxotere (RP56976, NSC 628503), a Taxol analogue. *Cancer Res* 51:4845–4852, 1991.

▶ Taxotere, an analog of taxol, has a broad spectrum of antitumor activity in experimental systems. It is produced in a semisynthetic process using a renewable source (the needles of yew trees). Phase I trials are in progress.

Frankfurt OS, Seckinger D, et al: Intercellular transfer of drug resistance. *Cancer Res* 51:1190–1195, 1991.

▶ Metabolic cooperation between cells may lead to intercellular transfer of resistance factors, such as glutathione. Inhibition of cell cooperation may potentiate the cytotoxicity of chemotherapy.

Rowinsky EK, Gilbert MR, et al: Sequences of Taxol and cisplatin: A phase I and pharmacologic study. *J Clin Oncol* 9:1692–1702, 1991.

▶ The sequence of cisplatin before taxol produced more toxicity. Pharmacologic studies demonstrated that cisplatin decreased taxol clearance rates. It is recommended that, in clinical trials of this combination, taxol should precede administration of cisplatin.

17 Complications of Cancer

Infections

Cytomegalovirus Infection Causes Delayed Platelet Recovery After Bone Marrow Transplantation

Verdonck LF, de Gast GC, van Heugten HG, Nieuwenhuis HK, Dekker AW (Univ Hosp Utrecht, The Netherlands)

Blood 78:844–848, 1991 17–1

Background.—Cytomegalovirus (CMV) infection after bone marrow transplantation (BMT) can cause CMV pneumonia, hematologic abnormalities, or graft failure. The effect of CMV infection on the hematopoietic recovery after marrow transplantation was studied retrospectively in 87 recipients of autologous BMT and 56 recipients of allogeneic BMT.

Methods.—The patients were divided into 2 groups based on CMV-positive or CMV-negative status before transplantation. Patients who tested negative for CMV were kept negative by the local transfusion policy.

Results.—Platelet recovery in the patients who underwent allogeneic BMT was significantly slower in the patients who were positive for CMV than in those who were negative for CMV. This difference remained when patients with acute graft-vs.-host disease greater than grade 1 were excluded. In patients with autologous BMT, the negative effect on platelet recovery was seen in patients with lymphomas, especially in CMV-positive patients compared with those who were not infected. Patients with acute leukemias had delayed recovery of platelets and granulocytes after autologous BMT, irrespective of CMV status. Cytomegalovirus infection had no effect on the recovery of granulocytes in autologous or allogeneic BMT.

Conclusions.—Cytomegalovirus infection caused delayed platelet recovery in patients after both autologous and allogeneic BMT. However, in recipients of autologous BMT, acute leukemia was more determinant than CMV infection for hematopoiesis after BMT. A deliberate transfusion policy that prevents transmission of CMV to CMV-negative BMT recipients may have a major impact on morbidity and mortality.

▶ Cytomegalovirus is not a very serious pathogen in immunocompetent individuals, because virus-infected cells are normally recognized by the host T cells and are eliminated. However, in recipients of allogeneic bone marrow, the donor-type T cells may be less effective at identifying CMV-infected cells, and the infection may spread. Cytomegalovirus is a very important cause of interstitial pneumonitis in transplant recipients. In this paper, the authors demonstrate that the virus can significantly retard platelet recovery in recipients of either allogeneic or autologous bone. The effects of the virus were relatively selective, and they are thought to represent specific cytotoxicity to megakaryocytes based on a murine model of CMV infection (1).—D.L. Longo, M.D., F.A.C.P.

Reference

1. Petursson SR, et al: *J Lab Clin Med* 104:381, 1984.

A Randomized, Controlled Trial of Prophylactic Ganciclovir for Cytomegalovirus Pulmonary Infection in Recipients of Allogeneic Bone Marrow Transplants

Schmidt GM, Horak DA, Niland JC, Duncan SR, Forman SJ, Zaia JA, City of Hope-Stanford-Syntex CMV Study Group (City of Hope Natl Med Ctr, Duarte, Calif; Stanford Univ, Stanford, Calif)

N Engl J Med 324:1005–1011, 1991 17–2

Introduction.—Cytomegalovirus (CMV)-associated interstitial pneumonia is the most common infectious cause of death after allogeneic bone marrow transplantation (BMT). Combined therapy with ganciclovir and intravenous immune globulin has been shown to improve survival in patients with CMV pneumonia. Whether prophylactic ganciclovir administration could prevent interstitial pneumonia in allogeneic BMT recipients with asymptomatic pulmonary CMV infection was determined in a randomized, controlled clinical trial.

Patients.—During a 3-year period, 104 patients with no evidence of respiratory disease after undergoing BMT underwent routine bronchoalveolar lavage on day 35 to determine the presence of pulmonary CMV. Sixty-four patients were negative for CMV. Of the 40 CMV-positive pa-

Rate at Which the 40 Patients Positive for CMV by Culture of Lavage Fluid Obtained on Day 35 had CMV Interstitial Pneumonia or Died. According to Treatment Assignment

Treatment Assignment	No. of Patients	Patients Who Died or Had Pneumonia*	Relative Risk (95% CI)†	P Value‡
		no. (%)		
Patients who could be evaluated				
Group 1 (ganciclovir)	18	4 (22)	0.33 (0.13–0.85)	0.015
Group 2 (observation)	15	10 (67)		
All randomized patients				
Group 1 (ganciclovir)	20	5 (25)	0.36 (0.16–0.80)	0.010
Group 2 (observation)	20	14 (70)		

*Data for patients who could be evaluated include 2 cases of CMV pneumonia and 2 deaths in group 1, and 10 cases of CMV pneumonia in group 2. The data for all randomized patients include 3 cases of CMV pneumonia and 2 deaths in group 1, and 13 cases of CMV pneumonia and 1 death in group 2.

†Indicates the risk of CMV pneumonia or death among the patients receiving ganciclovir, as compared with those under observation.

‡By 2-tailed Fisher's exact test. When step-wise logistic regression was used to adjust for severe graft-vs.-host disease at day 35, a significant treatment effect was still observed ($P = .001$).

(Courtesy of Schmidt GM, Horak DA, Niland JC, et al: *N Engl J Med* 324:1005–1011, 1991.)

tients, 20 were randomly assigned to prophylactic ganciclovir, and 20 were assigned to observation only. Intravenous ganciclovir was given twice daily at a dose of 5 mg of ganciclovir per kg for 2 weeks, and for 5 times per week thereafter until day 120 after BMT.

Results.—Five of the 20 CMV-positive patients (25%) treated with prophylactic ganciclovir died or had CMV pneumonia before day 120, compared with 14 of the 20 untreated, CMV-positive patients (70%) (table). None of the patients who received the full course of ganciclovir prophylaxis had CMV interstitial pneumonia. In 12 (22%) of the 55 evaluable CMV-negative patients, CMV pneumonia developed. In all, 31 patients had CMV interstitial pneumonia by day 120. Cytomegalovirus positivity of lavage-fluid and CMV-positive blood culture obtained on day 35 after BMT were the strongest predictors of CMV interstitial pneumonia.

Conclusions.—Asymptomatic pulmonary CMV infection is a major risk factor for CMV interstitial pneumonia in allogeneic bone marrow recipients. Prophylactic ganciclovir effectively prevents the development of CMV interstitial pneumonia in patients with asymptomatic CMV infection.

▶ Interstitial pneumonia produced by CMV is a common and serious complication of allogeneic BMT. A large review of the problem by the Seattle Group indicated that the overall incidence of CMV pneumonia was 16.7% and, in those patients, the mortality rate was 85%. A variety of techniques have been explored to reduce the morbidity and mortality of this complication, and studies with ganciclovir and intravenous immune globulin have previously been documented to improve survival in patients with this complication. This study explores the potential of prophylactic ganciclovir treatment in patients who have been documented to have persistent culture positivity but have no clinical symptoms of disease. Routine bronchoalveolar lavage was used, and patients with positive cultures were treated. Although the number of patients documented to have positive cultures was small (20 in each group), the mortality was clearly reduced by ganciclovir prophylaxis. Nevertheless, it is frustrating to see that 25% of the patients in the treatment group still had CMV pneumonia and died. Although the approach is not completely successful, prophylactic treatment with 5 mg of ganciclovir per kg, given intravenously twice daily for 2 weeks and then 5 times weekly until day 120, was associated with minimal toxicity—mostly mild increases in serum creatinine levels. It was also associated with neutropenia, which required dose modification in the maintenance phase. A vast majority of the patients tolerated this therapy without significant side effects. The use of prophylactic ganciclovir in culture-positive patients after BMT is effective in reducing the incidence of CMV interstitial pneumonia.— R.C. Young, M.D., F.A.C.P.

Use of Leukocyte-Depleted Platelets and Cytomegalovirus-Seronegative Red Blood Cells for Prevention of Primary Cytomegalovirus Infection After Marrow Transplant

Bowden RA, Slichter SJ, Sayers MH, Mori M, Cays MJ, Meyers JD (Univ of Washington; Puget Sound Blood Ctr, Seattle)

Blood 78:246–250, 1991 17–3

Introduction.—Cytomegalovirus (CMV) pneumonia remains a significant cause of infectious deaths after marrow transplantation. Because CMV-seronegative blood is not universally available, alternative ways of protecting against primary CMV infection are needed.

Objective.—A prospective study was carried out in 77 CMV-seronegative marrow transplant recipients. Those given standard unscreened blood products were compared with those who received both leukocyte-depleted platelets and CMV-seronegative red blood cells. A majority of the patients had transplantation for hematologic malignancy.

Outcome.—There were 7 CMV infections in the control group and none in the patients given leukocyte-depleted platelets, a significant difference. One patient had CMV pneumonia. Comparable amounts of red cells and platelets were given to patients in the 2 study groups.

Conclusions.—Leukocyte-depleted platelets are an effective means of preventing transfusion-associated CMV infection in marrow transplant recipients. Leukocyte depletion will likely be applied to the red cells as well, making it unnecessary to screen blood products for CMV positivity.

▶ The pathogenesis of CMV infections in bone marrow transplant patients is often passive inoculation through the infected leukocytes of CMV-seropositive-blood-component donors. This study clearly demonstrates that even a CMV-seropositive donor has little threat of infection if the blood components are depleted of leukocytes before transfusion. A variable fraction of normal donors is CMV-seropositive; 50% of the donors in the Seattle catchment area are seropositive.

The technique of depleting platelet collections of leukocytes is not technically demanding, and it requires neither specialized equipment nor fancy footwork. Blood is initially spun at 1,025 × g for 9 minutes; the supernatant is spun a second time at 3,000 × g for 20 minutes. The pellet of the second spin is highly enriched for platelets. It is resuspended in 50 mL of platelet-poor plasma, combined with other platelet concentrates, and then subjected to a final centrifugation at 400 × g before administration. The application of such a technical change may make it unnecessary to perform CMV screening in donor populations. It also promises to reduce the incidence of CMV infection from transfusion of contaminated blood products.—D.L. Longo, M.D., F.A.C.P.

Prophylactic Use of Ganciclovir in Allogeneic Bone Marrow Transplantation: Absence of Clinical Cytomegalovirus Infection

Atkinson K, Downs K, Golenia M, Biggs J, Marshall G, Dodds A, Concannon A (St Vincent's Hosp, Sydney, Australia)

Br J Haematol 79:57–62, 1991 17–4

Background.—Some, but not all, studies have shown that ganciclovir and cytomegalovirus (CMV) immunoglobulin decrease the mortality of CMV pneumonitis. Cytomegalovirus infection still causes many deaths. The administration of prophylactic ganciclovir to minimize the risk of CMV infection was studied in patients at high risk after undergoing allogeneic transplantation.

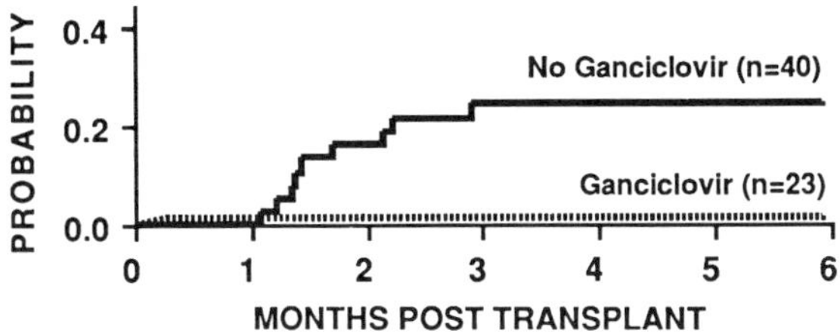

Fig 17–1.—A Kaplan-Meier plot of the probability of acquiring CMV infection in patients given prophylactic or no prophylactice ganciclovir who were immunosuppressed post-transplant with the cyclosporine/short methotrexate regimen and who received prophylactic acyclovir and the same blood product transfusion strategy. (Courtesy of Atkinson K, Downs K, Golenia M, et al: *Br J Haematol* 79:57–62, 1991.)

Methods.—Patients with hematologic malignancies were studied. There were 16 men and 9 women (age range, 20–44 years). In each case, either the recipient or the donor was CMV seropositive. Patients who were seropositive before transplantation received ganciclovir both before and after the procedure. Those who were seronegative before the transplant but had received seropositive marrow were given ganciclovir after the transplant. The dosage was 5 mg of ganciclovir per kg, given twice a day from day −8 to day −1 before the procedure, and resumed at day 21 or when the neutrophil count reached 1×10^9/L or more. The patients were compared with a group of 152 historic controls who did not receive prophylactic ganciclovir.

Results.—No patient showed nonhematopoietic toxicity; only 1 patient had treatment stopped because of renal impairment. Four of 19 evaluable patients had late reversible hematologic toxicity—2 had leukopenia and 1 each had thrombocytopenia and pancytopenia. There was no incidence of CMV interstitial pneumonitis (IP) or any other clinical CMV infection. At as long as 518 days after transplantation, 16 patients were alive. In the historic controls, 23% had clinical CMV infections and 17% had CMV IP. The incidence of clinical CMV infection was 24%, and the incidence of CMV IP was 13% when the analysis included only patients receiving the same cyclosporine/short methotrexate prophylaxis, the same acyclovir prophylaxis, and the same CMV- and leukocyte-filtered blood product transfusion technique (Fig 17–1).

Conclusions.—Pretreatment with ganciclovir appears to decrease the likelihood of CMV infection in patients receiving allogeneic bone marrow transplants. This is true even for those patients who receive immunosuppression regimens sufficient to control graft-vs.-host disease. The adverse hematopoietic effects appear to be reversible.

▶ Neither this study nor that outlined in Abstract 17–3 was randomized prospectively, but when one institutes a change that reduces the risk of CMV infection from 25% to zero, it may not take a randomized trial to be convinced. However, if you want a randomized trial, Goodrich and colleagues from Seattle (1) have provided such a trial in a slightly different subset of patients. Those patients undergoing bone marrow transplantation were screened for CMV excretion by culture of throat swabs, blood, urine, or bronchoalveolar lavage fluid. When a patient was found to be excreting virus, he/she was randomized to receive either placebo or 5 mg of ganciclovir per kg twice daily for 1 week, and then 5 mg/kg daily. The CMV disease developed in 1 of 37 ganciclovir-treated patients (3%) and in 15 of 35 placebo-treated patients (43%). The ganciclovir-treated patients also had improved survival compared with patients receiving placebo. The major toxicity was neutropenia, which reversed after discontinuation of the drug.

At day 35, Schmidt and colleagues (2) randomized transplantation patients with CMV-positive bronchoalveolar lavage fluid to ganciclovir or no therapy, and they found that ganciclovir reduced the incidence of CMV pneumonia by 77%. Pneumonia developed in only 15% of the patients with CMV-positive lavage fluid treated with ganciclovir, compared with 65% of those who were not treated. The difference in efficacy may be related to the relatively late initiation of therapy in the study by Schmidt et al.

The suppression of CMV disease by ganciclovir is dependent on continued treatment or reconstitution of CD8+ T cells capable of recognizing CMV-infected cells. In the Goodrich et al. study, ganciclovir was discontinued at day 100, and CMV disease developed in 4 patients after that point. In some patients, CMV disease develops without the virus being shed in a fashion detectable by periodic surveillance. In some patients, CMV develops resistance to ganciclovir. Administration of immunoglobulin (3), particularly immunoglobulin with high titers of antibody to CMV (4), may reduce the incidence of resistant disease. Foscarnet, which inhibits the DNA polymerase of CMV, may be effective in ganciclovir-resistant disease (5), but the results are largely anecdotal at this point.

The major clinical benefit that is documented with the use of prophylactic ganciclovir would appear to justify its use in all CMV-seropositive patients. The neutropenia it produces is of concern, but the effects of G-CSF or GM-CSF in this setting may ameliorate this problem. Perhaps one third of CMV-seropositive patients do not excrete the virus during the first 10 weeks post-transplant. Thus, most of this subset of patients would not benefit from prophylaxis. However, CMV is sufficiently serious in its effects that the use of prophylactic therapy would appear to be justified.

The recent report of transplant patients in whom interstitial pneumonitis is apparently induced by the CMV-related herpesvirus-6 may create another therapeutic problem (6). However, herpesvirus-6 appears to be sensitive to ganciclovir in vitro. The magnitude of the problem with herpesvirus-6 and the features that put patients at risk require further study.—D.L. Longo, M.D., F.A.C.P.

References

1. Goodrich JM, et al: *N Engl J Med* 325:1601, 1991.
2. Schmidt GM, et al: *N Engl J Med* 324:1005, 1991.
3. Emanuel D, et al: *Ann Intern Med* 109:777, 1988.
4. Reed EC, et al: *Ann Intern Med* 109:783, 1988.
5. Drobyski WR, et al: *Transplantation* 52:155, 1991.
6. Carrigan DR, et al: *Lancet* 338:147, 1991.

Nosocomial Pneumonia in Adult Patients Undergoing Bone Marrow Transplantation: A 9-Year Study

Pannuti CS, Gingrich RD, Pfaller MA, Wenzel RP (Univ of Iowa, Iowa City)

J Clin Oncol 9:77–84, 1991 17–5

Introduction.—Pneumonia is a major cause of morbidity and mortality in patients undergoing bone marrow transplantation (BMT). The incidence and etiology of nosocomial pneumonia that occurred in the first hospitalization period was defined in a group of patients with BMT.

Observations.—A group of 275 consecutive patients (age, 16 years and older) treated wtih BMT during a 9-year period was studied. Fifty-five patients (20%) had nosocomial pneumonia within 100 days of the transplant. The crude mortality during hospitalization was 74.5%. A cause could be established in 67% of the episodes (table). *Aspergillus* species, alone or in association with others, was responsible for 36% of the cases. *Aspergillus pneumonia* was associated with a crude mortality of 95%. Eliminating 90% of the *Aspergillus* cases would have reduced the overall attack rate to 13.4%, and the associated crude mortality to 43.4%.

Discussion.—These findings are consistent with the high mortality associated with pneumonia reported in other series of patients who had BMT. In the BMT unit studies, eliminating 90% of the *Aspergillus* cases, as might be expected with high-efficiency particulate air filtration and unidirectional airflow in patients' rooms, would have markedly reduced the overall pneumonia attack rate and crude mortality.

▶ The spectrum of pneumonias occurring after BMT varies not only in time, but also by institution. Many BMT programs now cite CMV as the major cause of pulmonary infection. These investigators from the University of Iowa found

Etiologic Agents and Methods of Diagnosis in 55 Episodes of Nosocomial Pneumonia in Adult Patients With BMT

Etiologic Agent	Number of Cases	Sputum	Sputum + Blood	BAL	OLB	Skin Biopsy	Nose Biopsy	Autopsy
Aspergillus species	20 (36.4%)	6		4	5	2	3	11
C albicans	3 (5.4%)							3
Cryptococcus neoformans	1			1				
Histoplasma capsulatum	1				1			
P carinii	3 (5.4%)	1		2				
Chlamydia trachomatis	1				1			
L pneumophila	2			2				
Pseudomonas aeruginosa	1		1					
Xanthomonas maltophilia	1		1					
Klebsiella pneumoniae	1		1					
CMV	7 (12.7%)			4	1			4
RSV	3 (5.4%)	2		1				1
Not identified	18 (32.7%)							

Abbreviation: OLB, open lung.
Note: Six patients had 2 agents isolated at time of pneumonia.
(Courtesy of Pannuti CS, Gingrich RD, Pfaller MA, et al: *J Clin Oncol* 9:77–84, 1991.)

Aspergillus pneumonia to be their most common infection. It is not only common, but remains lethal. The crude mortality in their patients with *Aspergillus* infections was 95%, and this infection was the primary reason for the high overall crude mortality (75%). Although the investigators propose the use of high-efficiency particulate air filtration and unidirectional airflow to reduce *Aspergillus* infections, the extent to which an approach would be successful remains unclear. The summary of their cases found in the table illustrates the wide variety of fungal, bacterial, and viral infections contributing to nosocomial pneumonia; it also highlights the unusual and changing patterns responsible for serious disease.—R.C. Young, M.D., F.A.C.P.

Herpes Simplex Virus Infection in the Immunocompromised Cancer Patient

Bustamante CI, Wade JC (Univ of Maryland, Baltimore)

J Clin Oncol 9:1903–1915, 1991 17–6

Background.—Patients wtih immunocompromised cancer continue to have severe herpes simplex virus (HSV) invasions. Herpes simplex infections now appear as a major cause of morbidity and mortality in this patient population. The current data and outlook were studied for viral infections in general and for HSV in particular.

Methods.—The medical and scientific literature determined the pathogenesis, clinical parameters, and present prophylactic and therapeutic protocols for treatment of HSV infections in immunocompromised patients.

Results.—The major causes of herpes infection include HSV-1 and HSV-2, which affect the mucosal and extramucosal locations in the body (including the eye, the viscera, genitals, skin, face, CNS, and peripheral nervous system). Herpes simplex virus-1 infections occur chiefly in children aged 2–10 years, but adults also can contract the disease. Herpes simplex virus-2 infections primarily affect adult genital areas. The normal immune system counters most invasions of the herpes virus strains, but the immunocompromised patient often has recurrent infection by these viruses. Those patients undergoing bone marrow transplant have an 80% chance of HSV reinfection that is usually severe, frequent, and long-term. Such HSV infections appear in the nasolabial, esophageal, and genital mucocutaneous locations. After chemotherapy, HSV infections occur in the oral cavity. If the nasal areas are infected with HSV, a secondary bacterial invasion can overwhelm the respiratory areas. Disseminated HSV occurs infrequently. Management and treatment of HSV infections usually involve acyclovir, but the drug's toxic and problematic side effects must be monitored carefully. However, acyclovir prophylaxis has shown promise in avoiding the reactivation of the HSV infection in the immunocompromised patient. Viral strains resistant to acyclovir have been documented.

Conclusions.—The effective treatment of HSV infections in immunocompromised patients requires the development of new antiviral agents to counter the development of viral resistance to acyclovir and to further reduce the mortality from these recurrent infections.

▶ Herpes simplex virus infections continue to be a serious cause of morbidity and, sometimes, mortality in immunocompromised patients with cancer. This comprehensive review of the problem highlights the clinical spectrum of disease, the currently available diagnostic techniques, and the available treatments. Ordinarily, diagnosis can be made on clinical grounds and can be confirmed with HSV titers and culture. Both oral and intravenous acyclovir are effective in the treatment of acute and chronic infections in immunosuppressed patients, although rapid recurrence of the disease often occurs after acyclovir is discontinued. Resistance to acyclovir appears to be relatively rare, although resistant strains are now being reported.—R.C. Young, M.D., F.A.C.P.

Detection of Circulating *Candida* Enolase by Immunoassay in Patients with Cancer and Invasive Candidiasis

Walsh TJ, Hathorn JW, Sobel JD, Merz WG, Sanchez V, Maret SM, Buckley HR, Pfaller MA, Schaufele R, Sliva C, Navarro E, Lecciones J, Chandrasekar P, Lee J, Pizzo PA (Natl Cancer Inst, Bethesda, Md; Duke Univ, Durham, NC; Wayne State Univ, Detroit; Johns Hopkins Med Insts, Baltimore; Becton Dickinson Advanced Diagnostics, Baltimore; et al)

N Engl J Med 324:1026–1031, 1991 17–7

Introduction.—Invasive candidiasis can be difficult to diagnose, yet is an important cause of morbidity and death in cancer patients. The value of blood enolase as a marker for invasive candidiasis was examined in 170 patients at high risk because of cancer and neutropenia. Twenty-four of the patients did in fact have invasive candidiasis that manifested as tissue infection in 13 cases and as fungemia in 11.

Methods.—Antigen testing was done in a blind manner by using a double-sandwich liposomal immunoassay for *Candida* enolase in serial serum specimens. The control subjects included 50 patients with candidal colonization and 96 who lacked evidence of candidiasis.

Findings.—More than half of the serum samples from patients with proven invasive candidiasis were positive; the assay was 54% sensitive. Multiple sampling was positive in 85% of the patients with proven deep tissue infection and in 64% of the patients with fungemia. The assay was 96% specific. Enolase antigenemia was seen in all but 1 of 5 patients in whom invasive disease was established by tissue diagnosis alone.

Discussion.—The presence of *Candida* enolase in the blood may be a useful indicator of deep infection in patients with cancer who are neutropenic. Limiting testing to those at high risk of invasive disease will maximize its specificity and help control costs.

▶ Invasive fungal disease has long been a serious complication in immunosupressed patients with cancer. Although invasive candidiasis is the most common fungal complication in such patients, the diagnosis has been difficult, and the distinction between candida colonization and invasive visercal disease has been problematic. Although the presence of either *Candida* pseudohyphae in biopsy tissue or persistent fungemia documents the disease, investigators have long sought more noninvasive diagnostic tools. These authors document the usefulness of detecting circulating *Candida* enolase as a marker for candidiasis. They document that 94% of the patients with superficial candidiasis are negative for antigen. The specificity is 96%, and the sensitivity is 85%. Unfortunately, there are significant false negatives, and multiple blood samples are required to achieve their sensitivity. Whereas the presence of *Candida* enolase antigenemia does indicate the presence of invasive candidiasis, the absence of the marker does not.—R.C. Young, M.D., F.A.C.P.

Amphotericin B vs High-Dose Ketoconazole for Empirical Antifungal Therapy Among Febrile, Granulocytopenic Cancer Patients: A Prospective, Randomized Study

Walsh TJ, Rubin M, Hathorn J, Gress J, Thaler M, Skelton J, McKnight J, Browne M, Narshall D, Cotton D, Hiemenz J, Longo D, Wesley R, Pizzo PA (Natl Insts of Health, Bethesda, Md)

Arch Intern Med 151:765–770, 1991 17–8

Background.—In patients with cancer with granulocytopenia, fungal infections may cause serious illness or death. Amphotericin B is an effective empirical antifungal agent, but its toxicity makes therapeutic alternatives desirable. A randomized, prospective study compared amphotericin B and ketoconazole in persistently or recurrently febrile granulocytopenic patients.

Methods.—Ninety-seven patients were eligible for empirical antifungal therapy, but 20 (21%) were ineligible for randomization to ketoconazole because they were unable to tolerate oral medications. A total of 72 patients was eligible for randomization; of these, 64 were assessable. The dose of ketoconazole was 200 mg/day for patients weighing less than 10 kg, 400 mg/day for those weighing between 10 and 39.9 kg, and 800 mg/day for those weighing more than 40 kg. The dose of amphotericin B was .5 mg/kg/day after an initial test dose of 1 mg.

Results.—Of the 6 patients with proved fungal infections who were randomized to receive ketoconazole, 5 had to cross over to amphotericin B because of progressive infection. Four patients in the amphotericin B group had to cross over to ketoconazole because of bronchospasm or progressive renal failure. The mean time to an afebrile state was 4 days with ketoconazole, compared with 3 days with amphotericin B, a nonsignificant difference. The patients in the ketoconazole group had a higher frequency of increased transaminase, whereas those in the amphotericin B group had a higher frequency of azotemia. Ketoconazole had unpredictable bioavailability.

Conclusions.—High-dose ketoconazole is not appropriate for empirical antifungal therapy in granulocytopenic patients because it cannot be given parenterally, is ineffective against proved mycoses, and has unreliable bioavailability. Thus, amphotericin B continues to be the drug of choice for this purpose. Alternatives to conventional amphotericin B should be developed.

▶ Sometimes good ideas just don't work. Fungal infections in patients with cancer who are febrile and granulocytopenic continue to be a serious problem. A series of careful studies has demonstrated the effectiveness of sequential application of prophylactic antibiotics followed by prophylactic antifungals if fever persists. Amphotericin B has long been the antifungal therapy of choice, but few physicians are satisfied with it. Its side effects, which include fever, renal toxicity, and liver function abnormalities, make new therapeutic alternatives highly desirable.

These investigators have carried out a straightforward, randomized prospective study comparing empirical amphotericin B therapy with high-dose ketoconazole (800 mg/kg/day orally). They document that the patients treated with prophylactic ketoconazole frequently required crossover to resolve their fever effectively. They appropriately conclude that amphotericin B remains the drug of choice for fungal prophylaxis in such patients, despite its side effects. Unfortunately, the study also documents the inability of either approach to eliminate the problem of invasive fungal disease. A total of 6% of the patients receiving high-dose ketoconazole, and 9% of the patients receiving amphotericin B died of fungal infections, despite prophylaxis. Although amphotericin B remains the drug of choice, it is still toxic and incompletely effective. We still need better drugs.—R.C. Young, M.D., F.A.C.P.

Lack of Association Between Neutropenia and the Incidence of Bacteremia Associated with Indwelling Central Venous Catheters in Febrile Pediatric Cancer Patients

Gorelick MH, Owen WC, Seibel NL, Reaman GH (George Washington Univ School of Medicine, Washington, DC)

Pediatr Infect Dis J 10:506–510, 1991 17–9

Background.—Infections, including those that develop into bacteremia, continue to cause morbidity and death in children with malignant diseases. Children undergoing cytotoxic chemotherapy appear to be at particular risk for these infections, which are usually marked by fever. The outcomes of 67 pediatric patients with cancer with indwelling catheters were evaluated. The patients had experienced 140 episodes of fever.

Methods.—Pediatric oncology records were reviewed retrospectively for data on all children with indwelling catheters who were admitted for fever between January 1989 and October 1989. The definitions for infection included an absolute neutrophil count of greater than $500/mm^3$ for neutropenia and a positive blood culture from the catheter (with or without a positive blood culture from a peripheral site) for bacteremia.

Results.—Of the 67 patients, 46 had at least 1 febrile episode related to neutropenia, and 37 had fever without the signs of neutropenia. Sixteen patients belonged to both of these groups. Six patients had a Portacath catheter, whereas the remainder had Broviac catheters. Of the 140 instances of fever, 55 (39%) occurred while the patient was not neutropenic, and 85 (61%) developed during neutropenia. Thirteen (23.6%) of the 55 non-neutropenic fevers were bacteremic, and 8 (9.4%) of the 85 neutropenic fevers were bacteremic, for a significant difference. The episodes of fever occurred twice as often in patients with exit-site infections in the non-neutropenic group than in the neutropenic group; however, the difference was not significant. Gram-positive organisms were the most common isolates in both neutropenic and non-neutropenic patients.

Implications.—These results indicate that an indwelling catheter may lead to increased risk of infection and sepsis in these young patients. The immediate administration of empiric antibiotics to all pediatric patients with cancer and both fever and an indwelling venous catheter is recommended.

▶ This interesting report raises the red flag. One cannot rely on neutropenia as an indicator of greater susceptibility to the development of infection from indwelling central venous catheters. The authors suggest an aggressive use of antibiotics when fever develops in patients with these catheters. This is certainly the practice in most cancer centers. Indwelling central venous catheters have become so common they are often taken for granted, and a central principle of nosocomial infection is often forgotten: the catheter is a foreign body and an obvious nidus for infection.—J.V. Simone, M.D.

Management

Greenfield Filter as Primary Therapy for Deep Venous Thrombosis and/or Pulmonary Embolism in Patients With Cancer

Cohen JR, Tenenbaum N, Citron M (Long Island Jewish Med Ctr; Albert Einstein College of Medicine, New Hyde Park, NY)

Surgery 109:12–15, 1991 17–10

Introduction.—Anticoagulation is associated with a high complication rate in patients with cancer and deep venous thrombosis (DVT) and/or pulmonary embolism (PE).

Methods.—The use of Greenfield filters (GFs) as primary treatment instead of anticoagulation was evaluated in 18 patients wtih cancer and DVT and/or PE who had received a GF since 1985. In the same 4-year period, 11 patients with cancer with DVT and/or PE were given anticoagulation treatment.

Results.—Major complications occurred in 4 patients who received anticoagulation therapy and in none who received a GF. The 4 complications in the anticoagulation group were 3 bleeding episodes and 1 PE. In each patient, anticoagulation was adequate. Two patients died of their complications. Each of the patients with bleeding complications required a transfusion of more than 3 units of blood. All 4 patients with complications had metastatic disease.

Conclusion.—Greenfield filter placement appears to be safer than anticoagulation for the treatment of DVT or PE in patients with cancer, especially those with metastatic disease. Insertion of GFs may be superior to anticoagulation as the primary treatment.

▶ This is a small, nonrandomized, retrospective study. As such, no firm conclusions about the superiority of GF compared with anticoagulation are possible. However, the complete absence of any complications after insertion of the GF is noteworthy.—R.F. Ozols, M.D., Ph.D.

Ondansetron (GR 38032F): A Novel Antiemetic Effective in Patients Receiving a Multiple-Day Regimen of Cisplatin Chemotherapy

Hainsworth JD, Omura GA, Khojasteh A, Bryson JC, Finn AL (Vanderbilt Univ, Nashville; Univ of Alabama, Birmingham; Ellis Fischel Cancer Ctr, Columbia, Mo; Glaxo, Inc, Research Triangle Park, NC)

Am J Clin Oncol 14:336–340, 1991 17–11

Background.—Patients with cancer who are receiving cisplatin have problems with nausea and vomiting. The selective serotonin type-3 antagonist ondansetron is effective in patients receiving both single- and multiple-day courses of cisplatin. A phase II trial of ondansetron's antiemetic efficacy was conducted in patients receiving several days of cisplatin therapy.

Methods.—The multicenter, open-label trial included 42 patients receiving their first course of cisplatin therapy. The doses of cisplatin ranged from 20 to 40 mg/m^2/day for 4–5 days. There were 28 men and 14 women (median age, 51 years) with a wide variety of tumor types. In 31 patients, ondansetron, .15 mg/kg, was given intravenously in 3 daily doses every 6 hours, with the first dose given 30 minutes before cisplatin was begun. The other 11 patients followed the same schedule, with a fourth daily dose added 17.5 hours after cisplatin administration. The patients received no other antiemetics.

Results.—Of the 40 patients in whom efficacy was evaluable, 13 had no vomiting during the 5 days of the study. On a daily basis, 50% to 75% of patients were completely free of emesis, and 65% to 93% had 2 or fewer episodes of emesis. Treatment failure occurred most commonly on days 3 and 4. Only minor and transient side effects, with no extrapyramidal side effects, were seen.

Conclusions.—In patients undergoing multiple-day courses of cisplatin therapy, ondansetron appears to be a safe and effective antiemetic treatment. Its efficacy is comparable to that of high-dose metoclopramide, and it has no extrapyramidal side effects. Randomized clinical trials are underway.

▶ Nausea and vomiting associated with platinum-based chemotherapy—as well as other intensive combination chemotherapies—have been an extremely unpleasant part of cancer treatment. Although physicians may have grown used to the reality of this side effect, patients have not. Nausea and vomiting remain 2 of the major fears and complaints about modern cancer chemotherapy. This multicenter trial studied ondansetron, a serotonin receptor antagonist, in patients receiving platinum-based chemotherapy. A third of the patients had no vomiting at any time during their treatment, and major protection, which was defined as less than 2 emetic episodes, occurred in 65% to 93% of the patients. Although this result is similar to the results of earlier studies with high-dose metoclopramide, ondansetron does not have the troublesome extrapyramidal side effects found in many patients receiving metoclopramide. Although the drug is not cheap, it does appear to be highly effective.—R.C. Young, M.D., F.A.C.P.

Comparison of Ondansetron and Ondansetron Plus Dexamethasone as Antiemetic Prophylaxis During Cisplatin-Containing Chemotherapy

Smith DB, Newlands ES, Rustin GJS, Begent RHJ, Howells N, McQuade B, Bagshawe KD (Charing Cross Hosp, London; Mount Vernon Cancer Centre, Northwood, Middlesex, England; Glaxo Group Research Ltd, Greenford, Middlesex, England)

Lancet 338:487–490, 1991 17–12

Introduction.—High-dose cisplatin chemotherapy for cancer results in particularly severe nausea and vomiting. Because the use of ondansetron alone does not control these particular cisplatin side effects, the efficacy of ondansetron plus dexamethasone as an antiemetic prophylaxis was compared with ondansetron alone.

Methods.—A double-blind, randomized, crossover design was used to study 30 men and 1 woman who had metastatic germ-cell tumors. Their 4-day chemotherapy included cisplatin. Ondansetron (8 mg/hour) was given to all patients for the first 8 days of chemotherapy to ensure control of delayed emesis from cisplatin. The patients were given either dexamethasone or placebo every 8 hours starting 2 hours before cisplatin (on day 4). During the second chemotherapy course beginning 14 days later, the patients received ondansetron plus placebo.

Results.—Twenty-seven of the original 31 patients were evaluable. Complete or major control of emesis was reported in 78% of the patients taking ondansetron plus dexamethasone, compared with 30% of those taking ondansetron plus placebo. Ondansetron plus dexamethasone demonstrated a significant advantage in controlling nausea and emesis in the crossover analysis. The side effects were minimal.

Conclusions.—Ondansetron plus dexamethasone was very effective in controlling the nausea and emesis associated with high-dose cisplatin chemotherapy. The combination can be given orally, and it causes no sedation or toxicity.

▶ We are on the constant look-out for effective controls of emesis caused by chemotherapy. Ondansetron is an effective agent and, as this study demonstrated, when combined with dexamethasone, it was even more effective. This is a promising combination that has the enormous advantages of oral administration and minimal to no toxicity. One hopes that the oral formulation of odansetron will become available in the marketplace. At present, only the very expensive parenteral form is available in this country.—J.V. Simone, M.D.

Phase I-II Trial of Erythropoietin in the Treatment of Cisplatin-Associated Anemia

Miller CB, Platanias LC, Mills SR, Zahurak ML, Ratain MJ, Ettinger DS, Jones RJ (Johns Hopkins Oncology Ctr, Baltimore)

J Natl Cancer Inst 84:98–103, 1992 17–13

Background.—Anemia may result from many causes in patients receiving cisplatin-containing chemotherapy, but erythropoietin deficiency seems to play an important role. Animal studies suggest that recombinant human erythropoietin (epoetin) can reverse cisplatin-associated anemia. The safety and effectiveness of epoetin treatment were evaluated in a phase I–II clinical trial.

Methods.—The study sample comprised 21 patients in whom anemia developed in association with cisplatin chemotherapy. There were 14 men and 7 women (mean age, 51 years) with cancers in a wide variety of sites. All had a hemoglobin level of less than 110 g/L. The patients were given escalating intravenous doses of 25, 50, 100, or 200 units of epoetin per kg, 5 times a week for 4 weeks.

Results.—In the patients receiving the 2 largest doses, the hemoglobin levels increased significantly after 4 weeks of treatment; there was a 19 g/L increase in the group given 100 units of epoetin per kg, and a 24 g/L increase in the group given 200 units of epoetin per kg. Twelve patients achieved a clinical response, which was defined as an increase greater than 10 g/L. Their mean increase was 25 g/L higher than the level at the same point in their chemotherapy cycle preceding epoetin treatment. The response to epoetin could not be predicted by either the serum erythropoietin level or the hemoglobin level. The treatment was well tolerated, with no severe dose-dependent side effects. There were 2 cases of hypertension that responded to standard antihypertensive therapy.

Conclusions.—Epoetin has promise as a safe and effective treatment for reversal of cisplatin-associated anemia. The best response is achieved at doses of 100 and 200 units of epoetin per kg. A phase III trial has been begun to assess epoetin's effects on transfusion requirements in patients receiving chemotherapy.

▶ Historically, hematologic toxicity has been the major dose-limiting toxicity associated with chemotherapy. Furthermore, anemia, thrombocytopenia, and neutropenia have frequently limited studies of dose escalation in patients with cancer. It is somewhat ironic that most of the progress that has been made in pharmacologically reversing hematologic toxicity has been made toward overcoming drug-induced anemia, the 1 hematologic toxicity that already is usually well controlled by administration of human blood products (in this case, packed cells), and that is rarely—if ever—dose-limiting. On the other hand, neutropenia and, particularly, thrombocytopenia remain major dose-limiting toxicities. Both G-CSF and GM-CSF have helped to decrease the consequences of neuropenia, but they essentially have no effect on thrombocytopenia. Newer cytokines (interleukin [IL]-3, IL-1 alpha, IL-6, and stem-cell factor) are in clinical and/or preclinical development based on their potential to stimulate earlier precursors of megakarocytes. It seems probable that, in the near future, either a cytokine or a combination of cytokines will be available that can completely reverse tri-lineage chemotherapy-induced hematologic toxicity and can permit a more detailed exploration of the relationship of dose intensity and survival in cancer.—R.F. Ozols, M.D., Ph.D.

Intrapleural Therapy for Malignant Pleural Effusions: A Randomized Comparison of Bleomycin and Tetracycline

Ruckdeschel JC, Moores D, Lee JY, Einhorn LH, Mandelbaum I, Koeller J, Weiss GR, Losada M, Keller JH (Albany Med College, Albany, NY; Univ of Alabama, Birmingham; Indiana Univ, Indianapolis; Audie Murphy VA Hosp, San Antonio, Tex; Bristol Myers US Pharmaceutical Group, Evansville, Ind)
Chest 100:1528–1535, 1991 17–14

Introduction.—Malignant pleural effusion remains a frequent complication of advanced cancer. In 1985, at 13 United States centers, the efficacy of tetracycline was compared with that of bleomycin in the treatment of this disorder.

Patients and Treatment.—Eighty-five patients were randomized to receive either low-dose (60 units) bleomycin therapy or a dose of tetracycline, 1 g, instilled via chest tube. All the patients had a cytologically pos-

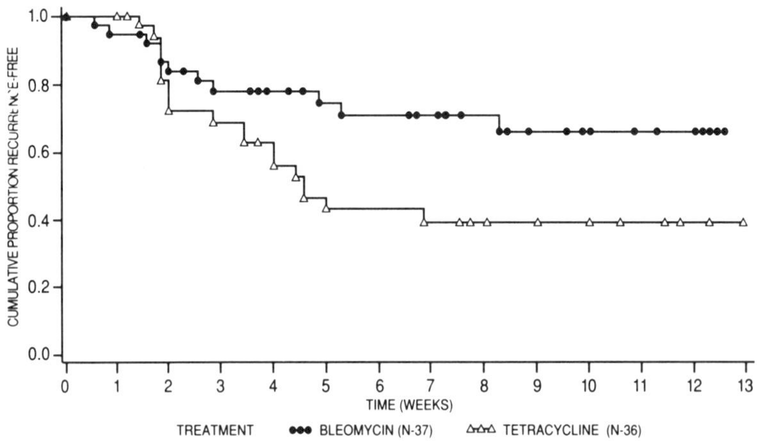

Fig 17–2.—Time to recurrence for all evaluable patients. One patient receiving each treatment was completely lost to follow-up. Bleomycin-treated patients had recurrence significantly later (P = .037). Consideration of all "eligible" (as opposed to all "evaluable") patients gave virtually identical results. (Courtesy of Ruckdeschel JC, Moores D, Lee JY, et al: *Chest* 100:1528–1535, 1991.)

itive pleural effusion and a good performance status. The lung reexpanded after tube thoracostomy, and drainage did not exceed 100 mL per 24 hours. None of the patients had previously received intrapleural treatment or systemic bleomycin.

Results.—In the 74 evaluable patients, the overall survival was similar in the 2 treatment groups. The median time to recurrent or progressive effusion was 32 days in the tetracycline group and at least 46 days in the bleomycin-treated patients (Fig 17–2). Recurrence rates within 30 days of treatment were 67% and 36%, respectively. At 3 months, 30% of the bleomycin-treated patients and 53% of those given tetracycline had recurrences. Toxicity was comparable in the 2 groups, although more tetracycline-treated patients had severe or life-threatening adverse effects.

Implication.—Controlling malignant pleural effusion is a palliative measure. Only one less day in hospital offsets the added cost of bleomycin therapy.

▶ This study clearly demonstrates that intrapleural bleomycin is more effective than tetracycline in the management of malignant pleural effusions.—R.F. Ozols, M.D., Ph.D.

Inhibition of Fluorouracil-Induced Stomatitis by Oral Cryotherapy

Mahood DJ, Dose AM, Loprinzi CL, Veeder MH, Athmann LM, Therneau TM, Sorensen JM, Gainey DK, Mailliard JA, Gusa NL, Finck GK, Johnson C, Goldberg RM (Cedar Rapids Oncology Project, Cedar Rapids, Iowa; Siouxland Hematology-Oncology Associates, Sioux City, Iowa; Oncology Research Association, Des Moines, Iowa; St Luke's Hospitals, Fargo, ND; Geisinger Clinic and Med Ctr, Danville, Pa; et al)

J Clin Oncol 9:449–452, 1991 17–15

Introduction.—Oral mucositis is a major dose-limiting complication of fluorouracil (5-FU) chemotherapy, particularly when given together with leucovorin. Oral cryotherapy at the time of 5-FU injection might reduce the blood flow to the oral mucous membranes, thereby protecting the oral mucosa from exposure to high concentrations of 5-FU.

Patients.—Of 95 patients undergoing their first cycle of chemotherapy with 5-FU and leucovorin, 50 were allocated randomly to oral cryotherapy at the time of the 5-FU infusion; 45 received no intervention. Those patients allocated to oral cryotherapy sucked on ice chips for approximately 30 minutes.

Results.—Oral cryotherapy given during infusion of 5-FU plus leucovorin significantly reduced subsequent mucositis as judged by the patients themselves and by their attending physicians.

Conclusion.—Cryotherapy is a simple, inexpensive, and generally well-tolerated means of decreasing 5-FU–induced mucositis.

▶ Oral ulcerations resulting from chemotherapy are not only painful, but they interfere with nutrition and can lead to infectious complications as well. The simple preventive measure of sucking on ice chips for 30 minutes with each dose of bolus 5-FU appears to be very effective in decreasing mucositis, and it should be routinely used. This simple technique also warrants further study with other mucositis-producing drugs.—R.F. Ozols, M.D., Ph.D.

Surgical Management of Pericardial Effusion in Patients With Malignancies: Comparison of Subxiphoid Window Versus Pericardiectomy

Park JS, Rentschler R, Wilbur D (Loma Linda Univ, Loma Linda, Calif)

Cancer 67:76–80, 1991 17–16

Introduction.—The best surgical technique for symptomatic pericardial effusions in patients with malignancies is a subject of controversy. Subxiphoid pericardial drainage is safe and effective, but many surgeons prefer to create a larger pericardial window (and thus ensure adequate drainage) by anterior thoracotomy or partial or total pericardiectomy. The effectiveness of these palliative techniques for symptomatic pericardial effusion was retrospectively assessed in 28 consecutive patients with advanced malignancies who underwent pericardial surgery for symptomatic pericardial effusions.

Methods.—Subxiphoid window formation was performed in 10 patients, with an average of 3.4 × 3.4 cm of pericardium resected. Another group of 18 patients was treated by the transthoracic approach, 12 with median sternotomy and 6 with left anterior thoracotomy.

Results.—The survival rates of the 2 groups were the same (Fig 17–3). The median survival was 2.67 months in the pericardial window group,

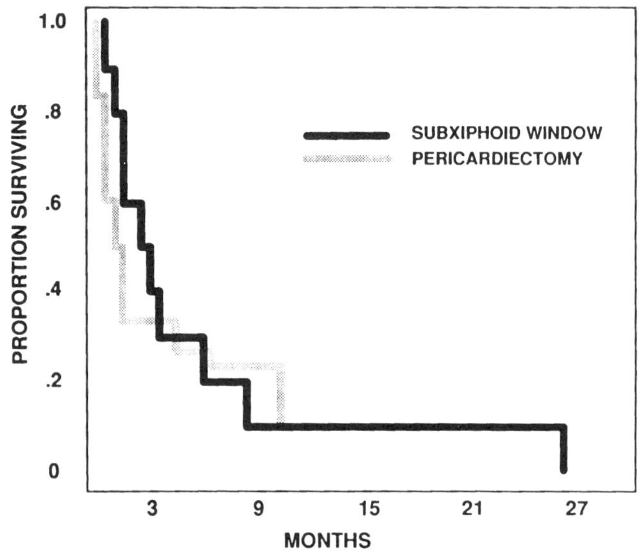

Fig 17–3.—A Kaplan-Meier analysis of survival of patients with subxiphoid window formation and pericardiectomy. (Courtesy of Park JS, Rentschler R, Wilbur D: *Cancer* 67:76–80, 1991.)

compared with 1.23 months in the pericardiectomy group. However, 67% of the pericardiectomy group had postoperative morbidity compared with only 10% of the pericardial window group. The major complications in the pericardiectomy group included superior vena cava thrombosis, persistent tamponade, acute renal failure, pneumonia and sepsis, massive pulmonary embolism, and myocardial failure.

Conclusion.—Because of its lower morbidity, supxiphoid pericardial window formation is preferred for palliation of symptomatic pericardial effusion in patients with malignancy. The higher rate of morbidity with pericardiectomy may be explained by the predominance of patients with already compromised respiratory function. Creating a generous-sized window may prevent failure of the subxiphoid window.

▶ Pericardial tamponade is most frequently observed in metastatic lung and breast cancer. Survival in most cases is short (median survival, less than 6 months), and palliation is the primary goal of therapy. The pericardial window is the treatment of choice because of its relative simplicity and low complication rate. There should be no enthusiasm to perform a randomized comparison of pericardiectomy vs. subxiphoid window based on the results of this and other retrospective studies that fail to document a survival advantage for the more invasive procedure with its higher complication rate. Furthermore, pericardiectomy with the instillation of an antitumor drug or sclerosing agent may be effective palliation (see Abstract 17–17).—R.F. Ozols, M.D., Ph.D.

Pericardiocentesis for Symptomatic Malignant Pericardial Effusion: A Study of 36 Patients

Celermajer DS, Boyer MJ, Bailey BP, Tattersall MHN (Royal Prince Alfred Hosp, Sydney, Australia)

Med J Aust 154:19–22, 1991 17–17

Background.—Many patients with cancer have neoplastic involvement of the heart and pericardium, although this condition is usually silent clinically. The best management of malignant pericardial effusion is controversial. A series of 36 symptomatic patients with this condition who were treated by pericardiocentesis was reviewed.

Patients.—The patients were 23 women and 13 men (mean age, 49 years) treated during an 8-year period. Most had underlying lung or breast carcinoma. Dyspnea was the presenting cardiovascular symptom in all but 2 cases; all had elevated jugular venous pressure; and most had fatigue, malaise, and anorexia. The median time from initial diagnosis of cancer to presentation wtih pericardial disease was 44 months. Pericardial effusion was confirmed by M-mode and 2-dimensional echocardiography. All patients had pericardiocentesis under electrocardiographic or echocardiographic guidance using a subxiphoid or apical approach.

Outcome.—The procedure was successful in 34 patients; 1 died during the procedure, and another required subxiphoid incision and drainage of the effusion (table). Twenty eight patients had intrapericardial sclerother-

Results of Pericardiocentesis in 36 Patients With Symptomatic Malignant Pericardial Effusion

	No. of patients
Technique	
Fluoroscopy electrocardiographic-guided pericardiocentesis	15 (42%)
Echocardiographic-guided pericardiocentesis	21 (58%)
Subxiphoid pericardiocentesis	28 (78%)
Apical pericardiocentesis	7 (19%)
Tube insertion and drainage	1 (3%)
Complications	
Death	1 (3%)
Transient atrial fibrillation	1 (3%)
Nil	34 (94%)
Results of cytological examination (35 patients)	
Positive	28 (80%)
Equivocal	2 (6%)
Negative	5 (14%)
Recurrence after initial pericardiocentesis (35 patients)	
Nil	28 (80%)
Single repeat pericardiocentesis	4 (11%)
Surgical decompression	2 (6%)
Recurrent failed pericardiocentesis	1 (3%)

(Courtesy of Calermajer DS, Boyer MJ, Bailey BP, et al: *Med J Aust* 154:19–22, 1991.)

apy, and only 3 needed repeat pericardiocentesis. Symptomatic effusion recurred in 4 of 7 patients who did not have sclerotherapy initially. The median survivals after this pericardiocentesis were 10 months for the patients with breast cancer and 4 months for all other patients.

Conclusions.—For patients with cancer with symptomatic malignant pericardial effusion, pericardiocentesis with intrapericardial sclerotherapy with tetracycline usually yields good local control. However, survival is poor, particularly for patients with malignancies other than breast cancer. Prospective controlled studies are needed to establish the best local and systemic treatment for these patients.

▶ The initial management of pericardial tamponade is pericardiocentesis, which is successful in relieving symptoms in the vast majority of patients. Sclerotherapy is effective in preventing recurrences, particularly if it is performed at the time of initial diagnosis of a pericardial effusion. In this study from Australia, approximately 50% of the patients with cardiac tamponade had lung cancer or an adenocarcinoma of unknown primary. The median survival for these patients was 2 months. One third of the patients had breast cancer; these patients had a median survival of 12 months after diagnosis of a pericardial effusion, reflecting a modest benefit of subsequent therapy. For survival to be improved in patients with pericardial effusion, more effective systemic therapy—and not merely a better local procedure—is needed.—R.F. Ozols, M.D., Ph.D.

Acute Complications

Treatment of Hypercalcemia of Malignancy With Intravenous Etidronate: A Controlled, Multicenter Study

Singer FR, for the Hypercalcemia Study Group (Univ of Southern California, Los Angeles)

Arch Intern Med 151:471–476, 1991 17–18

Introduction.—Hypercalcemia is a potentially life-threatening disorder in patients with cancer. If rehydration and diuresis are ineffective, drugs such as steroids and calcitonin may be tried; however, they are not consistently effective.

Methods.—The diphosphonate etidronate, which inhibits osteoclastic bone resorption, was investigated in patients with confirmed malignancy and a serum calcium at least .25 mM/L above the upper normal limit in a prospective, double-blind study. The patients were assigned to receive an infusion of either etidronate disocium in saline, 7.5 mg/kg, or saline alone. Hydration was done as needed, and furosemide was used to prevent fluid overload.

Results.—Nearly two thirds of the etidronate-treated patients regained normocalcemia within 1 week, compared with one third of the patients given saline alone. After 1 week, the treated patients had a mean serum calcium level of 2.67 mM/L compared with 2.94 mM/L for controls (Fig 17–4). More marked responses were seen in patients with higher baseline serum calcium levels. In no patient did side effects require with-

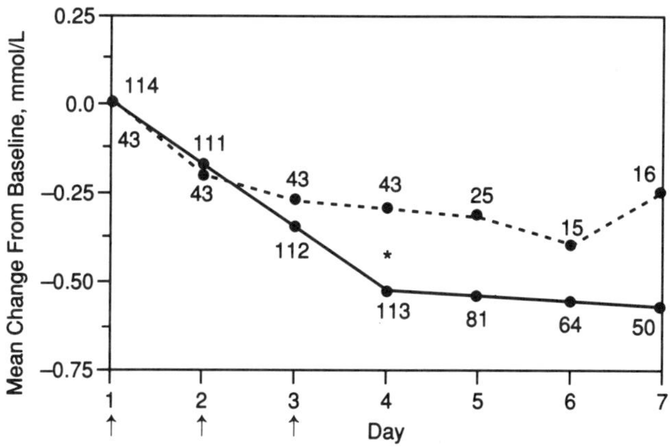

Fig 17–4.—The mean changes from baseline in the total serum calcium level in patients with hypercalcemia of malignancy receiving intravenous treatment with etidronate disodium *(solid line)* or saline *(broken line)*. The *arrows* denote infusion dosing. The daily number of patients in each treatment group is noted. The *asterisk* indicates $P < .001$. (Courtesy of Singer FR, for the Hypercalcemia Study Group: *Arch Intern Med* 151:471–476, 1991.)

drawal of treatment. Some patients had an increase in serum creatinine levels, and hypocalcemia developed in some, but with no serious clinical consequences.

Conclusion.—Intravenously administered etidronate is an effective means of countering hypercalcemia of a malignancy when combined with saline hydration, and with furosemide diuresis if necessary. The treatment may be more effective if prolonged.

▶ The initial approach to management of acute hypercalcemia of a malignancy is hydration and diuresis, which leads to enhanced renal calcium excretion. In most cases, this therapy is inadequate, and drugs such as steroids, calcitonin, mithramycin, and bisphosphonates are often necessary. The bisphosphonates, which are potent inhibitors of osteoclastic bone resorption, are effective in the acute treatment of hypercalcemia of malignancy. They also are particularly noteworthy for their absence of serious side effects. However, as with the other drugs that have been used to treat hypercalcemia, the duration of normocalcemia is transient. Unless effective antitumor therapy is instituted, most patients will have a recurrence of symptomatic hypercalcemia within 4–5 weeks. The bisphosphonate etidronate was recently compared with gallium nitrate (which also inhibits bone resorption). In a randomized double-blind study (1), gallium nitrate was judged to be superior because of a significantly longer duration of normocalcemia.—R.F. Ozols, M.D., Ph.D.

Reference

1. Warrell RP, et al: *J Clin Oncol* 9:1467, 1991.

The Influence of Intraoperative Hypotension and Perioperative Blood Transfusion on Disease-Free Survival in Patients With Complete Resection of Colorectal Liver Metastases

Younes RN, Rogatko A, Brennan MF (Sloan-Kettering Cancer Ctr, New York)
Ann Surg 214:107–113, 1991 17–19

Introduction.—Surgical resection of metastatic liver disease from colorectal cancer has recently become accepted. Although low operative morbidity and mortality rates with long-term survival have been reported, not all patients benefit from this approach. The clinical prognostic factors that influence outcome have not been defined conclusively.

Methods.—To identify the prognostic determinants and perioperative factors that affect disease recurrence and survival data on 133 patients who underwent complete hepatic resection during a 2-year period were reviewed. Evaluable data were available for 116 patients. Follow-up was for .6–31.4 months (median follow-up, 13.2 months).

Results.—The median time to second recurrence after complete hepatic resection for metastatic disease was 9.03 months. The overall disease-free survival rates were 49.4% at 1 year and 21.2% at 2 years. The overall survival was 91% at 1 year and 75% at 2 years. The median survival was not reached. Univariate analysis identified primary colorectal tumor site, preoperative carcinoembryonic antigen level, size and number of metastases, duration of operation, percentage mean arterial pressure, number and duration of hypotensive episodes, and whole blood transfusion as factors that significantly affect recurrence rates. However, only primary tumor site, carcinoembryonic antigen level, number of metastases, and number of intraoperative hypotensive episodes remained significant determinants of outcome after multivariate analysis. The number of hypotensive episodes was the single most significant factor affecting disease recurrence after resection.

Conclusion.—Because it is the most significant determinant of disease-free survival in these patients, careful intraoperative hemodynamic management is a fundamental requirement to avoid hypotensive episodes during hepatic resection in patients with colorectal liver metastases is a fundamental requirement.

▶ Liver metastases is the major cause of mortality from colorectal cancer. Surgical resection is currently the only effective treatment for selected patients with liver metastases. Although controversy remains regarding the specific clinical criteria needed to select appropriate candidates for hepatic resection, it is generally accepted that patients with a larger tumor burden (elevated carcinoembryonic antigen level; numerous and large metastases) are more likely to have a shorter disease-free interval after surgery. It has also been previously suggested that intraoperative transfusions of whole blood have led to shorter disease-free survival as well. This study demonstrates that hypotensive episodes during hepatic resection are likewise an adverse prognostic factor. Both transfusion and hypovolemic shock have experimentally been shown to have adverse immunologic effects that can lead to enhanced tumor proliferation. Both careful hemodynamic management to avoid hypotensive episodes and judicious use of blood products are clearly indicated in those patients who have the potential for cure after complete hepatic resection of colorectal metastases.—R.F. Ozols, M.D., Ph.D.

High Energy Neutron Treatment for Pelvic Cancers: Study Stopped Because of Increased Mortality

Errington RD, Ashby D, Gore SM, Abrams KR, Myint S, Bonnett DE, Blake SW, Saxton TE (Clatterbridge Hosp, Wirral, England; Univ of Liverpool, England; Med Research Council Biostatistics Unit, Cambridge, England)

BMJ 302:1045–1051, 1991 17–20

Background.—Since the development of hospital-based cyclotrons, registry-based evidence suggesting that high-energy neutron treatment could decrease morbidity in patients with locally advanced pelvic tumors has emerged. A comparative study of high-energy fast neutron treatment and conventional megavoltage photon treatment for such tumors was stopped because of increased mortality.

Methods.—The randomized study included 151 patients with locally advanced, nonmetastatic pelvic cancers. Twenty-seven patients had cervical cancers, 69 had bladder cancers, 7 had prostatic cancers, and 48 had rectal cancers. The patients were randomized to neutron or photon treatment in an unstratified manner and in a 3-to-1 ratio for the first 2 years of the study. For the next 2 years, they were randomized in a 1-to-1 ratio and stratified by tumor site. Comparable dose distributions were achieved for both forms of treatment. The main outcome measures were patient survival and cause of death in relation to metastasis and treatment-related morbidity.

Results.—After adjustment for tumor site and other important prognostic factors, such as T stage, N stage, and Karnofsky index, the relative risk of mortality was .66 in the photon group compared with the neutron group. The most common causes of death were metastasis and local tumor progression. The 2 study groups had similar short- and long-term complications. Because of the increased mortality noted in the neutron group, the trial was halted.

Conclusions.—High-energy neutrons apparently should not be used in the treatment of locally advanced cervical, bladder, or rectal carcinomas. This conclusion may not apply to locally advanced prostatic adenocarcinoma. Future trials of this type should have a data-monitoring committee.

▶ Neutrons have been with us for 50 years now, and their story is complex. Even so, their role in treatment is controversial. The advantage of neutrons is that they have a greater biological impact on neoplastic cells and do not recognize hypoxia as a limiting factor in controlling tumors. Investigators have long been interested in using neutrons in the treatment of cancer, because they should be more effective than x-rays. On the other hand, as this study shows, neutrons are difficult to collimate. This particular study was terminated—not because of the poor results as far as cancer was concerned, but because of the morbidity and mortality related to treatment. Conceivably, neutron studies in the modern era have taken place without actually determining the real "tolerance" for these neutron beams before beginning the study. Even so, this particular paper emphasizes that enthusiasm for eliminating the cancer is not enough; considerable attention has to be paid to the morbidity associated with the treatment as well.—E. Glatstein, M.D.

Autocrine Effects of Fibroblast Growth Factor in Repair of Radiation Damage in Endothelial Cells

Haimovitz-Friedman A, Vlodavsky I, Chaudhuri A, Witte L, Fuks Z (Mem Sloan-Kettering Cancer Ctr, New York; Hadassah-Hebrew Univ Hosp, Jerusalem; Columbia Univ, New York)

Cancer Res 51:2552–2558, 1991 17–21

Introduction.—Although mammalian cells are often able to repair radiation damage to DNA, not all lesions are reparable; others may or may not be repaired, depending on the competing processes of repair and lethal fixation. Little is known about the enzymatic paths involved in the repair of radiation lesions in eukaryotic cells.

Study Plan.—The previously suggested possibility that basic fibroblast growth factor (bFGF) may have a role in the regulation of repair of radiation damage in bovine aortic endothelial cells was assessed by generating radiation dose-survival curves for bovine aortic endothelial cells using culture dishes precoated with HR9-bFGF/ECM (extracellular matrix) for a colony formation assay. This natural basement membranelike ECM is enriched with ECM-bound bFGF.

Observations.—Under conditions of enrichment, the repair of radiation damage was greater than in cells plated on a bFGF-free isotype of the ECM. Delayed plating studies affirmed that the cells repaired potentially lethal radiation damage and regained clonogenic ability. Irradiated cells secreted bFGF into their conditioned medium.

Conclusions.—Basic fibroblast growth factor is a strong inducer of repair after the induction of potentially lethal radiation damage in endothelial cells. The use of intravenously administered bFGF for radioprotection deserves consideration.

▶ This is a very provocative paper dealing with the investigations of bFGF, which apparently can induce the repair of radiation damage in endothelial cells. The authors have done an enormous amount of work that suggests a potential clinical use of bFGF as a means of potentially protecting against radiation injury to the microvasculature (which is usually credited with a major role in normal tissue tolerance). This kind of study suggests a wide variety of potential uses of this substance to protect against radiation injury. Obviously, a great deal of additional work needs to be done.—E. Glatstein, M.D.

---

p53 Gene Mutations and Abnormal Retinoblastoma Protein in Radiation-Induced Human Sarcomas

Brachman DG, Hallahan DE, Beckett MA, Yandell DW, Weichselbaum RR (Univ of Chicago; Massachusetts Eye and Ear Infirmary, Boston)

Cancer Res 51:6393–6396, 1991 17–22

Background.—Therapeutic irradiation is potentially carcinogenic. Second malignancies, usually sarcomas, are known to originate in or at the edge of the radiation field several years after the initial radiation exposure. Whether changes of the tumor suppressor genes retinoblastoma (*RB*) and *p53* are associated with human radiation-induced sarcomas was determined.

Methods.—Tumor cells from 7 radiation-induced tumors were analyzed for abnormalities in tumor suppressor genes *p53* and *RB* at the DNA sequence and/or protein level. The *p53* mutations were studied by exon-specific polymerase chain reaction amplification and single-strand conformation polymorphism analysis of exons 5–8, followed by direct genomic sequencing of tumors with a variant pattern. Western immunoblotting was used for retinoblastoma gene analysis.

Results.—Three of the 6 sarcomas studied had an abnormal *p53* gene. Retinoblastoma protein was underphosphorylated in 3 of 7 tumors. This protein was absent in another tumor. Overall, 6 of 7 radiation-induced tumors had abnormalities of 1 or both suppressor genes.

Conclusions.—Sarcomas developing after ionizing radiation exposure contain abnormalities in tumor suppressor genes *p53* and *RB*. The x-ray inactivation of these and/or other genes may contribute to radiation carcinogenesis.

▶ This provocative paper from an excellent group of investigators suggests that radiation carcinogenesis may be related to the inactivation of tumor suppressor genes. Several patients with radiation-induced tumors were studied for abnormalities in *p53* and *RB* tumor suppressor genes. The *p53* gene was abnormal in 3 of 6 patients, and the RB protein appeared abnormal in 3 of 7 patients. Of 7 patients, 6 had some abnormality of 1 or both suppressor genes. This kind of work is expected to yield insight into the general area of radiation carcinogenesis.—E. Glatstein, M.D.

Paraneoplastic Pemphigus: An Autoimmune Mucocutaneous Disease Associated with Neoplasia.

Anhalt GJ, Kim SC, Stanley JR, Korman NJ, Jabs DA, Kory M, Izumi H, Ratrie H III, Mutasim D, Ariss-Abdo L, Labib RS (Johns Hopkins Univ, Baltimore; Natl Cancer Inst, Bethesda, Md; Ohio State Univ, Columbus)

N Engl J Med 323:1729–1735, 1990 17–23

Introduction.—Pemphigus is the mucocutaneous disease characterized by intraepithelial blisters induced by a loss of normal cell-cell adhesion (acantholysis). These conditions are associated with autoantibody production against cell-surface proteins of the stratified squamous epithelia. Data on 5 patients with cancer who also had painful mucosal ulcerations and polymorphous skin lesions on the trunk and extremities were reviewed.

Case Report.—Man, 62, had malignant follicular large-cell lymphoma that initially responded to chemotherapy. Nearly 1 year later, a pruritic urticarial skin lesion erupted. Considered an allergic reaction to diltiazem, the lesion did not resolve after stopping the drug. Skin biopsy specimens demonstrated necrosis of the epidermis that was consistent with severe erythema multiforme or toxic epidermal necrolysis. The skin condition worsened, and staphylococcal sepsis developed. The patient became febrile and debilitated, with denuded skin areas seen predominantly on the trunk. Prednisone and azathioprine treatments were discontinued, and imipenem was started; however, on hospital day 11, new oral and conjunctival eruptions appeared. A skin biopsy specimen showed an acantholytic intraepidermal blister that was consistent with pemphigus vulgaris. The patient's lymphoma was considered incurable, and the skin lesions improved slightly with prednisone. The patient died 1 year after the first skin eruption.

Methods.—Specimens from all 5 patients were studied by histologic and electron-microscopic techniques. The serum samples were analyzed by conventional methods, immunofluorescence, immunoprecipitation, and autoantibody testing.

Results.—In all 5 patients, there were persistent, painful erosions of the oropharynx and vermilion border of the lips that were resistent to usual therapy. Skin and mucosal samples had variable histologic results dominated by suprabasilar intraepithelial acantholysis, necrosis of the individual keratinocytes, and vacuolar-interface change. Immunofluorescence testing showed autoantibodies binding to the desmosome-containing tissue surface. A complex of 4 polypeptides (MW 250, 230, 210, and 190 kd) immunoprecipitated from all serum samples. The 250-kd polypeptide comigrated with desmoplakin I, and the 230-kd antigen comigrated with the antigen of bullous pemphigoid. In mice injected with the autoantibody, cutaneous blisters, a positive Nikolsky's sign, and epidermal and esophageal acantholysis developed.

Conclusion.—These patients had a new acantholytic mucocutaneous disease characterized by autoantibodies that are pathogenic on passive transfer. It is suggested that this disease be called "paraneoplastic pemphigus."

▶ The paraneoplastic diseases mediated by autoantibodies include Eaton-Lambert (myasthenia) syndrome, sensory polyneuropathies, cerebellar degeneration, and an acute loss of visual acuity. These neurologic syndromes are characterized by autoantibodies that cross-react with tumor and neuronal tissue. This report characterizes a new paraneoplastic syndrome, paraneoplastic pemphigus, in which autoantibodies against squamous epithelia produce a blistering mucocutaneous disease. The malignancies associated with this syndrome include malignant lymphoma, chronic lymphocytic leukemia, and sarcoma.—R.F. Ozols, M.D., Ph.D.

Acute Tumor Lysis Syndrome After Intrathecal Methotrexate Administration

Simmons ED, Somberg KA (Harbor-Univ of California Los Angeles Med Ctr, Torrance, Calif)

Cancer 67:2062–2065, 1991 17–24

Introduction.—Patients with a variety of neoplasms may have acute tumor lysis syndrome after systemic chemotherapy. Intracellular phosphates, urates, and other cellular debris are released as a result of rapid cell proliferation and the sensitivity of the tumor cells to chemotherapy. Data on a patient who had acute tumor lysis syndrome after intrathecal administration of methotrexate were reviewed.

Case Report.—Man, 44, was evaluated for progressive weakness, anorexia, and fevers for 3 months. After examination and laboratory testing, cefotaxime was administered because of blood cultures positive for *Salmonella* group C. On bone marrow biopsy, the marrow space was found to be completely replaced by small-noncleaved-cell lymphoma, high-grade B-cell type. The next day, preservative-free methotrexate, 15 mg, was administered intrathecally along with cranial irradiation. His serum phosphate level increased to 7.9 mg/dL within 48 hours; his serum creatinine level increased and his serum calcium level decreased. Small bilateral pleural effusions, pelvic ascites, and a necrotic mass in the left pelvic sidewall were seen on abdominal CT. Vigorous intravenous hydration and phosphate binders were initiated immediately. The phosphate level returned to normal in 6 days, whereas the creatinine level continued to increase, finally returning to normal at 11 days. Subsequently, methotrexate was administered intrathecally with oral leucovorin rescue. Systemic chemotherapy was administered with no recurrence of renal insufficiency or other abnormalities.

Conclusion.—Potentially toxic systemic methotrexate levels may occur with intrathecal administration of methotrexate. The duration of these levels and the peripheral effects of the drug may be increased by active CNS lymphoma. Leucovorin rescue may prevent side effects; it is not known whether it could prevent tumor lysis syndrome.

▶ Both the toxicity and the therapeutic effect of methotrexate are dependent upon the concentration and duration of exposure. Rapidly proliferating tumors are theoretically more sensitive, because a larger number of tumor cells pass through S-phase and are exposed to cytotoxic drug levels. Intrathecal methotrexate leads to persistent levels of plasma methotrexate for several days as a result of slow absorption from the CNS. Furthermore, meningeal disease may lead to an impairment of clearance, producing a further prolongation of plasma levels. In this case report, the classic presentation of acute tumor lysis syndrome was likely the result of the alteration in methotrexate pharmacokinetics in a highly sensitive, rapidly proliferating, B-cell lymphoma.—R.F. Ozols, M.D., Ph.D.

Coronary Artery Spasm Induced by 5-Fluorouracil

Luwaert RJ, Descamps O, Majois F, Chaudron J-M, Beauduin M (Hôpital de Jolimont, Haine-Saint-Paul, Belgium)

Eur Heart J 12:468–470, 1991 17–25

Background.—Although the ischemic cardiac toxicity of 5-fluorouracil (5-FU) has been studied extensively, it is an uncommon complication of unclear pathophysiology. In 1 patient, a 5-FU–induced coronary artery spasm was demonstrated angiographically.

Case Report.—Man, 70, had stage III, T3NO squamous carcinoma of the palate. He was free of angina, but he was a smoker and had been treated for arterial hypertension. He was to receive monthly cycles of carboplatin, 400 mg/m^2, on day 1, and 5-FU, 1,000 mg/m^2, daily for 4 days. His cardiovascular examination was normal on admission. Rest angina developed 72 hours after 5-FU therapy was begun (Fig 17–5). Infusion was discontinued, and chest pain and repolarization abnormalities disappeared with nitrate administration. At the second course of treatment, the same chest pain and ECG abnormalities appeared, and the infusion was stopped again. On angiography, the left ventricle was normal and there was no significant coronary artery stenosis. There was no response to ergonovine

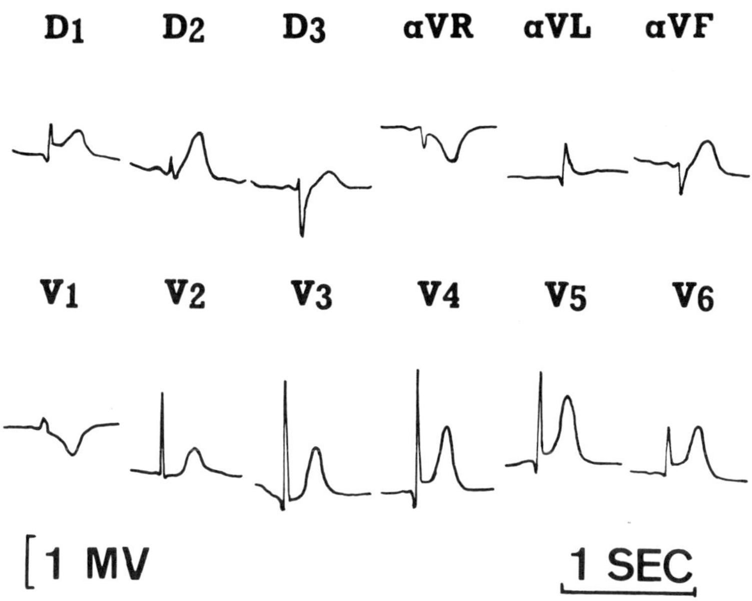

Fig 17–5.—Electrocardiogram during chest pain, showing ST-segment elevation in leads I,aVL, V4-6, and II,II,aVF. (Courtesy of Luwaert RJ, Descamps O, Majois F, et al: *Eur Heart J* 12:468–470, 1991.)

maleate, but 2 intravenous doses of 250 mg of 5-FU caused chest pain and 70% narrowing of the circumflex artery, which disappeared with injection of isosorbide dinitrate. Treatment with 5-FU was abandoned, and chest pain did not recur.

Discussion.—The patient had a coronary spasm resulting from administration of 5-FU. The mechanism is unclear, but vasospasm may be one of the mechanisms of ischemic cardiac toxicity of 5-FU.

▶ Cardiac toxicity of 5-FU is rare. In most patients with 5-FU–induced cardiac toxicity, coronary vasospasm has been believed to be the etiology, because patients most frequently are seen with chest pain, localized electrocardiogram abnormalities, and normal stress tests and angiograms. This report is an actual angiographic demonstration of coronary artery spasm induced by intravenous 5-FU. The mechanism of this toxicity is unclear, although endothelial damage by 5-FU leading to impaired vasodilation is a leading hypothesis.—R.F. Ozols, M.D., Ph.D.

Cardiac Disturbances During the Administration of Taxol

Rowinsky EK, McGuire WP, Guarnieri T, Fisherman JS, Christian MC, Donehower RC (Johns Hopkins Med Insts, Baltimore; Natl Cancer Inst, Bethesda, Md)

J Clin Oncol 9:1704–1712, 1991 17–26

Introduction.—Taxol is a new antimicrotubule drug that has a unique antineoplastic and antitumor mechanism. However, its clinical development has been slow, obstructed by a high incidence of serious hypersensitivity reactions (HSRs) and a limited supply of the drug. A variety of cardiac disturbances were observed in previous studies.

Methods.—The characteristics of these taxol-associated cardiac disturbances occurring in 4 phase I and II clinical trials of taxol performed during a 7-year period were reviewed.

Results.—Asymptomatic bradycardia was common. In one phase-II study of ovarian cancer, 29% of the patients who received the maximum-tolerated dose of taxol had this disturbance. A wide range of more serious disturbances was also seen, including atrioventricular conduction blocks, left bundle-branch block, ventricular tachycardia, and cardiac ischemia. There were 7 such incidences in 140 (5%) patients. One patient with hypertension and hypercholesterolemia died of myocardial infarction 19 hours after treatment with taxol was initiated. Other cardiac effects included bigeminy, trigeminy, increased premature ventricular contractions, and chest pain.

Conclusion.—Patients who receive taxol may have a variety of cardiac disturbances. Most have no serious sequelae, but there appears to be a significant causal relationship with taxol. Until the clinical risk factors, frequency, and significance of these effects are determined, patients who receive taxol should be monitored carefully.

▶ The actual cardiac toxicity of taxol remains to be established. It is not even clear whether the cardiac disturbances reported are a result of taxol or its Cremophor EL (polyoxyethylated castor oil) formulation, which is likely responsible for the hypersensitivity reactions reported after taxol administration. It is also of note that virtually all the serious cardiac toxicities occurred in patients who received the combination of taxol and cisplatin. When taxol alone is administered, there does not appear to be a need for cardiac monitoring, because the only cardiac toxicity of any regard is likely to be an infrequent case of asymptomatic bradycardia. Cardiac monitoring should be considered when taxol is used with cisplatin.—R.F. Ozols, M.D., Ph.D.

Ifosfamide-Related Acute Encephalopathy: Clinical and Radiological Aspects

Merimsky O, Inbar M, Reider-Groswasser I, Scharf M, Chaitchik S (Ichilov Hosp, Tel-Aviv, Israel)

Eur J Cancer 27:1188–1189, 1991 17–27

Introduction.—Ifosfamide, which is used in patients with a variety of malignancies, has side effects including nausea and vomiting, myelosuppression, and CNS toxicity. The manifestations of CNS toxicity in a small group of patients treated with ifosfamide were reviewed.

Patients.—Five of 18 patients had CNS toxicity develop 2–7 days after beginning treatment; none of the patients had any brain or neurologic symptoms before treatment. The manifestations varied, including personality changes, pathologic reflexes, and incontinence. Brain CT scans were normal in all patients but 1, who had a pre-existing asymptomatic metastasis. The CNS toxicity did not appear to result from tumor lysis. There were bulky tumors of the lower abdomen and pelvis in 4 women; 2 patients who had previous cisplatin therapy and were treated with ifosfamide, 5 g/m^2, for 24 hours died, as did another patient. The severity of encephalopathy and the width of the ventricles and sulci were unassociated. Pancytopenia developed in all patients, which further worsened their condition. When CNS toxicity was diagnosed, treatment was interrupted, CNS depressants were avoided, pH and electrolyte imbalance were corrected, and supportive treatment was given.

Conclusion.—A fractionated schedule should be used in patients undergoing treatment with ifosfamide, particularly in women with lower abdominal masses or patients undergoing cisplatin treatment. It is necessary to exclude other causes of CNS toxicity.

▶ This paper describes some of the clinical factors that appear to increase the risk of ifosfamide-related acute encephalopathy. It does not identify a history of prior cisplatin therapy as a risk factor. In other studies (1), a total dose of 600 mg of cisplatin per m^2 increased the risk of most ifosfamide-related toxicities (renal, hematologic, and CNS). Although this study suggests that the schedule may be important for CNS toxicity, a prospective trial would be necessary to take into account all the other factors that can influence ifosfamide toxicity.—R.F. Ozols, M.,D., Ph.D.

Reference

1. Goren MP, et al: *Cancer Res* 47:1457, 1987.

Intrathecal Vincristine: A Fatal Chemotherapeutic Error With Devastating Central Nervous System Effects

Bain PG, Lantos PL, Djurovic V, West I (Inst of Psychiatry; United Med and Dental Schools of Guy's and St Thomas's Hosps, London)
J Neurol 238:230–234, 1991 17–28

Introduction.—Vincristine is widely used in the treatment of many malignancies, because it produces virtually no myelosuppression. It is always fatal when injected intrathecally, because of its acute central neurotoxic effects. Data were reviewed on a patient in whom vincristine was accidentally injected intrathecally.

Case Report.—Man, 56, was undergoing maintenance chemotherapy, which was supposed to consist of vincristine administered intravenously, and he was accidentally given vincristine, .3 mg, intrathecally. The fluid was aspirated immediately and, because adverse effects were thought to be unlikely, the patient was sent home. He woke up 11 hours later with urinary frequency, intermittent lumbar pain, and limb weakness. He was admitted with meningism, moderate flaccid paralysis, absent reflexes, and diminished pain sensations in the L5 dermatomes and extensor plantar reflexes. His condition deteriorated, with lessening responses, increasing weakness, and progressive cranial nerve involvement. Respiratory arrest occurred 9 days later, and a wide range of complicating conditions developed until all signs of CNS activity ceased at 28 days. An autopsy showed that the most prominent damage was in the spinal cord, brain stem, and cerebellum, with the greatest severity in neurons nearest to the CSF. Petechial hemorrhages were seen in the cortex of the cerebellar vermis, and there was a remarkable degree of astrocytosis. Abundant corpora amylacea was found throughout the brain. Aggregated material noted in the perikarya and process of the anterior horn cells was accumulated neurofilaments.

Conclusion.—Such accidents are possible because of the neurotoxicity of vincristine and its use in complicated chemotherapy regimens. It is the responsibility of the physician to prevent such accidents.

▶ All 7 reported cases of the fatal consequences of inadvertent administration of intrathecal vincristine have followed the same unfortunate scenario. All patients had leukemia and were to receive intrathecal methotrexate and intravenous vincristine; however, intrathecal vincristine was administered by mistake. There have been no reports of patients surviving the erroneous administration of intrathecal vincristine. Such a tragedy can only be prevented by physician awareness of the fatal consequences of a mistaken route of administration. Meticulous safeguards must be in place and must be followed religiously.—R.F. Ozols, M.D., Ph.D.

Late Complications

Thyroid Diseases After Treatment of Hodgkin's Disease

Hancock SL, Cox RS, McDougall IR (Stanford Univ, Stanford, Calif)
N Engl J Med 325:599–605, 1991 17–29

Background.—Patients wtih Hodgkin's disease who have been treated with irradiation commonly have thyroid disease, especially hypothyroidism. A series of patients was studied to obtain more information on the spectrum and incidence of benign and malignant thyroid disease in these patients.

Methods.—The records of 1,787 patients with Hodgkin's disease treated between 1961 and 1989 were examined. Treatment consisted of radiation therapy alone in 810, radiation and chemotherapy in 920, and chemotherapy alone in 57. The patients were followed up for a mean of 9.9 years. At last follow-up, 1,533 were alive. Thyroid irradiation was done in 1,677 patients.

Findings.—The actuarial risk of hypothyroidism in 1,787 patients treated for Hodgkin's disease is shown in Figure 17–6. A total of 573 patients had clinical or biochemical signs of thyroid disease. Those who had thyroid irradiation had an actuarial risk of thyroid disease of 52% at 20 years and 67% at 26 years. Hypothyroidism was found in 513 patients. A group of 486 patients received thyroxine treatment for increased

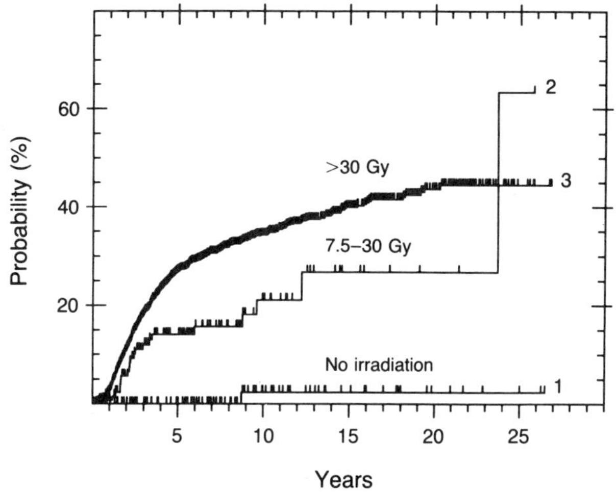

Fig 17–6.—Actuarial risk of hypothyroidism in 1,787 patients treated for Hodgkin's disease from the time of initial therapy. Curve 1 represents the risk in 110 patients who did not undergo irradiation of the thyroid. Curve 2 shows the risk in 140 patients who received 7.5–30 Gy. Curve 3 represents the risk in 1,537 patients who received more than 30 Gy. The differences between curves 1 and 2 (P = .0001), curves 2 and 3 (P = .0083), and curves 1 and 3 (P < .0001) were all significant by the Gehan test. (Courtesy of Hancock SL, Cox RS, McDougall IR: *N Engl J Med* 325:599–605, 1991.)

serum thyrotropin levels and either low free thyroxine or normal free thyroxine values. Twenty-seven had transient serum thyrotropin level increases that were not treated. Of the 30 patients who had Graves' hyperthyroidism, 17 had ophthalmopathy. The risk of having Graves' disease was 7.2–20.4 times that for healthy individuals. Six patients had silent thyroiditis with thyrotoxicosis. Of the 44 patients with single or multiple thyroid nodules, 6 had papillary or follicular cancers. The actuarial risk of thyroid cancer developing was 1.7%; the risk of thyroid cancer was 15.6 times that expected.

Conclusions.—The high risk of thyroid disease persists for more than 25 years after patients are treated with radiation therapy for Hodgkin's disease. Therefore, continued clinical and biochemical follow-up is needed in such patients. These patients have an increased risk of thyroid cancer and Graves' disease as well as hypothyroidism.

▶ In addition to the serious risk of permanent thyroid damage, the risk of malignancy of the thyroid is more than 15 times greater than expected. The risk of thyroid cancer is likely to have been significantly underestimated, because the latent period for thyroid cancer after radiation therapy is often 20 years or longer, and the median follow-up of this cohort is approximately 10 years. Thus, even more thyroid cancers can be expected.

Other radiation therapy-related risks have been identified in the Stanford patient population (1). Although a widely read original paper reported little increased mortality in patients with Hodgkin's disease who were successfully treated with radiation therapy compared with age-matched controls without

Hodgkin's disease (2), the control population in the original paper had a lower estimated survival than it should have had (67% compared with the correct 91%). As a result of using the correct control curve, the relative risk of death from a second cancer among patients with Hodgkin's disease treated with radiation therapy was 9.3. In addition, the risk of a fatal myocardial infarction was 3.2 times the normal risk, and the risk of death from all causes was increased 5.3-fold. These risks were not different between patients who had received combined-modality therapy and those who had received radiation therapy alone. Thus, these serious late risks appear to be related to the use of radiation therapy. Similar data on the survival of patients treated with chemotherapy alone are being collected in other centers.

Another set of risks that must be evaluated before opting for surgical staging and radiation therapy is those associated with exploratory laparotomy. The procedure has a low mortality in experienced hands, but the infectious consequences of splenectomy may lead directly to the death of 5% to 10% of patients during the course of years. Furthermore, approximately one third of patients undergoing laparotomy will require chemotherapy for advanced stage disease, and another 25% of the patients will require salvage chemotherapy after relapsing from radiation therapy-induced complete response. Thus, 50% or more of the patients with clinical early stage disease will require chemotherapy to control their disease. The bottom line is that 100 patients undergo laparotomy to cure approximately 50 with radiation therapy.

The toxicities of chemotherapy vary with the regimen; for MOPP treatment (Mustargen, Oncovin, procarbazine, and prednisone), in addition to the acute hematologic toxicity, there is an approximate 2% risk of acute leukemia developing, and the other major long-term toxicity is infertility. Both the infertility and the leukemia seem to be significantly lower when ABVD (Adriamycin, bleomycin, vinblastine, and dacarbazine) is used as chemotherapy. However, long-term follow-up of ABVD-treated patients has not yet been reported. There is no reason to think that patients treated with ABVD would be more likely to have late relapses, but it would be reassuring to see survival curves extended to 15 years; this should certainly be available from the Milan experience.

Another treatment option would be Ch1VPP (chlorambucil, vinblastine, procarbazine, and prednisone) (3), a regimen that was originally described by McElwain and colleagues (4) and was subsequently tested and verified in a variety of treatment centers. It is less acutely toxic than MOPP and may have a lower leukemia risk.

The physician now has several reasonable options for the treatment of patients with clinical early stage Hodgkin's disease.—D.L. Longo, M.D., F.A.C.P.

References

1. Hancock SL, et al: *Ann Intern Med* 114:810, 1991.
2. Hancock SL, et al: *Ann Intern Med* 109:183, 1988.
3. Vose JM, et al: *J Clin Oncol* 9:1421, 1991.
4. McElwain TJ, et al: *Br J Cancer* 36:276, 1977.

Discrete Pigmentation After Chemotherapy

Singal R, Tunnessen WW Jr, Wiley JM, Hood AF (Johns Hopkins Univ, Baltimore; Children's Hosp of Philadelphia)

Pediatr Dermatol 8:231–235, 1991 17–30

Background.—Many chemotherapeutic agents can cause diffuse hyperpigmentation of the skin, but there has been only 1 previous report of localized hyperpigmentation in areas of skin occluded by adhesive materials. Such a response developed in 2 children after chemotherapeutic ablation of metastatic sarcoma with cyclophosphamide, etoposide, and carboplatin before autologous bone marrow transplantation.

Case Report.—Boy, 6 years, had surgery for removal of a large clear cell sarcoma of the right kidney. Recurrences in a rib, adjacent pleura, and the frontal lobe of the brain developed 10 months after his initial chemotherapy. They responded to another course of chemotherapy, and the boy was admitted for bone marrow harvest, ablative chemotherapy, and autologous marrow reinfusion. A week after the start of chemotherapy, erosion and surrounding hyperpigmentation were seen on removal of electrocardiographic monitor pads (Fig 17–7). There was a diffuse, reddish-brown eruption on the anterior trunk, groin, hands, and auricles. There were 2 sites of discrete, annular pigmentation over previously bandaged marrow aspiration sites, as well as a linear patch of hyperpigmentation at the site of adhesive tape. The hyperpigmentation decreased over several weeks. Histologically, the pigmented areas showed hyperkeratosis, altered polarity of the keratinocytes, basal vacuolization, and a scant perivascular infiltrate in the papillary dermis. Melanin granules were increased throughout the epidermis and stratum corneum and in the upper dermis.

Conclusions.—Discrete hyperpigmentation appearing under areas of occlusion in patients undergoing chemotherapy may result from accumulation of the drug on the skin by sweating. This side effect is asympto-

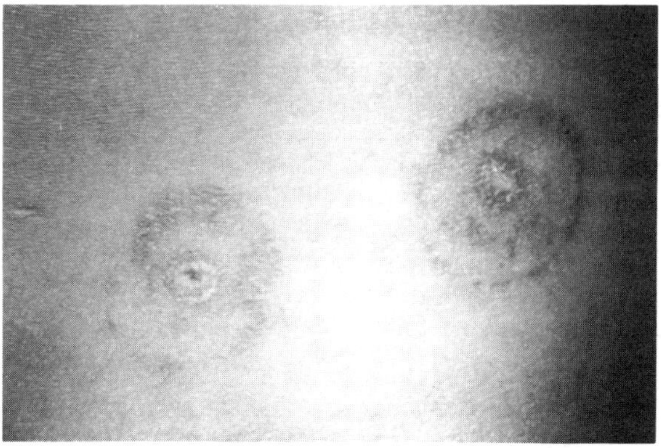

Fig 17–7.—Annular pigmentation and erosion at sites of cardiac monitor pads. (Courtesy of Singal R, Tunnessen WW Jr, Wiley JM, et al: *Pediatr Dermatol* 8:231–235, 1991.)

matic and causes no physiologic problems, but it should be prevented by measures such as reducing the accumulation of sweat under bandages and daily changing of monitor pads.

▶ This brief report has immediate practical value. Although it seemingly is a minor issue, hyperpigmentation in patients undergoing chemotherapy is an annoying side effect. The authors suggest that this can be prevented by reducing the sweat under occlusive bandages and by changing dressings more frequently, as well as by more frequent cleansing and showering; a small contribution to the improvement of the quality of life of patients with cancer.—J.V. Simone, M.D.

A Prospective Comparison of Neuropsychologic Performance of Children Surviving Leukemia Who Received 18-Gy, 24-Gy, or No Cranial Irradiation

Mulhern RK, Fairclough D, Ochs J (St Jude Children's Research Hosp, Memphis; Univ of Tennessee-Memphis)

J Clin Oncol 9:1348–1356, 1991 17–31

Introduction.—Children with acute lymphocytic leukemia (ALL) require adequate CNS prophylaxis to avoid the morbidity and mortality associated with this disease. The CNS therapies usually include cranial irradiation (CRT) with or without accompanying intrathecal methotrexate (IT MTX). A prospective study was undertaken to assess the neuropsychological performance of children with ALL treated with 18-Gy, 24-Gy, or no cranial irradiation.

Methods.—A total of 77 patients participated in the study. After attaining complete remission from ALL, the children were stratified into 2 groups for CNS prophylaxis: IT MTX and 18-Gy CRT or IT MTX and high-dose MTX. Twenty-eight patients who had received 24-Gy CRT were compared with these 2 groups. During remission, the children participated in psychological testing, either annually or biannually.

Findings.—No significant differences for Verbal, Full Scale, or Performance IQ assessments were observed between the 3 CNS therapy groups at 4 intervals (after 30 months of therapy, 0–35 months without therapy, 36–47 months after therapy, and 48 months or more after therapy). The final evaluation demonstrated a small but significant Verbal vs. Performance IQ difference for all 3 groups. The only reliable trend was the effect of sex on Verbal IQ, with 4 (11%) of 36 males showing significantly less decline in Verbal IQ scores (a decrease of 15 points or more) than the 18 (46%) of 38 females. Figure 17–8 presents the results of analyses of the Reading, Spelling, and Arithmetic scores. These results indicate that all 3 therapy groups experienced a significant decline in academic achievement over time.

Conclusions.—Female children appear to have more potential risk of deterioration in the Verbal IQ assessments than do male children. The risk factors associated with any other intellectual or achievement decreases found in this study could not be determined.

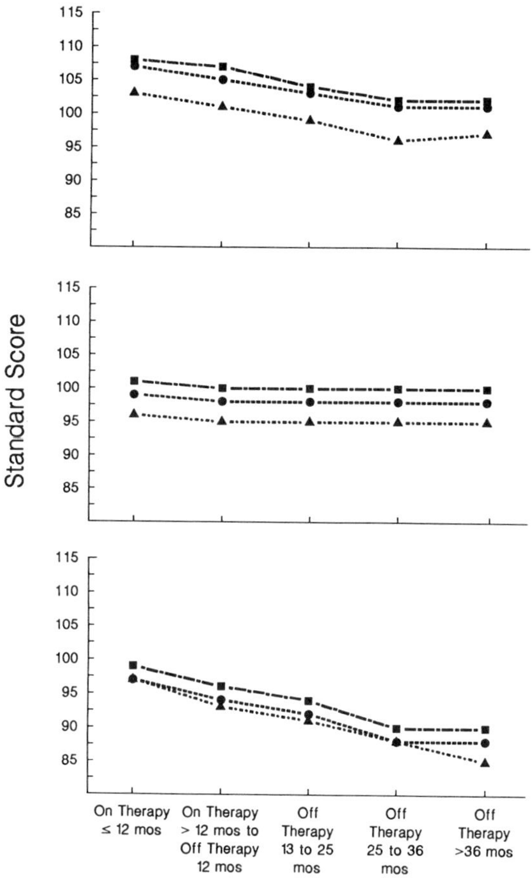

Fig 17–8.—Mean Reading, Spelling, and Arithmetic achievement of children receiving 18 Gy *(circles)* or 24 Gy *(triangles)* CRT, or MTX alone *(squares)* as CNS prophylaxis. (Courtesy of Mulhern RK, Fairclough D, Ochs J: *J Clin Oncol* 9:1348–1356, 1991.)

▶ There has now been voluminous literature on the effect of CNS irradiation on neuropsychological function in children with leukemia. Most studies suggest that there is a decrease in neuropsychological function that ranges from mild to severe (depending on the particular study, the instruments used for examination, and the population of patients being studied). The authors report the first *prospective* controlled study of this issue in patients given either 1 of 2 dosage levels of CRT or no irradiation. The surprising result was that there was a small but significant decline in Performance I.Q. for all 3 groups. This is shown graphically in the figure. The other surprising result of this study was that female children were at greater risk for deterioration in verbal I.Q. than were males. The decline in Arithmetic achievement was distributed evenly. This study has punctured some preconceived notions that I—and others—have held. The patients who were given no radiation therapy had received IT MTX and high-dose systemic MTX. One must speculate that MTX has an effect similar to that of radiation on neuropsychological function, or that other facets of the treatment for leukemia and its sociological milieu have such an effect. Another possibility is that the meningeal invasion known to occur in virtually every child somehow compromises cerebral circulation either by itself or synergistically with chemotherapy or radiation. This study forces us to rethink our ideas on this matter.—J.V. Simone, M.D.

Linear Growth in Children With Acute Lymphoblastic Leukemia Treated Without Cranial Irradiation

Katz JA, Chambers B, Everhart C, Marks JF, Buchanan GR (Univ of Texas Southwestern Med Ctr, Dallas; Children's Med Ctr, Dallas)

J Pediatr 118:575–578, 1991 17–32

Introduction.—The linear growth of children with acute lymphoblastic leukemia (ALL) who received cranial irradiation (CI) has previously been studied. A group of children with newly diagnosed non–T-cell, non–B-cell ALL received treatment without CI. The patients' growth patterns were monitored during a 5-year period.

Methods.—Thirty children met the requirements for inclusion in the study. The patients received CNS prophylaxis with intrathecal methotrexate, hydrocortisone, and cytarabine, but no CI. The duration of therapy was 3 years. Height determinations were made at diagnosis, 8–12 times each year during the 3 years of treatment, 3 or 4 times during the fourth study year, and semiannually during the last study year. Growth velocity was calculated at 12-month intervals from the time of diagnosis.

Results.—During the first year after diagnosis, the patients had decreases in standardized height percentile, and growth velocity was significantly less than that of normal children. Between years 3 and 4, both height and growth velocity showed significant gains, and by the end of 5 years, both parameters were similar to those of normal children. No differences were demonstrated between boys and girls.

Discussion.—Cranial irradiation has been reported to decrease linear growth during and after treatment, and it has also been associated with intellectual and neuropsychologic dysfunction. Many current regimens of chemotherapy have eliminated CI as a component of CNS prophylaxis. Minimal effects on linear growth were found for ALL treatment programs using only intrathecal medications as CNS prophylaxis. Further multicenter studies are recommended.

▶ It has long been known that irradiation of the CNS impairs linear growth in children, whether the treatment is given for leukemia or for brain tumors. The degree of impairment is related to age, i.e., the younger the child at the time of irradiation, the greater the impairment. Some growth catch-up is exhibited, but (as shown in this study) it is common for the ultimate height achieved to be less than what would normally be anticipated. Fortunately, irradiation of the CNS has become necessary for only a small proportion of patients with leukemia. Once again, we are reminded that a growing child differs from the mature adult in terms of the impact of any form of cancer therapy.—J.V. Simone, M.D.

Effects of Radiation on Testicular Function in Long-Term Survivors of Childhood Acute Lymphoblastic Leukemia: A Report From the Childrens Cancer Study Group

Sklar CA, Robinson LL, Nesbit ME, Sather HN, Meadows AT, Ortega JA, Kim TH, Hammond GD (New York Univ; Univ of Minnesota, Minneapolis; Univ of Southern California, Pasadena; Children's Hosp of Philadelphia; Children's Hosp of Los Angeles)

J Clin Oncol 8:1981–1987, 1990 17–33

Introduction.—Gonadal dysfunction in children who have undergone therapy for acute lymphoblastic leukemia (ALL) is generally caused by direct gonadal damage resulting from chemotherapy and radiotherapy (RT) rather than occurring as a secondary consequence of hypothalamic-pituitary injury from cranial RT. Ovarian dysfunction has been noted in girls treated for ALL with low-toxicity chemotherapy (no alkylating agents) and RT that included the gonadal area. The effects of identical therapy on subsequent testicular function were assessed in 60 boys (mean age, 14.5 years) who were an average of 4.5 years of age at diagnosis of ALL, and who had completed therapy an average of 5 years earlier.

Methods.—All patients underwent the same chemotherapy regimen (one of low gonadal toxicity) and the identical maintenance therapy; thus, their therapy differed only in the RT phase. Craniospinal RT (24 Gy) extending into the abdominal field (12 Gy; including gonads) was administered to 11 boys; 23 had craniospinal RT alone (24 Gy in 19; 18 Gy in 4), and in 26 boys, RT was limited to the cranium (24 Gy in 21; 18 Gy in 5).

Results.—Boys who had craniospinal RT extending to the abdomen differed significantly from those who had cranial RT alone because plasma follicle-stimulating hormone levels were increased (50% vs. 0%), and testicular size was reduced to less than the 10% percentile for age and pubertal stage (50% vs. 0%). Craniospinal RT alone resulted in intermediate levels of damage. There were no significant differences in these measures between the groups based on age at diagnosis, interval since radiation, or length of duration of maintenance chemotherapy. In 9% to 13% of the boys in each group, puberty was delayed. In 48 of the 50 boys tested, plasma luteinizing hormone and testosterone levels were normal.

Conclusion.—Germ-cell dysfunction as indexed by plasma follicle stimulating hormone levels and testicular size may result from scattered radiation from craniospinal RT, as well as from direct RT of the gonads. However, in most boys treated for ALL with cranial RT and low-toxicity chemotherapy, normal testicular function was preserved. Although Leydig cell failure has previously been reported in boys who received testicular RT with 20-Gy fractionated doses, 12 Gy did not significantly affect the normal plasma levels of luteinizing hormone and testosterone in this study.

▶ The take-home message from this study is very simple: the older practice of giving craniospinal irradiation for prophylaxis of CNS leukemia should no longer be used, because of both the reason outlined in this study and the availability of alternative regimens. There is sufficient scatter of irradiation in boys to sterilize the gonads or at least reduce gonadal function. Fortunately, craniospinal irradiation is seldom necessary, except in rare circumstances in which there is already active CNS leukemia or in some regimens for poor-risk patients. This is another example of the fine-tuning of leukemia therapy for nontherapeutic reasons.—J.V. Simone, M.D.

Acute Myeloid Leukemia in Children Treated With Epipodophyllotoxins for Acute Lymphoblastic Leukemia

Pui C-H, Ribeiro RC, Hancock ML, Rivera GK, Evans WE, Raimondi SC, Head DR, Behm FG, Mahmoud MH, Sandlund JT, Crist WM (St Jude Children's Research Hosp, Memphis)

N Engl J Med 325:1682–1687, 1991 17–34

Background.—The semisynthetic podophyllotoxin derivatives etoposide and teniposide are widely used in the treatment of malignancies. However, this treatment has been associated with the development of acute myeloid leukemia (AML) in children and adults. The importance of potential risk factors in the development of secondary AML in children treated with these epipodophyllotoxins was studied.

Methods.—The study sample comprised 734 consecutive children with acute lymphoblastic leukemia who achieved complete remission. The patients were seen during a 10-year period. They were entered into 1 of 2 therapy studies based on their risk of recurrence, and they were then randomized to receive various maintenance therapy regimens. The dosage of teniposide ranged from 0–5,100 mg/m^2, and the dosage of etoposide was either 0 or 9,000 mg/m^2. For protocols including epipodophyllotoxins, the dose schedule ranged from induction only to twice weekly. The follow-up included cytochemical studies, immunologic cell typing, and cytogenetic studies.

Results.—Twenty-one patients had secondary AML; in 17 patients, it was the initial adverse event. There was an independent association between prolonged epipodophyllotoxin administration on a twice weekly or weekly basis and the development of secondary AML. At 6 years, the overall cumulative risk was 3.8%; however, twice-weekly administration carried a 12.3% risk, and weekly administration had a 12.4% risk. Among the other groups, the highest cumulative risk was 1.6%. The total dose appeared to be unrelated to development of secondary AML after adjustment for the frequency of treatment. No conclusions could be drawn as to the relative risk of etoposide compared with teniposide. Thirteen patients achieved remission of AML, but only 2 remained in remission.

Conclusions.—In children with acute lymphoblastic leukemia treated with epipodophyllotoxins, the risk of having secondary AML appears to depend on the frequency of administration. No important role is noted for cumulative epipodophyllotoxin dose, radiotherapy, or the initial biological features of the leukemic blast cells. The mutagenic effects must be minimized while the therapeutic value is maximized, and children at increased risk of AML must be identified.

▶ This study identifies another risky agent used in the treatment of childhood leukemia. A high frequency of AML was observed in a subpopulation of patients given epipodophyllotoxins. It appeared that the frequency of administration was a key factor in determining the patients in whom this complication would develop. With anthracyclines, the cumulative dosage seems to be the major factor. Although one is relieved to learn that there are schedules of epipodophyllotoxin administration that do not appear to be associated with a high frequency of secondary AML, that this agent can cause such a dire complication is worrisome, because it may be deadly in the "safe" dosage if combined with another factor. Also, a long period of follow-up of the surviving and apparently unaffected patients will be necessary to be comfortable with continued therapy.—J.V. Simone, M.D.

Late Cardiac Effects of Doxorubicin Therapy for Acute Lymphoblastic Leukemia in Childhood

Lipshultz SE, Colan SD, Gelber RD, Perez-Atayde AR, Sallan SE, Sanders SP (Children's Hosp; Dana-Farber Cancer Inst; Harvard Med School; Harvard School of Public Health, Boston)

N Engl J Med 324:808–815, 1991 17–35

Introduction.—Cardiotoxicity has been associated with doxorubicin treatment. The long-term effects of this agent, however, have not been established. The cardiac status of 115 children in continuous remission who were treated for acute lymphoblastic leukemia with doxorubicin 1–15 years earlier was assessed.

Methods.—A single dose of doxorubicin was administered to 18 children, and multiple doses were administered to 97. The single doses totaled 45 mg of doxorubicin per m^2 of body-surface area, and multiple doses totaled 228–550 mg of doxorubicin per m^2 (median, 360 mg/m^2). A median of 6.4 years had elapsed since the end of treatment.

Results.—Abnormalities of left ventricular afterload or contractility occurred in 57% of the children. The most significant predictor of abnormal cardiac function was the cumulative dose of doxorubicin. Of those patients given 1 dose, 17% had slightly increased age-adjusted afterload, and none had reduced contractility. However, 65% of those given at least 228 of doxorubicin had increased afterload and/or reduced contractility. Increased afterload resulted from decreased ventricular wall thickness, not from hypertension or ventricular dilation. According to a multivariate analysis of patients given at least 228 mg of doxorubicin, the only significant predictors were a higher cumulative dose, which predicted reduced contractility, and age younger than 4 years at the time of treatment, which predicted increased afterload. In 24 (71%) of the 34 patients assessed serially, afterload increased progressively. Symptoms did not correlate well with indexes of exercise tolerance or ventricular function. Congestive heart failure occurred within 1 year of doxorubicin treatment in 11 children, 5 of whom had recurrent heart failure 3–10 years after completing doxorubicin therapy; 2 needed heart transplantation. None of the children had late heart falure as a new event.

Conclusion.—The treatment for 1 potentially fatal childhood disease may cause another serious and potentially fatal disease. There was an unexpectedly high incidence of late cardiovascular abnormalities in these patients. The contribution of doxorubicin to the cure of children with cancer must be balanced against the later effects of treatment and the influence on the child's quality of life.

▶ This is the kind of paper that makes all cancer therapists shudder, particularly those that treat children. An astonishing 57% of the children in this study had detectable abnormalities of left ventricular function. The most disturbing statistic is that 65% of those patients who were given at least 228 mg of doxorubicin per m^2 had abnormalities. This dosage is well within the range of what was considered "safe" in the early years; in fact, doxorubicin, 500 mg/m^2, was considered the upper limit of safety. The sophisticated investigations by these authors indicate that a much lower dose can cause measurable difficulties. The implications for these children as they become adults and are subject to coronary artery disease are not known, but they certainly give one pause. However, one must not lose sight of the fact, that these authors have had enormous success in the cure of childhood acute lymphoblastic leukemia. They—and we—are on the horns of a dilemma when it comes to modifying very successful therapy in the hopes of reducing the potential late effects.—J.V. Simone, M.D.

Exercise Echocardiography in the Detection of Anthracycline Cardiotoxicity

Weesner KM, Bledsoe M, Chauvenet A, Wofford M (Wake Forest Univ, Winston-Salem, NC)

Cancer 68:435–438, 1991 17–36

Background.—Long-term survival for children with cancer has improved, partly as a result of the use of anthracycline antineoplastic therapy. Children treated with anthracycline, however, may develop cardiac dysfunction, which often appears during exercise. The use of echocardiography and exercise to diagnose myocardial dysfunction was assessed in children previously treated with anthracycline.

Methods.—Twenty children who were asymptomatic long-term survivors of cancer participated in the study. Resting heart rate, blood pressures, and echocardiographic measurements were recorded. Eighteen patients had a pulse Doppler study of the left ventricle for mitral flow assessment.

Results.—Of the 20 patients in the study, 10 (4 females and 6 males; mean age, 14 years) had received anthracyclines (mean dose, 291 mg/m^2). Ten long-term survivor patients (5 females, 5 males; mean age, 16 years) had not received anthracyclines. No statistical differences were found for resting heart rate or systolic and diastolic blood pressures between the 2 patient groups. After exercise, the shortening fraction in the echocardiographic measurement was significantly less in the anthracycline group than in the nontreated patients. A significant difference between the 2 groups occurred at rest for the left ventricular filling measurement, with 1 of 9 anthracycline-treated patients and none of 9 non–anthracycline-treated patients showing an A wave with a greater peak velocity than the E wave. After exercise, 3 of 9 anthracycline-treated children and 1 of 9 nonanthracycline-treated children had an A wave greater than the E wave.

Implications.—Exercise echocardiography can identify subtle myocardial abnormalities in children treated with anthracyclines who have survived the childhood cancer for a long time. Further study is needed to support the use of exercise echocardiography in these patients.

▶ This paper is complementary to the one by Lipshultz et al. (Abstract 17–35). It indicates that routine testing for cardiac function in long-term survivors of cancers who were given anthracyclines may not detect abnormalities. Exercise studies may be necessary. Of course, the long-term practical implications of these findings are not known, which makes long-term follow-up clinics increasingly important.—J.V. Simone, M.D.

Congenital Anomalies in Children of Patients Who Received Chemotherapy for Cancer in Childhood and Adolescence

Green DM, Zevon MA, Lowrie G, Seigelstein N, Hall B (Roswell Park Cancer Inst, Buffalo, NY)

N Engl J Med 325:141–146, 1991 17–37

Background.—Children and adolescents frequently receive chemotherapeutic agents for their cancers. When these cancer survivors reach adulthood, many become concerned about the mutagenic effects of the anticancer drugs on their future children. The frequency of congenital anomalies in the children of parents who had received cancer therapy as a child or adolescent was determined.

Methods.—The medical records of 1,239 consecutive patients who were younger than 20 years of age between January 1960 and December 1984, and who received chemotherapy for cancer were reviewed. A subpopulation of 383 former patients who were currently 18 years of age or older was chosen for further study. Of these 383 patients, 100 responded to a questionnaire by mail. Of the 202 pregnancies reported, 17 ended in spontaneous abortions, 4 ended in therapeutic abortions, and 1 was an ectopic pregnancy; there also were 4 stillbirths, 13 premature deliveries, and 163 full-term live births.

Results.—Among the male respondees, 25 reported the birth of 39 offspring (23 girls, 16 boys), which included 1 stillbirth. Two of the live-birth youngsters had birthmarks, and 1 had a skin tag, demonstrating a 7.9% minor anomaly rate in infants born after chemotherapy. No relationship was found between the congenital anomalies in infants of fathers who had chemotherapy and the drug, father's age at diagnosis, or length of time after treatment. For female patients, 63 children (26 girls and 37 boys) included 1 stillbirth, 6 premature births and 57 live births. Five of the 57 livebirths (8.1%) had congenital anomalies (1 each of tetralogy of Fallot, a hydrocele, a ventricular septal defect, and a hemangioma). The ventricular septal defect occurred significantly more often in the children patients with cancer who had had chemotherapy. The tetralogy of Fallot occurred more frequently among the male children of the white female patients with cancer. Structural congenital cardiac defects were found in 10% of the children born to women who had received dactinomycin. Neither the number of mutagens used nor the cumulative dose corresponded to the congenital defect frequency.

Implications.—Patients who undergo cancer chemotherapy as children or adolescents do not have an increased frequency of congenital defects in their offspring. The possible adverse effect of dactinomycin in the children of these parents requires further analysis and research.

▶ For anyone who treats children with leukemia and other forms of cancer, this is a wonderful paper. We have worried for years that all the treatment regimens we use have the potential for causing germ-cell mutations that might result in congenital anomalies in the offspring of our surviving patients. We can breathe a little bit easier now. Although we are certainly not out of the woods, within the framework of this study, it appears that there is no major impact. Until we can eliminate all potentially mutagenic forms of therapy, this type of study will be most helpful in gauging the adverse risks of our regimens.—J.V. Simone, M.D.

Additional Reading

Fraschini G, Ciociola A, et al: Evaluation of three oral dosages of ondansetron in the prevention of nausea and emesis associated with cyclophosphamide-doxorubicin chemotherapy. *J Clin Oncol* 9:1268–1274, 1991.

▶ Oral ondansetron was shown to be an effective antiemetic for patients receiving a noncisplatin cyclophosphamide-doxorubicin-based chemotherapy.

Eguiguren J, Ribiero RC, Pui C-H, et al: Secondary non-Hodgkin's lymphoma after treatment for childhood cancer. *Leukemia* 5:908–911, 1991.

▶ In this large series, secondary non-Hodgkin's lymphoma occurred most often in children with Hodgkins disease; it carries a very poor prognosis.

Neglia JP, Meadows AT, Robison LL, et al: Second neoplasms after acute lymphoblastic leukemia in childhood. *New Engl J Med* 325:1330–1336, 1991.

▶ The strongest observation of this study is that children with acute lymphoblastic leukemia, especially those who received brain irradiation before 5 years of age, have a greatly increased risk of having a brain tumor develop.

Rubin CM, Arthur DC, Woods WG, et al: Therapy-related myelodysplastic syndrome and acute myeloid leukemia in children: Correlation between chromosomal abnormalities and prior therapy. *Blood* 78:2982–2988, 1991.

▶ Alkylating agents and epipodophyllotoxins appear to be the primary culprits in the development of this complication.

Cheruku R, Tapazoglou E, et al: The incidence and significance of thromboembolic complications in patients with high-grade gliomas. *Cancer* 68:2621–2624, 1991.

▶ This study confirms the high incidence of thromboembolic complications in patients with high-grade glioma. Even responding patients are at risk for death from pulmonary embolism. However, the optimum approach to management is unclear, because anticoagulation has been associated with a significant complication rate.

Becker DM, Philbrick JT, et al: Axillary and subclavian venous thrombosis. *Arch Intern Med* 151:1934–1943, 1991.

▶ As determined in this article, axillary and subclavian vein thrombosis can lead to pulmonary embolism and death, with incidences of 9.4% and 1.2%, respectively. Appropriate therapy in most patients is systemic anticoagulation with surgery; thrombolytic therapy is reserved for refractory cases.

18 Supportive Care

Physician Attitudes

Burnout Syndrome in the Practice of Oncology: Results of a Random Survey of 1,000 Oncologists

Whippen DA, Canellos GP (Editorial Office of the Journal of Clinical Oncology; Dana-Farber Cancer Inst, Boston)

J Clin Oncol 9:1916–1921, 1991 18–1

Introduction.—Burnout resulting from stress can occur in any profession and impair performance. The extent of burnout among American oncologists was surveyed.

Methods.—A questionnaire was mailed to 1,000 randomly selected physician subscribers to the *Journal of Clinical Oncology*.

Results.—The majority of the surveys were returned completed. Overall, there was a 56% rate of professional burnout reported. There was a significantly lower rate of burnout among those oncologists practicing in an institution or university. The most frequent definition of the nature of burnout was frustration or sense of failure, whereas lack of personal and vacation time was the most cited reason for burnout (table).

Conclusions.—Considering the high rate of burnout that was reported voluntarily, further work on the subject is warranted.

▶ "Doctor, I don't know how you do it." How often have each of us heard that statement from patients, friends and family. We generally shrug and respond blandly. Indeed, it is a good question. How *do* we do it? The results of this study suggest that we don't do it very well. Of the 1,000 American oncologists who were surveyed, almost 60% experienced some burnout in their professional lives. Interestingly, there was little significant difference between the in-

Suggestions for Burnout Alleviation by Respondents by Year of Completion of Training and Overall

Suggestion	Before 1970 (%)	1970-1979 (%)	1980 or Later (%)	Overall (%)
More vacation or personal time	66	68	71	69
Sabbaticals	49	49	34	43
More travel and conference attendance	32	35	36	34
Smaller patient load	28	33	35	33
Participation in cooperative clinical trials	25	15	26	21
More involvement in institutional health care policy making	26	26	13	21
More teaching	26	10	17	16

(Courtesy of Whippen DA, Canellos GP: *J Clin Oncol* 9:1916–1921, 1991.)

cidence of burnout amongst medical, surgical, and radiation oncologists. Institution- or university-based oncologists reported a lower incidence of burnout than did those in private practice. Frustration or sense of failure was the most frequent description of burnout, and insufficient personal or vacation time was the most frequent explanation. Almost 70% of the physicians indicated the need for more vacation or personal time to alleviate burnout. The high frequency of palliative or terminal care, heavy workload, and increasing reimbursement issues were contributing factors to burnout. Although the overall results suggest a pessimistic oncology environment, 80% of the oncologists said that their career had met their expectations. This curious paradox suggests that the oncologists apparently expected to experience burnout. It would appear that we need to study ourselves as much as our patients.—R.C. Young, M.D., F.A.C.P.

Oncologists Vary in Their Willingness to Undertake Anti-Cancer Therapies

Lind SE, Good M-J D, Minkovitz CS, Good BJ (Mass Gen Hosp; Harvard Med School, Boston)

Br J Cancer 64:391–395, 1991 18–2

Background.—Physicians' personal opinions of cancer treatments may affect the treatment of their patients and explain some of the variation in the treatment patterns detected. Whether differences exist in the opinions of oncologists on the value of various cancer therapies was determined.

Methods.—Interviews were conducted with 51 oncologists to determine whether they would undergo chemotherapy or radiation therapy for several common malignancies. Recommendations to a spouse or sibling were also assessed. The physicians' view of an experimental therapy was also examined.

Results.—There was considerable heterogeneity in the responses of the oncologists. In only 37% of the 30 cases involving standard therapies did at least 85% of the oncologists agree on treatment. The physicians were significantly more likely to recommend an experimental therapy to another individual than to accept it for themselves.

Conclusion.—There is a good deal of variation in the personal preferences of oncologists for cancer therapies for a variety of common malignancies. Further studies are needed to determine the relationship between personal preference and patient treatment.

▶ In the 1991 YEAR BOOK, we reviewed a paper by Slevin et al. that compared attitudes toward cancer treatment by doctors, nurses, and the general public (1). It suggested that patients themselves were considerably more enthusiastic than their doctors. This study makes similar conclusions. The authors asked radiation oncologists, surgical oncologists, and medical oncologists to evaluate therapy in several prototypical situations, and to assess whether they would accept therapy or recommend it to their families. In general, the oncologists were unenthusiastic about accepting experimental therapy, even in the absence of a satisfactory alternative. As in earlier studies, surgical oncologists were more likely to refuse therapy than either medical or radiation oncologists. Surprisingly, physicians in general were significantly mroe likely to recommend therapy for a spouse or sibling than to accept it for themselves. This study suggests that physicians, like characters from *Alice in Wonderland,* are becoming "curiouser and curiouser."—R.C. Young, M.D., F.A.C.P.

Reference

1. Slevin ML, et al: *BMJ* 300:1458, 1990.

Presenting a Diagnosis of Cancer: Patient's Views

Peteet JR, Abrams HE, Ross DM, Stearns NM (Dana-Farber Cancer Inst, Boston; Salem Hosp, Salem, Mass)

J Fam Prac 32:577–581, 1991 18–3

Background.—Little information is available either on the way American patients are informed of a cancer diagnosis or on their satisfaction with the method by which they were informed. Therefore, a study of 32 patients given a diagnosis of cancer was undertaken.

Method and Results.—A semistructured interview was performed by psychosocial clinicians. All patients had been informed of their diagnosis by a physician. The information was conveyed in person 84% of the time. The patients said that being informed with hope, information, caring, and respect for privacy were helpful. They also valued having a supportive person present. Almost 40% of the patients reported that their hopes were directed toward remission and quality of life rather than cure at the time of interview. Those patients who had had a misdiagnosis initially reported mistrust of information from physicians.

Conclusion.—When physicians are presenting a diagnosis of cancer, they must foster trust and provide hope for patients. Providing treatment information contributes more to hope than does cheerfulness. Those patients who have been given a misdiagnosis require special consideration to reestablish trust.

▶ It is encouraging to see studies that address the complex problem of improving doctor-patient interactions when the diagnosis of cancer is made. In the 1991 Year Book, we reviewed a paper by Blanchard et al. that illustrated that patient satisfaction depended upon the perception of how well the doctor outlined future treatment and treatment goals (1). The Blanchard study, which was based on a detailed interview of 32 patients (of whom half were treated at a comprehensive cancer center and half were treated in a community hospital), demonstrated similar findings. The vast majority of the patients who received this information from physicians in the context of appropriate cancer treatment information said that the interaction fostered trust and hope. Those patients who initially receive a misdiagnosis present a unique and difficult problem because of their persistent mistrust of information received from physicians.

More studies of this type should enable oncologists to better train young physicians in this important communication skill.—R.C. Young, M.D., F.A.C.P.

Reference

1. Blanchard CG, et al: *Cancer* 65:186, 1990.

Analysed Interaction in a Children's Oncology Clinic: The Child's View and Parent's Opinion of the Effect of Medical Encounters

Inman CE (Univ of Hull, England)

J Adv Nursing 16:782–793, 1991 18–4

Introduction.—Communication in a pediatric oncology setting can be difficult, especially as a result of attempts to provide these children with advanced medical care. Young patients usually receive systematic explanations of their diagnosis, treatment, and side effects. Advanced preparation and education can reduce anxiety and depression in children with cancer. Based on a pilot study, an interview process was developed for children with cancer and their parents.

Methods.—Ten children and their parents were interviewed at home or in the hospital using transcribed audio tapes, assessment of the child's gaze direction in relation to the doctor, and ethnographic notes recorded in the consulting room. Three of the child's brief, nonscheduled interviews were with an unaccompanied child.

Findings.—Eight of the 10 interviews resulted in relaxing the child and encouraging a discussion of his or her situation. Most of the patients recalled at least 1 "good" occurrence in the clinic visit, but most had low acknowledgment of interaction with the doctor. Most of the parent interviews, which occurred before the child's second appointment, were relaxed and resulted in a consistent association between the report of the children's attitude and behavior. The results of the clinical assessment and interaction showed the dominant role of the doctor. In 9 of 10 interactions, the doctor gazed more frequently at the child than the child did at the doctor. One doctor gazed at the clinic notes more often, which allowed the child to observe and watch the physician. The excess child-watching appeared to make the children more nervous, whereas the least amount of child-watching produced a more relaxed child.

Conclusions.—These findings indicate that using several methods of collecting information can broaden the knowledge of the young cancer patient. The outcome suggests that the appropriate positive interaction between clinic personnel and both the child with cancer and his or her parents can reduce the child's anxiety, especially if physicians lower the amount of time they watch the child.

▶ This is one of those studies that arrives at a conclusion that strikes the reader as being self-evident. The investigators found that clinic visits were more acceptable for children when the staff invested more personal attention, gave adequate explanations of procedures, and handled the children sensitively. My mother is not a physician, but she knew this a long time ago. I would venture to say that the same conclusion would be true for patients of any age, not just for children and their families.—J.V. Simone, M.D.

Effect of Patients' Expectations of Benefit With Standard Breast Cancer Adjuvant Chemotherapy on Participation in a Randomized Clinical Trial: A Clinical Vignette Study

Fetting JH, Siminoff LA, Piantadosi S, Abeloff MD, Damron DJ, Sarsfield AM (Johns Hopkins Oncology Ctr, Baltimore; Univ of PIttsburgh, Pa)

J Clin Oncol 8:1476–1482, 1990 18–5

Background.—Patients often appear to misunderstand the benefits of standard adjuvant therapy for breast cancer, which is frequently the control arm of a randomized trial. Patients' expectations may be overly optimistic, partly because of vague communication between them and their physicians. How the physician's description and the patient's expectations of the benefits of standard therapy influence participation in clinical trials was evaluated in a clinical vignette study.

Methods.—The study sample comprised 282 women with cancer (mean age, 51 years). Of the women, 83% had at least a high school diploma, and 86% had received chemotherapy; 39% had taken part in a clinical trial of cancer treatment. The patients were randomized to 1 of 2 versions of a clinical vignette in which a patient with breast cancer was to choose between standard cyclophosphamide, methotrexate, and 5-fluorouracil (CMF) treatment or a comparative trial of CMF and cyclophosphamide, doxorubicin, and 5-fluorouracil. The only difference between the vignettes was whether the results in terms of disease-free survival (DFS) were presented verbally or numerically; the patients were randomized 3:1 to the verbal vignette. After they had made their choice, the patients estimated the 10-year survival with standard CMF therapy.

Results.—Of the verbal vignette group, 52.4% chose the clinical trial compared with 34.7% of the numeric vignette group. As expected, the estimates of 10-year DFS varied considerably. Of the women in the longest third of DFS estimates in the verbal vignette group, 34.4% chose the trial—compared with 59.4% in the middle third and 58.5% in the shortest third. Other factors predicting selection of the trial were younger age, college education, and previous participation in a trial. On multivariate logistic regression, the expected benefit from CMF was a more important factor than the description of benefit.

Conclusion.—Physicians need to ensure that patients have realistic expectations of the benefits of standard adjuvant therapy. The most important predictor of choosing to participate in a trial is the patient's estimate of the long-term results with standard therapy. Educational materials for individual trials might be a useful adjunct to physician-patient communication.

▶ Some physicians have a difficult time getting their patients to enter clinical trials; others do not. The possible reasons for this difference were explored in this intriguing study from Johns Hopkins. A total of 282 patients was randomized to receive 2 different vignettes describing the potential benefit of CMF as an adjuvant chemotherapy. The vignettes were identical, except that 1 had a verbal description of CMF benefits and the other had a numerical presentation of the results. Those patients who received only the verbal description were significantly more likely to enter the clinical trial than those receiving the numerical vignette. One of the most surprising outcomes of the study was the tremendous variation in patient estimates of 10-year DFS. Approximately one third of the patients estimated 10-year survival to be from 0 to 47%; another third, from 47% to 68%; and the top third, from 68% to 100%. Not surprisingly, the likelihood of agreeing to a clinical trial was related to the patient estimates of success with CMF alone. As was frequently demonstrated in other trials, it is the patient's expectations about the benefit rather than the documented benefit that influences his or her decision. Those who believed that CMF alone was highly effective did not elect the trial; those who were pessimistic, did. The overall implications of this trial are that patients are exquisitely sensitive to small differences in the way therapeutic outcomes and clinical trials are presented.—R.C. Young, M.D., F.A.C.P.

Cost Effectiveness

Evaluation of a Home Intravenous Antibiotic Program in Pediatric Oncology

Wiernikowski JT, Rothney M, Dawson S, Andrew M (Chedoke-McMaster Hosps, Hamilton, Ont, Canada)

Am J Pediatr Hematol Oncol 13:144–147, 1991 18–6

Introduction.—Increasing health care costs have forced hospitals and physicians to examine and implement more cost-efficient treatment programs. A program of home intravenous antibiotic administration was begun for febrile neutropenic episodes in children with cancer.

Methods.—During a 6-month period, 13 children with malignant disease had courses of intravenous antibiotics administered at home. Children with indwelling right atrial catheters were eligible if they were afebrile for at least 48 hours after initiation of antibiotics in hospital; receiving appropriate antibiotics as determined by culture; clinically stable; and if their parents were able to reliably administer intravenous antibiotics as evaluated by a pediatric oncology nurse. The children were sent home with enough antibiotics and supplies for a 10- to 14-day regimen.

Results.—The 13 children and families that participated successfully treated 22 episodes of infection. The cost of the in-home program was considerably less than that of in-hospital treatment. Twelve days of inpatient therapy cost approximately $7416, and the cost of 13 days of home therapy was estimated at $2781. Parental feedback was uniformly positive.

Conclusions.—The in-home intravenous antibiotic treatment program for children with malignant disease is apparently convenient and cost effective. The treatment was highly successful when implemented by motivated and enthusiastic parents.

▶ The increasing pressure on physicians in health care institutions to reduce the number of inpatient hospital days has led to a number of innovations in outpatient care. What we are learning is that it is possible to give more care on an outpatient basis if one has the technology and supporting staff. Home infusion is one of those techniques. In this paper, antibiotics were the drugs given. However, in my own institution and in others, patients in an ambulatory setting are given a wide range of chemotherapeutic agents using portable pumps. No one likes inpatient hospitalization, especially children and their parents. They will cooperate in carrying out even complex procedures for the advantage of taking the child home or to the hotel in the evening. All it takes is a supportive system and the will of the staff to carry it out.—J.V. Simone, M.D.

Cardiopulmonary Resuscitation and the Patient With Cancer

Vitelli CE, Cooper K, Rogatko A, Brennan MF (Mem Sloan-Kettering Cancer Ctr, New York)

J Clin Oncol 9:111–115, 1991 18–7

Background.—Both patient and physician often consider cardiopulmonary arrest (CPA) to be a terminal event in a patient with cancer, especially if metastatic disease is present. There have been no reports of objective clinical parameters of patients who might benefit from resuscitation, and the decision to resuscitate is often left to the house officer on duty.

Methods.—A total of 750 had CPA while hospitalized at a cancer center during a 3-year period. Of these, 85% were admitted for supportive care only, and no resuscitation was attempted. The remaining 114 patients did receive cardiopulmonary resuscitation. Statistical analyses were done to identify the variables predicting final outcome in this group of patients.

Results.—Resuscitation was successful in 65.7% of the patients; however, only 12 patients, or 10.5%, were discharged alive from the hospital. These patients survived a median of 150 days after discharge. The patients who were discharged stayed for a mean of 11.3 days in the intensive care unit compared with 3.3 days for those who were not discharged. The patient's performance status at admission was the only variable that predicted the likelihood of being discharged alive after CPA. For patients who spent more than half their time in bed at the time of admission, the chance of being discharged alive after CPA was only 2.3%.

Conclusions.—The admission performance status of patients with cancer is the most powerful predictor of being discharged alive after CPA.

No correlations are noted between age and prognosis or the presence of metastatic disease and outcome. All patients should have assessment of cardiopulmonary resuscitation status at admission to obviate the need for emergency resuscitation decisions.

▶ Cardiopulmonary resuscitation is a resource-intensive, cost-intensive, labor-intensive effort that is clearly capable of saving lives. However, the ultimate success of such an effort becomes problematic when serious underlying diseases, such as cancer, exist. Several large retrospective reviews have documented essentially no long-term survivors after cardiopulmonary resuscitation of patients with cancer. A study from the Memorial Sloan-Kettering Cancer Center suggests that approximately 10% of patients with cancer can be successfully resuscitated and discharged from the hospital. The median survival after discharge was approximately 5 months. Although age, disease prognosis, and the presence of metastatic disease did not correlate with successful resuscitation, the patient's performance status clearly did. Only 2% of the patients who spent more than half of their time in bed on admission were successfully resuscitated and discharged. These authors suggest that performance status should be considered in discussions with patients and families regarding cardiopulmonary resuscitation status.—R.C. Young, M.D., F.A.C.P.

Pain

Intrathecal Narcotics for Relief of Pain from Head and Neck Cancer

Andersen PE, Cohen JI, Everts EC, Bedder MD, Burchiel KJ (Oregon Health Sciences Univ; St Vincent Hosp, Portland)
Arch Otolaryngol Head Neck Surg 117:1277–1280, 1991 18–8

Introduction.—Pain control remains an important part of therapy in patients with unresectable head and neck cancer. Secondary measures may be required in those who do not experience pain relief with conventional means. Based on the unexpected relief of pain in such a patient with cancer after placement of an epidural and then an intrathecal catheter for continuous fentanyl infusion to relieve abdominal discomfort, 9 additional patients with head and neck cancer were treated in the same manner.

Methods.—A retrospective review identified all patients who had not experienced pain relief with oral narcotic or non-narcotic analgesics for head and neck tumors. Candidates for the fentanyl treatment first underwent a trial of lumbar epidural narcotics.

Technique.—Implantation of the drug delivery pump usually occurs on the patient's right side. The intrathecal catheter is then inserted subcutaneously around the flank, connecting to the pump. The reservoir of the pump is filled with morphine sulfate. The pump delivers a constant infusion of 10% of the drug needed for pain relief during the epidural portion of the experiment.

Findings.—The mean preimplantation visual analog scale (VAS) score was 7.6/10 (Fig 18–1), which differed from the mean VAS scores for all

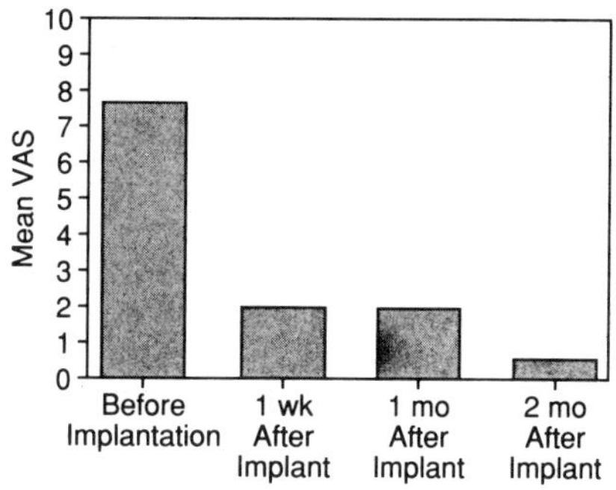

Fig 18–1.—The mean visual analog scale vs. time of implantation. (Courtesy of Andersen PE, Cohen JI, Everts EC, et al: *Arch Otolaryngol Head Neck Surg* 117:1277–1280, 1991.)

patients of 1.9/10, 2/10, and .5/10 at 1 week, 1 month, and 2 months, respectively, after pump implantation. All patients except for 1 required an increased infusion rate to maintain pain control. The mean morphine dose increased over time (Fig 18–2). Three complications occurred: 1 patient had chronic anticoagulation (because of a prosthetic heart valve), and a hematoma developed at the implantation site; 1 patient experienced self-limited urinary retention; and in 1 patient, an obstructive kink developed in the intrathecal catheter 1 month after implantation. Total pain therapy time ranged from 30 to 84 days.

Conclusions.—These findings indicate that an implantable pump that delivers intrathecal morphine can alleviate pain in patients with head and neck cancer. This method is safe and effective.

▶ A few cancer centers in this country have excellent pain control programs that run the gamut from treatment with oral analgesics to neurosurgical intervention. However, the average therapist is not personally familiar with these options. This study demonstrates another useful approach that may be required for patients with severe pain in the head and neck area, which would seem to be a more onerous site of pain than others. The approach outlined in this study, although requiring epidural placement of the catheter, was well tolerated and very effective. It had the additional advantage of being left in place for extended periods of time. Pain is a very lonely experience, and physicians

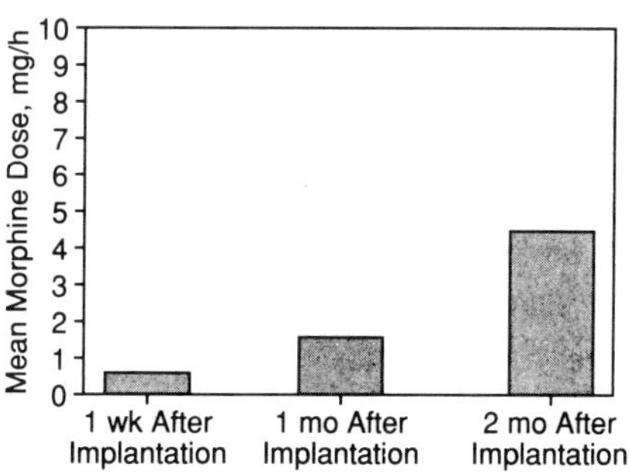

Fig 18–2.—The mean morphine dose vs. time after implantation. (Courtesy of Andersen PE, Cohen JI, Everts EC, et al: *Arch Otolaryngol Head Neck Surg* 117:1277–1280, 1991.)

often are less sensitive than they ought to be to taking aggressive measures to control pain.—J.V. Simone, M.D.

Patient Controlled Analgesia for the Young Pediatric Patient

Gureno MA, Reisinger CL (St Luke's Hosp, Cedar Rapids, Iowa)

Pediatr Nursing 17:251–254, 1991 18–9

Introduction.—Although children are assumed to experience similar postoperative pain as adults, studies have shown that children often receive inadequate pain control after operation. One reason is that pain in children is difficult to assess because a child may deny pain to avoid a feared injection. The safe use of patient-controlled analgesia (PCA) in children older than 10 years has previously been documented. The safety and efficacy of PCA was assessed in 15 children (aged, 3–11 years; mean age, 6 years) who were undergoing unilateal or bilateral ureteroneocystostomy.

Methods.—All children received PCA through a computer-controlled infusion pump attached to a primary intravenous line. A continuous background infusion of analgesics was administered through the pump to avoid peak and trough analgesia levels. The pump contained a lock-out mechanism to prevent overdosing. Mature children controlled the pump themselves, whereas younger children were assisted either by a responsible parent or by a nurse.

Results.—The average time of pump use was 82.7 hours. All the children maintained excellent pain control, as was apparent from their activities and self-report. Serious side effects or respiratory depression did not occur. The total amount of morphine received was 36–72 mg/kg/24 hours, which varied with each child. A written survey completed by the parents after their child's hospital discharge revealed a high level of satisfaction with this method of pain control. The use of PCA at this hospital has now been expanded to include pediatric patients undergoing appendectomy, hypospadias repair, orchiopexy, craniotomy, and orthopedic procedures.

Conclusion.—Patient-controlled analgesia is an effective method of pain control in children, even in those as young as 3 years of age.

▶ One of my pet peeves is the general lack of physician sensitivity to adequate analgesia in patients with cancer; this is even worse for children with cancer. I am also a strong proponent of patient-controlled analgesia when circumstances permit. This study is included to demonstrate that even pediatric patients can safely control analgesia. It is very impressive that the five 3-year-old children who were part of this study successfully used the system.—J.V. Simone, M.D.

A Clinical Survey of Controlled-Release Morphine Sulphate for Cancer Pain Relief in a Japanese Hospice

Tsuneto S, Hayashi A, Miyazaki M, Kashiwagi T (Yodogawa Christian Hosp, Osaka, Japan)

Postgrad Med J 67:79S–81S, 1991 18–10

Background.—Pain control is an essential part of hospice care for patients with cancer.

Patients and Results.—Seventy-six hospice patients received controlled-release morphine during a 5-year period. Forty-four were women and 32 were men, and the mean age was 61 years. A total of 46% had gastrointestinal tumors. The most common cause of pain was visceral, followed by bone pain, nerve pain, and soft tissue infiltration. The mean initial dose of controlled-release morphine was 81.4 mg, and the mean maximum dose was 178.6 mg. No increase from the initial dosage was needed for 61% of the patients. Of the remainder, 34% had an increase of 8% to 125%, and 4 patients had their dosage increased by more than 500%; the reason for this was nerve involvement. The total effectiveness of controlled-release morphine was 92%; a dosage of 240 mg of morphine per day or less was sufficient for pain control in 90% of the patients. The most common side effect was drowsiness, followd by nausea, vomiting, constipation, confusion, and hallucination.

Conclusions.—Controlled-release morphine appears to be an effective means of pain control for patients with cancer. The side effects are minimal, and most can be managed with appropriate measures.

▶ In a hospice setting, any mechanism of pain control that does not require injections is welcome. This study underscores an option available to physicians in an easily administered oral form. The main side effect was drowsiness in 21% of the patients and nausea in 11%. For the relief it provided without needles, this was a small price to pay.—J.V. Simone, M.D.

Psychosocial

Problems at Social Re-Integration of Long-Term Cancer Survivors

Greaves-Otte JGW, Greaves J, Kruyt PM, van Leeuwen O, van der Wouden JC, van der Does E (Erasmus Univ; Zuiderziekenhuis, Rotterdam, The Netherlands)

Eur J Cancer 27:178–181, 1991 18–11

Background.—Many patients with cancer who achieve a medical "cure" have difficulty readapting to society. To help in understanding the nature and extent of the problems, 849 patients who used to have cancer were surveyed.

Methods.—The patients, who had had no relapse of cancer for at least 5 years, were sent a 190-item questionnaire concerning background and medical information, everyday activities, pretreatment and post-treatment social characteristics, the perceived consequences of cancer and its treatment, relationships, leisure activities, and psychological aspects. A total of 76% of the subjects returned satisfactorily complete responses. Of this group, 72% were women (mean age, 55.5 years) and 28% were men (mean age, 51.5 years).

Findings.—More than half the respondents still had some symptoms attributable to their cancer or its treatment. For 62%, socioeconomic position had not changed since the time before their diagnosis. Of the respondents who were employed at the time of their diagnosis, 28% were now housekeepers; 99% of that group was female. There was no significant difference in absence from work (in days per year) between the time of the survey and the year before diagnosis. The respondents believed that their cancer had negatively affected their financial position and prospects for promotion. Of the subjects who tried to take out a new insurance policy or modify an existing one, 70% had problems—most commonly refusal by the insurance company. In comparison with the average population, the subjects had diminished well-being.

Conclusions.—Problems with work and finances, as well as insurance, are commonly experienced by long-term survivors of cancer. Psychosocial care for these patients should begin during cancer treatment and continue after treatment has ended.

▶ Oncologists have a tendency to believe that cancer problems are over once the disease is cured. This study from The Netherlands suggests otherwise. Although most of the patients were self-supporting and their socioeconomic position had not substantially changed, 70% of the patients who tried to take out insurance or modify an existing policy experienced refusal, higher premiums, or medical examinations. Their overall psychological well-being was lower than that of the average Dutch population, and there was diminished psychological well-being in these long-term survivors of cancer. This is not the first study to demonstrate similar results, and it emphasizes the continued need both for support and for efforts to address some of the societal hurdles placed in front of patients whose cancer was cured.—R.C. Young, M.D., F.A.C.P.

Quality of Life Assessment: An Independent Prognostic Variable for Survival in Lung Cancer

Ganz PA, Lee JJ, Siau J (Univ of California, Los Angeles)

Cancer 67:3131–3135, 1991 18–12

Introduction.—Quality of life (QL) assessment is being increasingly used in trials of cancer treatment. The patient assessment of outcome is added to the traditional measures of response.

Study Design.—The patient-rated QL was correlated with survival in a homogeneous sample of 40 patients with advanced metastatic lung cancer. The patients completed the Functional Living Index-Cancer (FLIC) instrument, a validated cancer-specific measure of QL. The patients had an average age of 62 years. Most had Karnofsky performance scores greater than 80 and had lost less than 5% of body weight.

Findings.—Because of a strong relationship between patient-rated QL and the Karnofsky score, survival and QL were related using the Cox proportional-hazards model. The initial patient-rated quality of life correlated significantly with survival. In addition, being married also was associated with significantly improved survival.

Conclusions.—Nonmedical factors such as patient related QL and marital status may have a role in survival after treatment of lung cancer. Demographic information should be acquired from all patients entering cancer treatment trials. In addition, systematic QL assesments should be an integral part of cancer management.

▶ There is a growing literature to suggest that the patient's attitude toward disease and self has an independent influence on the duration of survival. Such results are always hard to confirm because of the "soft" nature of that type of data and the difficulty of quantitation. The authors have taken a slightly different approach to the issue. Their results suggest that if a patient thinks he has a better QL, then he has a longer period of survival. Is this because he is in better shape and therefore is likely to live longer than a patient who isn't? Or is it because he feels better and takes a more positive outlook, thereby independently extending his life span? Although it is hard to know which reason is true, another finding in this study suggests that attitude and circumstance may, in fact, influence the duration of survival. The authors found that married patients had a longer survival than unmarried patients. If one is an optimist (as I am) who views marriage as a positive influence on the QL, then these factors may indeed prolong survival independent of the stage of disease and specific treatment. It would be nice if this were true.—J.V. Simone, M.D.

Relationships Between Emotional Control, Adjustment to Cancer and Depression and Anxiety in Breast Cancer Patients

Watson M, Greer S, Rowden L, Gorman C, Robertson B, Bliss JM, Tunmore R
(Inst of Cancer Research, Sutton, England)

Psychol Med 21:51–57, 1991 18–13

Introduction.—There is ongoing debate and controversy over the possible relationship between the psychological responses to breast cancer and disease outcome. Two parallel findings have been reported in the literature. Some studies have shown that emotional control is more common among women with breast cancer than among those with benign breast disease or among healthy controls. Other studies have found that a helpless or fatalistic attitude toward the disease might be related to a poor prognosis. Whether there is an association between these findings was examined in 359 women (aged 25–75 years) with early stage breast cancer.

Methods.—The women were seen individually between 1 and 3 months after diagnosis. All patients completed questionnaires assessing the relationships between emotional control, adjustment to cancer, and psychological morbidity.

Results.—There was a highly significant association between the tendency to control emotional responses and an attitude of fatalism toward the disease; there also was a significant association between control of anger and a helpless attitude. In addition, psychological morbidity was linked to the type of adjustment to cancer. The prevalence rates of significant psychological morbidity were 16% for anxiety and 6% for depression. Those levels of morbidity were lower than the levels previously reported, suggesting that some changes may be occurring in the clinical management of oncology patients and the support services that are now increasingly being offered.

Conclusion.—There is a significant association between emotional control and a fatalistic attitude, and to a lesser degree, between control of anger and feelings of helplessness toward cancer. Encouraging patients to ventilate their emotions may be beneficial for an enhanced quality of life.

▶ Much has been written about the effect on survival of the so-called "fighting spirit" vs. the pessimistic outlook. In the 1991 YEAR BOOK, we reviewed an article by Richardson et al. that was unable to confirm a relationship between psychological factors and survival in patients with hematologic malignancies or rectal cancer (1). This study focused on a population of patients with breast cancer, and it documents a significant association between the tendency to control one's emotional responses and a subsequent attitude of fatalism toward the disease. This may serve, in part, to explain the paradoxical observation that angry, outspoken, difficult-to-manage patients actually experience a better survival than those very compliant, stoic, and cooperative patients with cancer. Although this study does not resolve the question, it does suggest an association between suppressed emotional responses and a fatalistic attitude. Although we physicians are generally pleased when patients are compliant, cooperative, stoic and controlled, perhaps we shouldn't be.—R.C. Young, M.D., F.A.C.P.

Reference

1. Richardson JL, et al: *J Psychosom Res* 34:189, 1990.

Quality of Life

Late Effects of Adjuvant Chemotherapy and Postoperative Radiotherapy on Quality of Life Among Breast Cancer Patients

Berglund G, Bolund C, Fornander T, Rutqvist LE, Sjödén P-O (Karolinska Hosp, Stockholm; Univ of Uppsala, Sweden)

Eur J Cancer 27:1075–1081, 1991 18–14

Background.—The diagnosis of breast cancer and its subsequent treatment can cause persistent psychological problems for many patients. In the first year, chemotherapy appears to cause more problems with quality of life than does radiotherapy; however, there have been no comparative studies of the late effects of these 2 treatments. Quality-of-life issues were studied in patients who had undergone adjunctive radiotherapy or chemotherapy as many as 10 years earlier.

Methods.—The subjects were 448 women who were participants in a controlled study of treatment of breast cancer. All the women had primary modified radical mastectomy, after which they were randomly allocated to receive radiotherapy or adjuvant chemotherapy. Quality-of-life issues were assessed by a questionnaire, which addressed activities, symptoms, anxiety, depression, and satisfaction with life. The response rate was 83%.

Results.—Few differences were noted between groups in home and community activities and signs of anxiety and depression. Of patients who had radiotherapy, 75% reported decreased stamina vs. 61% of those receiving chemotherapy. Aversion to smells was a problem for 18% of the chemotherapy patients and 10% of the radiotherapy patients. Radiotherapy patients had significantly more symptoms related to their operative scar and more symptoms of anxiety. As a group, the chemotherapy patients rated their quality of life higher than did the radiotherapy patients; there was no relationship with age or time since treatment.

Conclusions.—Chemotherapy and radiotherapy for breast cancer do not appear to reduce quality of life significantly 2–10 years after treatment, and there are only small differences between the 2 types of treatment. The investigators' quality-of-life questionnaire should be tested for reliability and validity.

▶ Although everyone, including the Food and Drug Administration, is clamoring for studies on the impact of cancer therapy on quality of life, such studies are rare and difficult to perform. These Swedish investigators have looked at quality of life 2–10 years after either adjuvant chemotherapy or radiation therapy in 448 patients with breast cancer who were free of disease post treatment. They used a questionnaire structured quality-of-life assessment document in which patients were asked to rate (on a scale of 0–4) the extent that special activities, physical sequelae, and mood states altered their quality of life. It is reassuring to note that, in these patients whose breast cancer was cured, neither adjuvant treatment severely impaired life conditions; however, the patients who underwent radiotherapy, had decreased stamina and anxiety whereas those who had chemotherapy had persistent problems with smell aversion. Overall, the patients treated with chemotherapy scored higher quality-of-life estimates than those treated with radiation therapy. It is likely that a variety of quality-of-life assessments will be necessary before we can arrive at a technique for consistently analyzing these effects in a balanced way.—R.C. Young, M.D., F.A.C.P.

Sex or Survival: Trade-Offs Between Quality and Quantity of Life

Singer PA, Tasch ES, Stocking C, Rubin S, Siegler M, Weichselbaum R (Univ of Chicago; Univ of Toronto)

J Clin Oncol 9:328–334, 1991 18–15

Introduction.—Clinically localized prostate cancer may be treated with either radiotherapy or radial prostatectomy, but the comparative survival rates are controversial. Many physicians believe that, although surgery offers a higher survival rate, it may also produce a higher rate of impotence. A treatment-choice technique was used to assess how men value survival and sexual potency when asked to trade one for the other.

Methods.—Interviews were conducted with 50 men (aged 45–70 years) without known prostate cancer. The treatment-choice techniques used a hypothetical rate of survival of 90% at 5 years for surgery and an impotency rate of 90% for surgery and 40% for radiotherapy.

Results.—Of the respondents, 32% were unwilling to trade any survival, but 68% were willing to trade a 10% or greater advantage in 5-year survival to maintain potency by choosing radiotherapy. A willingness to trade survival for sexual potency was related to the level of education, but not to age, interest in sex, frequency of sexual intercourse, or ability to achieve erection. Those respondents with high educational status or those who were working full time or were retired were less willing to trade survival for sexual potency.

Conclusion.—Both quality and quantity-of-life considerations affect the hypothetical patient's choice between surgery and radiotherapy as treatment for localized prostate cancer. Physicians must understand the range of patient preferences regarding treatment of localized prostate cancer and be prepared to discuss all options with patients thoroughly.

▶ The debate between urologists and radiation therapists regarding the treatment of localized (stage A2 or B) prostate cancer has primarily focused on survival as the endpoint. Physician preference and patient selection factors have produced clinical trials from which survival rates cannot be directly compared. If there truly are differences in survival for comparable patients with localized prostate cancer treated with either radical prostatectomy or radiation therapy, they clearly are not of a great magnitude. Consequently, the toxicity of treatment becomes a major factor in the selection of therapy for an individual patient.

This study emphasizes how an individual patient's assessment of the importance of sexual function affects the choice of therapy. Some patients appear to be willing to accept a substantial risk of decreased survival to maintain potency. Of added interest in this study was the absence of age as a significant selection factor in this hypothetical trade-off between sex and survival. In contrast, educational level and employment status were independent predictors in selecting more for survival than for potency. To make a truly informed decision, the patient should be encouraged to discuss treatment options with both a urologist and a radiation therapist.—R.F. Ozols, M.D., Ph.D.

Quality of Life in Long-Term Survivors of CNS Tumors of Childhood and Adolescence

Mostow EN, Byrne J, Connelly RR, Mulvihill JJ (Natl Cancer Inst, Natl Insts of Health, Bethesda, Md)

J Clin Oncol 9:592–599, 1991 18–16

Introduction.—Brain and CNS tumors follow leukemia as the leading cause of cancer deaths in children less than 15 years of age. The survival rates do not often consider the quality of life in these young patients. The quality of life into adulthood of long-term survivors of children who had had CNS tumors was assessed.

Methods.—A total of 342 adults (or their proxies) who had CNS tumors was interviewed regarding quality of life. These individuals had the CNS tumors diagnosed before 20 years of age (between 1945 and 1974), had survived at least 5 years, and were 21 years old by December 31, 1979. Their medical records were also reviewed.

Findings.—The patients had an average age of 11.3 years at diagnosis of the tumor. At the last follow-up examination, the survivors averaged 32 years of age compared with a group of 479 matched controls who were 33.2 years of age. Surgery had contributed to all or part of the treatment in 94% of the survivors. Deaths had occurred before the interview in 47 survivors and 7 controls, and the survivors were more likely to die as adults or become mentally incompetent than controls at any time. The CNS tumor survivors had a higher risk for the adverse aspects of quality-of-life measurements, including unemployment, stopping work because of a health condition, inability to drive a car, or describing their health as poor. Male survivors experienced more unfavorable outcomes than did female survivors. The tumor site and treatment appeared to alter the quality of life of the survivors, particularly in those with supratentorial tumors and those receiving radiation therapy.

Conclusions.—These findings suggest that, although the interview questions were unrefined measures and highly subjective, much needs to be done to improve the quality of life of patients who survive CNS tumor treatment. The exploration of parent self-help groups, promotion of sibling and peer interactions, and identification of patient differences to minimize negative effects are recommended.

▶ In addition to having great difficulty treating CNS tumors successfully in children, one has the additional problem of worrying that some aspect of treatment—especially radiation therapy or surgery—might seriously compromise the quality of life in survivors. As this paper demonstrates, survivors of brain tumor have a significant reduction in quality of life as adults. The problems of unemployment and poor self-image were observed in a significant number of patients when compared with sibling controls. For example, 25% of the survivors of supratentorial tumors were never employed, and nearly half the patients had to change jobs or stop working because of their health condition. Still, 85% of the survivors had some employment, and 83% could still drive a car; 80% described their health as excellent or good. Not too bad considering the site of the tumors.—J.V. Simone, M.D.

Subject Index

A

D

E

F

G

H

P

Q

R

U

V

W

X

Y

Z

Author Index

A

B

C

D

H

M

S

T

U

V

W

Y

Z